普通高等教育"十一五"国家级规划教材

全国高等医药院校药学类专业第二轮实验双语教

U0297201

生理学实验与指导

（第 2 版）

主　　编　丁启龙　卢　娜

副 主 编　张小博

中文审校　王秋娟

英文审校　张彩铃

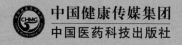

中国健康传媒集团

中国医药科技出版社

内容提要

本教材是"全国高等医药院校药学类专业第二轮实验双语教材"之一，全书包括42个实验，重点突出生理学实验中的基本操作、基本技能和基本理论。所列实验除少数可供选择的以外，在大多数院校生理实验室都有条件做到。本书还介绍了常用的实验动物、动物活体解剖技术以及生理实验的常用仪器设备，以供不同专业的教学需要。本教材为书网融合教材，即纸质教材有机融合电子教材、教学配套资源（PPT、微课、视频、图片等）、题库系统、数字化教学服务（在线教学、在线作业、在线考试），使教学资源更加多样化、立体化。

本教材主要供药学及相关专业使用。

图书在版编目（CIP）数据

生理学实验与指导／丁启龙，卢娜主编 . —2 版 . —北京：中国医药科技出版社，2020.6

全国高等医药院校药学类专业第二轮实验双语教材

ISBN 978 – 7 – 5214 – 1854 – 5

Ⅰ.①生… Ⅱ.①丁… ②卢… Ⅲ.①人体生理学 – 实验 – 双语教学 – 医学院校 – 教学参考资料

Ⅳ.①R33 – 33

中国版本图书馆 CIP 数据核字（2020）第 089499 号

美术编辑 陈君杞
版式设计 南博文化

出版 **中国健康传媒集团** ｜中国医药科技出版社
地址 北京市海淀区文慧园北路甲 22 号
邮编 100082
电话 发行：010 – 62227427 邮购：010 – 62236938
网址 www.cmstp.com
规格 889 × 1194mm $\frac{1}{16}$
印张 15 $\frac{3}{4}$
字数 350 千字
初版 2004 年 3 月第 1 版
版次 2020 年 6 月第 2 版
印次 2024 年 7 月第 3 次印刷
印刷 三河市万龙印装有限公司
经销 全国各地新华书店
书号 ISBN 978 – 7 – 5214 – 1854 – 5
定价 48.00 元

获取新书信息、投稿、为图书纠错，请扫码联系我们。

教学是学校人才培养的中心环节，实验教学是这一环节的重要组成部分。"全国高等医药院校药学类专业实验双语教材"是中国药科大学坚持药学实践教学改革，突出提高学生动手能力、创新思维，通过承担教育部"世行贷款21世纪初高等教育教学改革项目"等多项教改课题，逐步建设完善的一套与药学各专业学科理论课程紧密结合的高水平双语实验教材。

本轮修订，适逢"全国高等医药院校药学类专业第五轮规划教材"及《中国药典》（2020年版）、新版《国家执业药师资格考试大纲》出版，整套教材的修订强调了与新版理论教材知识的结合，与《中国药典》（2020年版）等新颁布的法典法规结合。为更好地服务于新时期高等院校药学教育与人才培养的需要，在上一版的基础上，进一步体现了各门实验课程自身独立性、系统性和科学性，又充分考虑到各门实验课程之间的联系与衔接，主要突出了以下特点。

1. 适应医药行业对人才的要求，体现行业特色，契合新时期药学人才需求的变化，使修订后的教材符合《中国药典》（2020年版）等国家标准及新版《国家执业药师资格考试大纲》等行业最新要求。

2. 更新完善内容，打造教材精品。在上版教材基础上进一步优化、精炼和充实内容。紧密结合"全国高等医药院校药学类专业第五轮规划教材"，强调与实际需求相结合，进一步提高教材质量。

3. 为适应信息化教学的需要，本轮教材全部打造成为书网融合教材，即纸质教材与数字教材、配套教学资源、题库系统、数字化教学服务有机融合，为读者提供全免费增值服务。

4. 坚持双语体系，强调素质培养教材以实践教学为突破口，采用双语体系编写有利于加快药学教育国际接轨，提高学生的科技英语水平，进一步提升学生整体素质。

"全国高等医药院校药学类专业第二轮实验双语教材"历经15年4次建设，在各个时期广大编者的努力下，在广大使用教材师生的支持下日臻完善。本轮教材的出版，必将对推动新时期我国高等药学教育的发展产生积极而深远的影响。希望广大师生在教学实践中对本套教材提出宝贵意见，以便今后进一步修订完善，共同打造精品教材。

吴晓明

全国高等医药院校药学类专业第五轮规划教材常务编委会主任委员

2019年10月

本教材是"全国高等医药院校药学类专业第二轮实验双语教材"之一，适用于高等院校药学类及相关专业的生理学实验教学。第一版自 2004 年 3 月出版，十几年来，在医药类高等院校作为本专科教材使用，实用性和适用性得到广大教师和学生的肯定，也得到很多有益的反馈与建议。为了适应高等院校教学改革的需要，根据当前高校教学模式和教学需求的变化，本次进行了第三次修订，本版修订侧重于建设纸质教材、数字化资源、教学平台三位一体的双语生理学实验立体化教材。本书包括 42 个实验，重点突出生理学实验中的基本操作、基本技能和基本理论。所列实验除少数可供选择的以外，在大多数医药院校生理实验室都有条件做到。本书还介绍了常用的实验动物、动物活体解剖技术以及生理实验的常用仪器设备，以供不同专业的教学需要。编者希望本教材及相关资源可以用于线上线下相结合的混合式教学，有利于学生在线进行课堂外的个性化、自主化学习。本次修订主要内容如下。

1. 对第 2 版中存在的部分不合理的内容进行纠正修改。与前版相比，本书增加了相应的英文译文。由于感觉器官系统的实验在药学专业类院校较少开展，故本版不再编入。生理现象或反应的记录以 BL-420 生物信号采集和分析系统为主，辅以二道生理记录仪，淘汰记纹鼓。为了避免重复，图片、表格均只出现在英文部分。

2. 建设书网融合教材，即纸质教材有机融合电子教材、教学配套资源（PPT、微课、视频、图片等）、题库系统、数字化教学服务（在线教学、在线作业、在线考试），使教学资源更加多样化、立体化。

参加本书编写的人员为中国药科大学生理教研室的丁启龙、卢娜、李运曼、吴玉林、郭青龙、傅纪华、印天华等老师。再版时卢娜负责全文错误修订，张小博负责 PPT 制作，丁启龙负责微视频制作。

由于编者水平所限，不妥之处恳请读者指正，以便再版时改进。

编　者
2019 年 12 月

第一章　总　论

第一节　生理学实验课的目的、要求和规则

一、生理学实验课的目的和要求

生理学实验是通过一些有代表性的实验，使学生初步掌握生理学实验的基本操作技术，了解获得生理学知识的科学方法，以及验证和巩固生理学的基本理论。逐步培养学生能够客观的对事物进行观察比较、综合分析和独立思考的能力，逐步树立对科学工作的严肃态度、严格要求、严密的工作方法和实事求是的工作作风。

（一）实验前的准备工作

1. 仔细阅读实验指导，了解本次实验的目的、要求、实验步骤和操作程序。

2. 结合实验内容复习有关理论，做到充分理解并预测该实验各个步骤应得的结果。

3. 熟悉所用仪器的性能及手术的基本操作方法。

4. 注意和估计实验中可能发生的误差。

（二）实验时的注意事项

1. 实验器材的安放力求整齐、清洁、有条不紊。

2. 按照实验步骤，以严肃认真的态度循序操作，不能随意更动，不得进行与实验无关的活动。要注意保护实验动物和标本，爱护并节省实验器材和药品。

3. 仔细、耐心地观察实验过程中出现的现象，随时记录并联系讲授内容进行思考。如：①发生了什么现象？②为什么会出现这种现象？③这种现象有什么生理意义等。

（三）实验后的整理

1. 实验用具整理。所用器械擦洗干净，如果损坏应立即报告指导教师。做好实验室的清洁工作。

2. 整理实验记录，做出实验结论，并写好实验报告。

二、实验结果的处理

在实验过程中将所观察到的结果变为可测量的指标，以便研究其各种变化规律。因此，实验中所得到的结果需要进行分析和整理。

凡属于测量性质的结果，如长短、高低、快慢、轻重等，均应以正确的单位和数值定量。

一般有曲线记录的实验结果，尽量用曲线记录。在曲线上应标注说明，要有刺激记号、时间记号等。

为了便于比较分析，有些实验测量出的结果可采用表格或绘图。制表格时可将观察的项目列在表内左侧；右侧顺序填写各项结果变化数值，亦可附简要说明。绘图时应注意以下几点。

1. 在图的旁边列出实验结果的数值表格。

2. 横轴表示各种刺激条件，纵轴表示所发生的各种反应。

3. 坐标轴适当注解，包括剂量或浓度单位。

4. 选择大小适宜的标度以便作图，根据图的大小确定坐标轴的长短。

5. 绘制经过各点的曲线或折线要光滑，如果不是连续性变化，亦可用柱形表示。

6. 在图下注明实验条件。

在实验中取得的数据，必要时需做统计学处理（详见附录三），求出均数、标准差及进行差异显著性检验，才能对实验结果进行评价。

三、实验报告

（一）写作要求

1. 示教实验或自己做的实验均要每人按时写出报告。

2. 按照每一实验的具体要求，认真写出实验报告，写报告应注意文字简练、通顺，书写清楚、整洁及正确使用标点符号，报告要求如下。

（1）注明姓名、班次、组别、日期、室温及气压。

（2）实验序号与题目。

（3）实验目的。

（4）实验方法一般不必描述，如果实验仪器与方法临时变动或操作技术影响观察的可靠性时，可做简要说明。

（5）实验结果是实验中最重要的部分，应将实验过程所观察到的现象真实、正确地记述，实验中的每项观察都应随时记录。实验结束后，根据记录填写实验报告，不可单凭记忆书写，否则容易发生错误和遗漏。实验结果的处理见前项要求。

（6）讨论和结论　实验结果的讨论是根据已知的理论知识对结果进行解释和分析。要判断实验结果是否为预期的，如果出现非预期结果，应该考虑和分析其可能的原因。还要指出实验结果的生理意义。实验结论是从实验结果中归纳出一般的、概括性的判断，也就是这一实验所能验证的概念、原则或理论的简明总结。结论中一般不罗列具体的结果。在实验讨论中，未能得到充分证据的理论分析不应写入结论。

实验讨论和结论的书写是富有创造性的工作，应该严肃认真，不应盲目抄袭书本。参考课外读物应注明出处。

（二）实验报告的一般格式

生理学实验报告

姓名_____班次_____组别_____日期_____室温_____气压_____

实验序号与题目_____

实验目的_____

实验方法_____

实验结果_____

讨论和结论_____

四、实验室规则

1. 遵守学习纪律，准时到实验室。在室内应穿实验衣。

2. 专心实验，不在实验室内做其他与实验无关的工作。

3. 保持实验室安静，切勿喧哗。

4. 养成爱好整洁的良好习惯，注意保持实验环境及器材等的整洁。零星动物尸体、碎片及残余物品应放置在指定的地方，不要随地乱丢。

5. 公用器材及药品用毕后，必须立即归还原处。

6. 公共仪器各组使用，决不能与别组互换。如果仪器损坏或机件不灵，应立即报告教师或仪器室管理员，以便修理、更换或报损。

7. 爱护公共财物，节约水电、药品、棉花、蒸馏水、溶液，爱护器材、家具及实验动物。如有不应有的损坏及过量消耗，按照具体情况由个人或小组赔偿。

8. 实验完毕后将仪器整理干净，物归原处，养成实习工作的良好习惯。

9. 值日学生应做好清洁卫生工作，负责处理动物尸体，关好水、电、门、窗。

第二节 活体解剖技术

生理学实验是以活的动物及其器官、组织或人体作为观察对象和实验材料的。在动物实验中，活体解剖技术对生理学实验的成败起着十分重要的作用。在实验过程中，学生应着重学习、掌握这些操作技术，以提高动手能力。

生理学实验一般可分离体实验和在体实验两类，后者又可分为急性实验和慢性实验两种。急性在体实验法是动物在麻醉或毁坏脑或脊髓的状态下，用手术暴露某一器官，观察研究其功能及变化规律。如在体心脏活动的观察、肾脏泌尿功能的研究等。急性离体实验法是将要研究的器官或组织从活的或刚处死的动物体上取出，置于接近正常生理条件的人工环境中，以观察研究其生理功能。如离体心脏灌流、离体肠管的活动以及用坐骨神经 – 腓肠肌标本研究神经肌肉的生理功能等。急性实验法不能持久，只能在一定时间内进行观察研究，而且实验后动物不能存活。慢性实验法是在特定条件下，以完整而清醒的动物为对象的实验方法，可以在较长时间内，连续的反复观察动物的某一生理功能。此法常需要先在动物体上实施某种无菌外科手术，如胃肠道瘘管术；或在机体的一定部位埋藏电极或切除某一器官等，需待动物恢复健康后方可进行实验。这种实验花费时间较长，动物需要特殊的护理。

扫码"学一学"

一、手术器械及用途

根据生理学实验需要，常用手术器械包括手术刀、手术剪、手术镊、蛙类毁髓针、玻璃解剖针等。

（一）手术刀

主要用于切开和解剖组织。可根据手术部位与性质，更换大小不同的刀柄。常用的执刀法有四种。

1. 执弓式 为最常用的一种执刀方式，动作范围广而灵活，用于腹部、颈部或股部的皮肤切口（图 1 –1）。

2. 执笔式 用于切割短小切口，用力轻柔而操作精细。如解剖血管、神经，做腹膜小切口等（图 1 –2）。

3. 握持式 用于切割范围较广，用力较大的切口。如截肢、较长的皮肤切口等。

4. 反挑式 用于向上挑开，以免损伤深部组织，如挑开脓肿。

（二）手术剪

手术剪主要用于剪皮肤或肌肉等粗软组织，也可用来分离组织，即利用剪刀的尖端插入组织间隙，分离无大血管的结缔组织。手术剪分尖头剪和钝头剪，其尖端有直、弯之别。另外还有一种小型手术剪，叫眼科剪，主要用于剪血管或神经等柔软组织，眼科剪也有直头与弯头之分。正确的执剪姿势如图1-3所示，即用拇指与无名指持剪，食指置于手术剪的上方。

（三）血管钳

血管钳主要用于钳夹血管或出血点，以达到止血的目的。也用于分离组织、牵引缝线、把持或拔出缝针等。执血管钳的姿势与执手术剪姿势相同（图1-4）。开放血管钳的手法是：利用右手已套入血管钳环口的拇指与无名指相对挤压，继而以旋开的动作开放血管钳。

血管钳按手术所需，分直、弯、有齿、长柄、无损伤以及大中小等各类型。例如直血管钳用于手术野浅部或皮下止血；弯血管钳用于较深部止血；蚊式血管钳用于精细的止血和分离组织。

（四）持针钳

持针钳用于把持缝针，缝合各种组织。使用时应利用持针钳的最尖端夹持缝针，而缝针被夹持的部位，应在缝针尾端和中部1/3交界处。执持针钳与执手术剪姿势相同，但为了缝合方便，可不必将拇指和无名指套入环口中，而把持于近端柄处（图1-5）。

（五）手术镊

手术镊主要用于夹持或提起组织，以便于剥离、剪开或缝合。手术镊分有齿和无齿两种。前者用于把持较坚韧的组织，如皮肤、筋膜、肌腱等。后者用于把持脆弱的组织，如血管、神经、黏膜。正确的执镊方法如图1-6，即以拇指对食指和中指，轻、稳和用力适当的把持组织。

（六）骨钳

骨钳主要用于咬切骨组织，如打开颅腔或骨髓腔等。骨钳分为剪刀式和小蝶式两种（图1-7），前者适用于咬断骨质，后者适用于咬切骨片。

（七）颅骨钻

颅骨钻主要用于开颅时钻孔（图1-8）。

（八）毁髓针

毁髓针是专门用来毁坏蛙类脑和脊髓的器械，分为针柄和针部（图1-9A）。

（九）玻璃解剖针

玻璃解剖针是专用于分离神经与血管的工具。有直头与弯头两种，尖端圆滑（图1-9B）。

（十）缝针

缝针用于缝合各种组织。缝针有圆针和三棱针两种，又有直型和弯型之别，而且大小不一。圆针多用于缝合软组织，三棱针用于穿皮固定缝合，弯针用于缝合深部组织。

（十一）动脉夹

动脉夹主要用于短期阻断动脉血流，如插动脉套管时使用。

二、活体解剖技术

（一）动物选择

常用的实验动物有狗、猫、兔、大白鼠、小白鼠、豚鼠、蟾蜍或蛙等，均需选用健康动物。一般说，健康的哺乳动物毛色有光泽，两眼明亮，眼和鼻无分泌物，鼻端潮而凉，反应灵活，食欲良好。健康的蛙或蟾蜍则皮肤湿润，喜爱活动，静止时后肢蹲坐，前肢支撑，头部和躯干部挺起等。

扫码"看一看"

动物种类的选择需根据实验内容而定，以期解剖和生理特点适合于预定实验的要求。如研究主动脉弓减压神经传出冲动的作用时，常选用兔为实验对象，因为兔的减压神经在颈部自成一束，与迷走神经伴行，易于寻找和分离。在研究心脏特殊传导组织电活动时，常选用狗的浦肯野纤维及兔的窦房结作为实验材料，因为狗的浦肯野纤维在心室内较为粗大，很容易解剖分离。在生理学的研究中，特别是基础理论研究中，合理选择实验动物，常常是实验成败的关键，但并非愈是高等动物愈好，应根据实验需要，因地制宜地加以考虑。

（二）动物的麻醉

在慢性或急性在体实验中，施行手术之前必须将动物麻醉。麻醉可减少动物在手术或实验过程中的疼痛，使其保持安静，从而保证实验顺利进行。麻醉剂种类繁多，作用原理不尽相同。除了麻痹中枢神经系统以外，还会引起其他生理功能的改变。因此，在应用时需根据动物种类及实验或手术的性质慎重选择。麻醉必须适度，过深或过浅均会给手术或实验带来不良影响。麻醉的深浅可从呼吸、某些反射消失、肌肉紧张程度及瞳孔大小加以判断。常用刺激角膜、夹捏后肢股部肌肉的简易方法来观察其反应，进而了解动物的麻醉深度。适宜的麻醉状态是呼吸深满而平稳，角膜反射与运动反应消失，肌肉松弛。

1. 常用麻醉剂的种类和用法 麻醉剂可分为局部麻醉剂和全身麻醉剂两种。局部麻醉常用0.5%～1.0%盐酸普鲁卡因或2%盐酸可卡因做皮肤或黏膜表面麻醉。在生理实验中，多采用全身麻醉剂，如挥发性的乙醚和非挥发性的巴比妥类，氨基甲酸乙酯等。

（1）乙醚 是一种呼吸性麻醉剂，适用于各种实验动物。在用乙醚麻醉猫、兔或鼠时，可将动物放在特制的玻璃钟罩内，同时放入浸有乙醚的脱脂棉，动物吸入后15～20秒开始发挥作用。在麻醉狗时，可用特制的麻醉口罩套在动物嘴上，慢慢将乙醚滴在口罩上，并注意让动物安定。

乙醚有刺激呼吸道黏液分泌的作用，为防止呼吸道堵塞，可用硫酸阿托品（0.1～0.3mg/kg）皮下或肌内注射。

乙醚麻醉易于掌握，比较安全，作用时间短，麻醉后容易苏醒，但要专人管理，以防过早苏醒或麻醉过量。

（2）戊巴比妥钠 适用于各类实验动物。常配制成5%水溶液，一般由静脉或腹腔注射。戊巴比妥钠作用开始快，一次给药的麻醉有效时间为2～4小时，不需特殊管理。如在实验中需要补充注射时，再由静脉注射1/5剂量，维持1～2小时。在麻醉过量时可产生严重的呼吸和循环抑制，导致动物死亡。

（3）乌拉坦　又名氨基甲酸乙酯或脲酯，易溶于水，常用浓度为 20% ~ 25%。适用于多种动物，如狗、猫、兔，多用于静脉或腹腔注射，蛙类用皮下淋巴囊注射。

非挥发性麻醉剂使用简便，维持时间较长，实验中无须专人照管，麻醉深度也较易掌握，因此大多数实验时采用，其缺点是苏醒缓慢。常用麻醉剂的剂量和用法见表 1 - 1。

表 1 - 1　常用麻醉剂的剂量和用法

麻醉剂	动物种类	给药途径	药物浓度	剂量（mg/kg 体重）	维持时间（小时）	备注
乙醚	各种动物	气管吸入	—	适量	较短	乙醚对呼吸道有刺激作用，可用阿托品皮下或肌内注射预防
戊巴比妥钠	狗、猫、兔	静脉	3%	30	2 ~ 4	麻醉较平稳，麻醉过量时，可用咖啡因，苯丙胺解救
	狗、猫、兔	腹腔		35		
	鼠类	腹腔		40		
	鸟类	肌肉		50 ~ 100		
乌拉坦	狗、猫、兔	静脉	20% ~ 25%	1000	2 ~ 4	易溶于水，对器官功能影响较小
	狗、猫、兔	腹腔		1000		
	鼠类	腹腔		1000		
	鸟类	肌肉		1250		
	蛙类	皮下淋巴囊		2000		
氯醛糖	狗、兔	静脉	1%	60 ~ 80	3 ~ 4	溶解度较低，可加温助溶，但不可煮沸，对呼吸及血管运动中枢影响较小
	猫	腹腔		60 ~ 80		
	鼠类	腹腔		80 ~ 100		
硫喷妥钠	狗、猫	静脉	2.5% ~ 5%	15 ~ 25	0.5 ~ 1.5	溶液不稳定，需使用前配制，刺激性较大，不宜作皮下或肌肉内注射。静脉注射对心血管及内脏损害较小，注射宜慢，以免麻醉过深
	兔	静脉		10 ~ 20		
苯巴比妥钠	狗、猫、兔	静脉	10%	80 ~ 100	24 ~ 72	麻醉诱导期较长，深度不易控制。不易作血压实验。麻醉过量可用苯丙胺，四氯五甲烷解救
	狗、猫、兔	腹腔		100 ~ 150		
	鸽	肌肉		300		

2. 麻醉剂的给药途径及方法　非挥发性麻醉剂的给药途径为注射给药法，主要有静脉、腹腔、肌内、皮下和淋巴囊注射。

（1）静脉注射　常用于麻醉狗、兔。狗在麻醉前必须安定，以防伤人。用粗棉带捆绑狗的嘴鼻部，即从下颌绕到上颌打一结，然后绕向下颌打一结，再将棉带引至头后，在颈部背面打第三个结，最后再打一活结（图 1 - 10）。狗最常用于注射和采血的静脉为前肢内侧的头静脉和后肢小腿外侧的小隐静脉。注射前，注射部位需剪毛，用手握压静脉近心端处，使血管充血膨胀。将注射针头顺血管方向先刺入血管旁皮下，然后再刺入血管，此时可见回血。注射者一手固定针头，一手缓慢进行推注（图 1 - 11）。

兔静脉注射的常用部位为耳缘静脉。兔耳的外缘血管为静脉，中央血管为动脉。注射前最好将动物放入兔箱内固定，使兔头露于箱外，以防注射时挣扎。先除去注射部位的被毛，用左手食指和中指夹住耳缘静脉近心端，使其充血，拇指和无名指固定兔耳。用右手持注射针头顺血管方向刺入静脉（图1-12），刺入后再将左手食指和中指移至针头处，协同拇指将针头固定于静脉内，缓缓注射。如注射阻力过大或局部肿胀，说明针头未刺入血管，应拔出重新刺入。首次注射应从静脉远心端开始，以便进行反复注射。

（2）腹腔注射　常用于麻醉猫和鼠类。给猫做腹腔注射时要紧紧抓住颈后皮肤皱襞，迅速将注射针头刺入腹腔，注射完毕后立即退出针头。猫是易怒动物，牙、爪均可伤人，为了安全，可将猫放入布制口袋内，封口后进行注射。给鼠类做腹腔注射时，也需注意安全。对小白鼠可采用手持法进行注射（图1-13），即用左手小指和无名指将鼠尾夹住迅速用其余三指抓住鼠耳及颈部皮肤，将腹部朝上，右手将注射针头刺入下腹部白线稍外侧处，注射针与皮肤呈45°夹角，若针头通过腹肌后抵抗消失，应保持针头不动，然后轻轻回抽，如无肠内容物、尿液或血液抽出，可轻轻注入麻醉剂。

（3）肌内注射　猴、狗、猫、兔多选用两侧臀部或股部进行肌内注射。固定动物后，右手持注射器，使之与肌肉成60°夹角，一次刺入肌肉。注射完毕后用手轻轻按摩注射部位，帮助药液吸收。

（4）皮下注射　在注射麻醉中不常用。小白鼠的皮下注射部位通常在背部，可将皮肤拉起，注射针刺入皮下。将针头轻轻向左右摇摆，容易摆动则表明已刺入皮下，然后注射药物。拔针时，可用手指轻轻压住注射部位，以防药液外漏。对大白鼠、豚鼠、兔、猫等，可选用背部、大腿内侧或臀部等皮下脂肪较少的部位进行皮下注射。

（5）淋巴囊注射　常用于麻醉蛙或蟾蜍。由于蛙类皮肤较薄，弹性较差，抽针后药液易自注射处外流，故宜用胸部淋巴囊注射。方法是针头刺入口腔黏膜，通过下颌肌层入皮下淋巴后囊（图1-14）再进行注射，一只动物一次可注射0.25~1ml溶液。

（三）急性动物实验的基市操作技市

1. 手术切口与止血　在哺乳动物身体上行皮肤切口之前，需将切口部位及其周围的毛剪去，用剪刀依次剪毛，剪时切忌提起毛，以免剪及皮肤。剪下的毛应放在盛有水的玻璃烧杯中，以免毛到处飞扬污染环境。做切口前，应注意切口大小和解剖结构，一般以少切断神经和血管为原则，同时应尽可能使切口与各层组织纤维方向一致。切口大小既要便于手术操作但也不可过大。切时用左手拇指和食指、中指将切口上端两侧的皮肤固定，右手持手术刀，用执弓式或执笔式，以适当的力量，一次全线切开皮肤和皮下组织，直至肌层。

手术过程中，要随时注意止血，以免手术野血肉模糊，难以分辨血管和神经，延误手术时间。止血方法视出血情况而定，微小血管出血，可用温热生理盐水纱布按压止血；较大血管出血，需先找到出血点，用止血钳夹住而后用线结扎；大血管破损，应准确而快速止血，否则失血过多影响实验。实验期间，应将创口暂时闭合，或用温热生理盐水纱布盖好，以免组织干燥。

2. 手术结　手术结不仅是外科手术的重要技术，也是急性动物实验的基本技术。手术结有多种，在生理学实验中以方结最为常用，打结有单手打结法、双手打结法、持钳打结法。单手打结法最为方便，但结线必须留的长些。持钳打结法适用于结线太短或结扎过深等情况。

3. 颈部手术

（1）气管分离术 将动物仰卧位固定，剪去颈部腹面的毛，用手术刀在紧靠喉头下部沿颈部正中切开皮肤。切口长度：兔、猫为 5 ~ 7cm，狗约 10cm，大鼠和豚鼠为 2.5 ~ 4cm。在气管正腹面用手或止血钳逐层分离皮下结缔组织，即露出覆盖于气管腹面的胸骨舌骨肌。用止血钳由正中线将胸骨舌骨肌分开，即可暴露气管。

（2）颈外静脉分离术 哺乳动物的颈外静脉粗大、壁薄，且分布很浅，位于颈部皮下，胸锁乳突肌（狗为胸头肌）外缘。分离该静脉时，用左手拇指与食指捏住切口一侧的皮肤，再向外翻，可将暗紫色的粗大静脉翻于食指上，用玻璃解剖针或细止血钳由静脉外侧分离结缔组织，即可将颈外静脉分离出来，然后穿线备用。

（3）颈总动脉的分离 颈总动脉位于气管外侧，腹面被胸骨舌骨肌和胸骨甲状肌所覆盖。分离时可用左手拇指和食指捏住已分离的气管一侧的胸骨肌，再稍向外翻，即可将颈总动脉以及神经束翻于食指上，用玻璃解剖针或止血钳轻轻分离动脉外侧的结缔组织，便可将颈总动脉分离出来，最后穿线备用。注意颈部神经与颈总动脉被结缔组织包绕在一起，形成血管神经束。在分离动脉时，应注意神经的部位与行走，切勿伤及与其伴行的神经。

（4）神经分离术 在分离颈总动脉的基础上，提起动脉即可看到粗细不同的神经，用玻璃解剖针小心分离其外的结缔组织，一般分离出 2cm 即可穿线备用。颈部的神经分布因动物种类不同而不同。兔颈部神经束内有 3 条粗细不同的神经，其中迷走神经最粗，呈白色，一般位于外侧；交感神经稍细，略成灰色，一般位于内侧；减压神经最细，位于迷走神经与交感神经之间，减压神经属于传入神经。猫的迷走神经与交感神经并行，迷走神经较粗，交感神经较细，减压神经并入迷走神经中。狗在颈总动脉背外侧有一条粗大的迷走 – 交感干，迷走神经的结状神经节与交感神经的颈前神经节相邻。迷走神经从第 1 颈椎下面进入颈部，与交感神经干并行，被一结缔组织鞘所包绕，形成迷走 – 交感神经干，在进入胸腔后，两条神经才分开。

4. 腹部手术 在动物实验中，腹白线系腹部切口的常用部位，是位于腹中线下面的白色腱膜线，从胸骨的剑突隆起直至耻骨联合，神经、血管分布极少。因此，通过腹白线所做的腹正中切口的长度因实验要求和动物种类而不同。如在观察兔胃和小肠运动实验中，需在胸骨下方做 8 ~ 10cm 的切口，才能充分暴露胃和小肠；而在兔尿形成的调节实验中，只需自耻骨联合向上做 2 ~ 3cm 的切口，即可将膀胱引出。

5. 股部手术 股部血管与神经在实验中也较常用，如插入心导管、测压、注射和采血等，股部血管和神经在股三角处通过。股三角为股部手术的常用部位，是耻骨肌与缝匠肌后部的后缘之间所形成的三角区。在股三角内有股动脉、股静脉和股神经通过。

血管与神经分离术：将动物仰卧固定，先用手指在股部内侧根部触摸动脉搏动部位，剪去该部位的被毛，用手术刀沿血管平行方向做一 4 ~ 5cm 切口，用止血钳分离皮下结缔组织，再将耻骨和缝匠肌的交点处分离，并将缝匠肌后部向外拉开，其下方可见筋膜包绕的神经血管束（图 1 – 15）。用蚊式止血钳小心分离其结缔组织，并穿线备用。血管神经的自然位置为股静脉位于内侧，股神经位于外侧，股动脉位于两者之间。

（四）采血技术

由于实验动物不同，实验需要和采血数量有别，所选用的采血方法也不相同。这里仅介绍几种实验动物的常用采血技术。

1. 兔和豚鼠

（1）心脏采血 将兔或豚鼠仰卧固定，剪去左侧胸部相当于心脏部位的被毛，用碘酒和酒精消毒皮肤，选择心脏跳动最明显处做穿刺。一般由胸骨左边缘外3cm处刺入兔的第3肋间隙，在豚鼠则刺入第4~6肋间隙。穿刺时，最好用左手触诊心脏，以作配合。当针头接近心脏时，会感到心脏的搏动，血液自然进入注射器。如认为针头已进入心脏，但抽不出血液，可把针头稍微退出或进入一点。心脏采血经6~7天后，可以重复进行。采血量在兔一次可取20~25ml，豚鼠可取6~7ml。

（2）兔耳中央动脉采血 将兔置于兔固定箱内，用酒精棉球擦揉兔耳片刻，使其充血。在兔耳中央有一条纵行、较粗、颜色鲜红的中央动脉。用左手固定兔耳，右手持注射器，在中央动脉末端，沿动脉平行地向心脏方向刺入动脉，轻轻抽动针筒，即可见血液进入注射器。一次可采血约15ml（采血后应注意止血）。采血一般使用6号针头，不可太细。需加注意的是，兔耳中央动脉易发生痉挛性收缩，因此，采血前必须使兔耳充血。当动脉扩张，未发生痉挛性收缩前立即进行抽血，时间过长，动脉会发生较长时间的收缩，采血难以进行。

此外，兔和豚鼠还可以从股静脉、颈静脉、股动脉、颈总动脉采血，一般需做、静脉分离术后取血。

2. 小白鼠和大白鼠

（1）尾静脉采血 将鼠置于固定箱内，露出鼠尾，可用二甲苯涂擦鼠尾，使尾静脉充血。用剪刀剪断尾尖（小白鼠1~2mm，大白鼠5~10mm）后，即可流出血液。如血流不畅，用手轻轻从尾根部挤压数次，可取到数滴血液。

如实验需要间隔一段时间而多次采血时，每次采血可将鼠尾剪去很小一段。采血后用棉球压迫止血，并立即用6%液体火棉胶涂于尾部伤口处，使之结一层火棉胶薄膜，以保护伤口。

（2）眼眶后静脉丛采血 先制作硬质玻璃吸管，管长7~10cm，一端管径为0.6mm，壁厚为0.3mm的毛细管。采血部位是眼球和眼眶后界之间的眼眶后静脉丛。采血时，用左手从背部捉住动物，以食指和拇指握住颈部，利用对颈部所加的轻压力，使头部静脉血液回流困难，眼球充分外突。右手持消毒吸管，将其尖端插入内侧眼角，并轻轻由鼻侧眼眶壁平行地对喉头方向推进4~5mm，即达眼眶后静脉丛。为防止血液凝固，采血前可用1%肝素溶液湿润吸管壁。采血后将吸管拔出，同时放松左手使出血停止。用此采血法一次可取小白鼠血液0.2ml，大白鼠0.5ml，一般不发生术后穿孔出血或其他合并症。还可根据实验需要，于数分钟后在同一穿刺孔重复采血。除大、小白鼠，豚鼠和兔也可以从眼眶后静脉丛采血（图1-16）。

（3）小白鼠摘眼球取血。

3. 狗和猫 可在前、后肢皮下静脉采血。其基本方法与静脉注射法相同。需加注意的是抽血时速度要慢，以防针口吸着血管壁。此法一般可抽取10~20ml血液。此外，还可从颈静脉、颈动脉、股动脉采血，基本方法见颈部手术和股部手术。如实验需要抽取大量血液，可用心脏采血法，其方法与兔的心脏采血相同。

（五）动物的处死方法

1. 脊椎脱臼法 用左手拇指和食指捏住小白鼠头的后部，并用力下压，右手抓住鼠尾，用力向后上方拉，即可使颈椎脱臼，瞬间死亡（图 1 – 17）。

2. 空气栓塞法 向动物静脉内注入一定量的空气，使之发生栓塞而死亡。猫、狗、兔和豚鼠均可用此法处死。兔一般选用耳缘静脉，狗有前肢或后肢皮下静脉注射。兔、猫等静脉内注入 20～40ml 空气，狗注入 80～150ml 空气即可致死。

（王秋娟）

第三节　生理学常用仪器

生理学仪器一般由四大部分组成，即刺激系统、探测系统、信号调节系统和记录显示系统。

为使机体或离体组织、细胞兴奋，需要给予刺激。常用的刺激装置为电子刺激器。当生理现象是生物电信号时，探测系统可以是引导电极，包括记录单细胞电活动的玻璃微电极和记录群细胞电活动的粗大金属电极。当生理现象为其他某种能量形式时，如机械收缩、压力和声音等，探测系统又可以是换能器。由于生物电信号较为微弱，仅 $10\mu V \sim 100mV$，所以必须经过放大器放大，才能在记录仪或示波器上记录或显示变化的波形。记录系统通常使用示波器或笔描式记录仪。图 1 – 18 表示这些仪器的配置。

一、刺激系统

多种刺激因素，如光、声、电、温度、机械及化学因素都能使可兴奋组织产生生理反应。实验生理学中应用最广泛的是电刺激，因为这种刺激易于控制刺激参数，对组织没有损伤或损伤较小。在常用的刺激系统中，我们主要介绍电子刺激器和各种刺激电极。

（一）电子刺激器

电子刺激器是一种能产生一定波形的电脉冲仪，所产生的波形大致有方波、正弦波和不对称的波形（如感应电波）。因方波波形简单，易于产生和严格控制，而且计算刺激量也比较容易，陡峭的前沿刺激电流也比较有效，故方波最为常用（图 1 – 19）。

刺激强度是指方波幅度，可用电压或电流强度表示。电流强度一般从几微安至几十毫安，电压可在 200V 以内。刺激强度过小，不能使细胞膜静息电位（绝对值）降低至阈电位而引起细胞兴奋；刺激强度过大，可引起组织内电解和热效应而使其损伤和破坏。故在实验中，过强、过弱的刺激均应避免。

刺激时间是指方波的持续时间，又叫波宽。一般刺激器的持续时间从几十微秒至数秒；采用单向方波刺激时，刺激时间不宜过长，否则将产生损伤效应。为了减少引起组织损伤的电解和热效应，应尽量缩短刺激时间，并采用正负双向方波刺激。另外，使用最佳刺激时间与刺激强度的大小密切相关。一般讲，使用 1ms 波宽的双向方波刺激时，方波振幅以 10V 为佳；若波宽减小至 0.5ms，振幅常需加大至 40～50V。

在连续刺激时，还可调节刺激频率。刺激频率是刺激方波的重复频率，一般少于 1000

次/秒。刺激频率过高时，可能有一部分刺激落于组织的不应期而无反应，使刺激与生理效应不能同步。刺激频率的选择随被刺激组织的不同而变化，生理实验中以60～100次/秒为佳。应用连续刺激时，还可根据实验需要调节"串长"。"串长"表示以重复频率不断输出刺激方波可持续的时间，即一连产生数个方波的时间。

电子刺激器除可调节上述刺激参数外，尚有其他功能可供使用。总周期是同步脉冲的周期，同步脉冲表示一次刺激的时间点。同步脉冲输送到整个实验系统中，使各仪器有共同的时间起点，以保持时间上的同步。从同步脉冲到出现刺激方波的时间称为"延时"。调节"延时"，可使方波或方波刺激所引起的生理反应出现在示波器荧光屏上合适的位置，以便观察和记录。

（二）刺激电极

刺激电极多用金属制成。根据其性能可分为普通电极、保护电极和乏极化电极等（图1-20）。本文介绍前两种电极。

普通电极和保护电极多用银丝或不锈钢丝制成，一般将两条金属丝镶嵌在有机玻璃或电木框套内，刺激端裸露，作为细胞外刺激用。保护电极的绝缘框套在刺激端弯曲成钩状，金属丝包埋其中，仅在钩内一面裸露，故可保护其周围组织免受刺激（图1-20A和B）。

二、探测系统

（一）玻璃微电极

微电极作为生理学仪器探测系统的一部分，广泛应用于单细胞电活动的测量。微电极包括金属微电极（可用不锈钢丝、钨丝、铂丝等制作）和玻璃微电极（图1-20C）。玻璃微电极的制备法有多种，可参考有关文献。

（二）换能器

换能器（传感器）是指将一种能量形式转变为另一种能量形式的装置。作为探测系统的组成部分，可将非电性质的生理现象，如机械、声、光、磁以及温度等能量形式转变为电信号。然后将这种电信号经过前置放大器放大，显示或记录在示波器或记录仪上。换能器的种类很多，如张力换能器、压力换能器、光电换能器、声电换能器以及温电换能器等。本文介绍前三种换能器。

1. 张力换能器和压力换能器 这两种换能器在生理学研究中应用最为广泛。张力换能器可以测量在体及离体组织或器官的舒缩活动情况。压力换能器可以测量机体的各种压力变化（血压、胸膜腔内压、肺内压、心腔内压及消化管内压等）。基本原理用应变片将力或位移等非电量生理现象转变为电变化。应变片有电阻丝应变片和半导体应变片两种，它们通常安装于惠斯登电桥的线路中。

2. 光电换能器 这类换能器主要用光敏元件——光电管或光电池制作，基本原理是将光线强弱的变化转变为电流的变化。此变化的电流转变为电位，可直接引进示波器或记录仪。这类换能器也可用来测量压力或位移变化，甚至测量小动物的自发活动及脉搏的变化等，如光电池制作的压力换能器及拉力换能器。

三、信号调节系统

动物组织受刺激时的兴奋反应，可用示波器进行观察。但因生物电信号常很微弱，仅靠示波器的放大有时尚不够，必须经过放大器的放大，才能在示波器或记录仪上显示或记录变化的波形。前置放大器的功能是将微弱的生物电信号进行初步放大，供主放大器再放大。

放大器的种类很多，按其用途可分为电压放大器、电流放大器和功率放大器；按其放大的频率可分为直流放大器（呼吸、脉搏等）、低频放大器（动作电位等）、高频放大器及视频放大器；按其耦合方法可分为直流耦合放大器、阻容耦合放大器和变压器耦合放大器等。下面将正确使用放大器的有关性能指标作一简单介绍。

1. 频率响应　放大器对不同频率的信号具有不同的放大倍数，只能对某一范围内的频率有基本相同的放大作用。其上限频率与下限频率之间的频率范围，就是放大器的频率响应范围，称为放大器的通频带。在选择放大器时，必须适合所要放大的生理信号的频率范围。一般生物放大器要求频率响应范围是：直流放大器 $0 \sim 100\mathrm{kHz}$。

2. 时间常数　时间常数的正确与否，对图形的清晰、正确、不失真起着极其重要的作用。在电生理实验中，为了适合记录各种快变化或慢变化电位，特在前置放大器的输入端或前极和后极放大器之间加装时间常数选择（即高、低频补偿或衰减）电路。在记录快变化电位时，时间常数可选小些（如 $0.001\mathrm{s}$）；而记录慢变化电位时，时间常数则需加大（一般为 $2\mathrm{s}$）。记录中枢神经系统电活动时，时间常数不应小于 $0.1\mathrm{s}$。时间常数的选择可参考表 $1-2$（见后）。

3. 放大倍数　表示放大器放大信号的能力，说明放大器灵敏度的高低。前置放大器主要是进行电压放大，可用电压放大倍数 Ku 表示。

$$\text{Ku（电压增益）} = \text{输出电压} / \text{输入电压}$$

可见，电压放大倍数是放大器输出电压与输入电压的比值，一般可用直接测量法测出输出与输入电压的大小来计算。在电生理实验中，放大器放大倍数的选择需根据所研究的生物电信号的大小而定。如记录神经或心肌纤维的跨膜电位时，灵敏度可调节在 $5 \sim 10\mathrm{mV/cm}$；记录在体神经的电活动时，则灵敏度应调至 $50 \sim 100\mu\mathrm{V/cm}$。

4. 信噪比　任何一个放大器，除把有用的生物电信号放大外，还同时把一些无规则变化的电压或电流加以放大。这样杂乱无规则的电压或电流叫作放大器的噪声。在电子学上，常用信号噪声比（信噪比）来表示放大器放大微弱信号时的这一性能。

$$\text{信噪比} = \text{信号功率} / \text{噪声功率}$$

可见，只有信噪比大于1，微弱信号才能有效地加以放大。否则，放大器的放大倍数再高也无济于事。因为信号和噪声都以同样的放大倍数放大，例如，人的脑电只有几十微伏，如果脑电图机的噪声与输入端的噪声等效，电压为 $100\mu\mathrm{V}$ 以上，则脑电波就被淹没在噪声之中，无法分辨。所以信噪比也是放大器性能的重要指标。一个良好的生物放大器，必须信噪比和放大倍数都大。

放大器的噪声来源有内源性噪声和外源性噪声两种。内源性噪声是放大器本身或附属设施所产生的，如晶体管和电阻等由于电子的热运动而产生的热噪声。外源性噪声来自外周的交变电磁场或电磁波辐射，一般把这种噪声称为干扰。区别放大器噪声和干扰的方法是输入端接地，示波器上留下的噪声电平是放大器噪声，而接地后所消除的噪声部分为外界干扰信号。

在电子设备中，抑制噪声和排除干扰的有效措施是屏蔽和接地。如对干扰源施加屏蔽，屏蔽实验仪器，特别是实验对象，均可有效地排除干扰。一般电生理实验最好在屏蔽室或屏蔽箱内进行，所用仪器均应为金属机壳，各仪器间的连接线都应用屏蔽线，特别是对放大器的输入线以及前放与主放之间连线，更应做好屏蔽，尽量缩小接头处的裸露部分。所有屏蔽都应有良好接地。接地就是将某个点和一个等电位点或等电位面用低电阻导体连接起来，以构成电路和系统的基准电位。因此该点电位即为大地电位。电生理实验均应采取接地系统，以保证安全，并为信号电压提供基准电位。对于接地的方式，一般认为电生理实验以采用并联一点接地的方式为宜。噪声与干扰是电生理实验的大敌，在实际工作中往往需要花费很大的精力和很长的时间去解决。但是，妥善地把屏蔽和接地结合起来，并认真考虑接地方式，就可以解决大部分噪声和干扰。

5. 输入阻抗与输出阻抗 阻抗匹配在放大器放大过程中亦占有很重要的地位，也是保证放大器从信号源将信号顺利地检出、放大和显示的一项主要指标。放大器的阻抗匹配关系好像电池的内阻一样，如果内阻很低，接上相应的灯泡就会很亮；内阻增大，灯泡变暗；内阻很高时，灯泡几乎不亮。在放大器中，也存在输入阻抗与输出阻抗之间的搭配关系。

一般说来，对于一个多级放大器，特别是生物放大器，要求输入阻抗较高（1MΩ以上），这可以减小信号源的负担、减少生物信号的损失。在微电极的研究工作中，由于微电极尖端极细（一般 0.5～1MΩ 或更高），内阻很高（一般 10～20MΩ 或更高），要求微电极放大器具有特别高的输入阻抗（一般高达 10000MΩ）。否则，信号源内阻很高，引起输出的微弱生物信号的电压大都降落在这个电阻上，使放大器真正得到的输入极小。所以必须进行阻抗变换，使放大器的输入阻抗提高并远大于微电极的输入阻抗才行。

四、记录与信息处理系统

（一）示波器

示波器是用来观察电压或电流变化情况和测定其数值大小的一种电子仪器。凡能变换为电压或电流的电学量或非电学量，均可用示波器进行观察与测量。

示波器的核心部分是电子示波管，另有扫描讯号发生器、放大器和电源。

1. 电子示波管 示波管由电子枪、偏转系统及荧光屏三部分组成（图 1-21）。

（1）电子枪 是产生电子束和赖以聚焦的特殊装置，由灯丝、阴极、控制栅极和三个阳极等组成。

灯丝和阴极的作用是发射电子，控制栅极可控制电子射线的强度，从而达到控制荧光屏上光点辉度的作用。第一阳极和第二阳极组合在一起，分别加一定的电压，起到电子透镜的作用，可使电子束在荧光屏上会聚成一点，起到聚焦的作用。所以第一阳极为聚焦阳极。板面上的"聚焦"旋钮，是改变第一阳极的电压来调节聚焦的。第三阳极为加速阳极，可加速电子运动的速度，并能吸收屏幕上被击出的二次电子。

（2）偏转系统 包括两对相互垂直的偏转板，即一对垂直偏转板（y 轴偏转板）和一对水平偏转板（x 轴偏转板）。垂直偏转板上的电压发生变化时，可使电子束做上下运动。水平偏转板可控制电子束的左右移位，并用以产生扫描基线。示波器面板上的"水平位移"和"垂直位移"旋钮，是分别调节这两对偏转板上的电压大小，来改变光点位置的。在电生理实验中，生物信号加在 y 轴上，x 轴代表时间，这样就可以使光点在荧光屏上随时间而做直线运动。

（3）荧光屏　为示波管底的玻璃屏幕，屏的内壁涂有一层荧光物质。当高速运动的电子束打到荧光屏上某点时，此点就发光。在单位时间内打到荧光屏上的电子数越多，发光就越强。常用的荧光物质有硅酸锌（产生绿光）和硫化锌（产生蓝光）。电子束打到荧光物质上发光，而电子束停止后，发光还持续一定时间才停止，这段时间称为余辉时间。一般说来，观察频率高的信号时，宜选用短余辉示波管；而观察频率低、变化缓慢的信号时，则用长余辉示波管为宜。

2. SBR－1型示波器的正确使用

（1）一般注意事项

①开机时板面各旋钮一般置于下列位置：辉度　中间位置；触发电平　自动或连续；x 轴作用　正常；灵敏度　20V/cm；垂直位置　中心位置。

②电源接通后，冷却风扇开始工作，仪器预热30分钟后，性能即趋稳定，可进行校正与使用，能连续工作8小时。

③如因散热不佳或机内故障，使机内温度达到55℃以上时，示波器自动停止工作，应查明原因，排除故障后再行使用。

④在使用或维修时，若切断电源，应待3分钟后再接通电源开关，否则易损坏电源部分。

（2）辉度与聚焦　辉度旋钮用以调节光点的亮度，顺时针旋转，光点逐渐变亮。实验时，光点亮度不宜过大，一般以利于观察即可。

聚焦的调节应在慢扫描时进行，因为此时光点清晰，易于辨别。将光点调到最圆最小即可。

标尺亮度旋钮用来控制荧光屏面板上的照明灯，其亮度愈大，标尺愈明亮。标尺横坐标用以测量信号的时间过程，纵坐标用以测量信号的电压。摄影时，标尺亮度应适中。否则给人以喧宾夺主的感觉。

（3）垂直放大系统与输入方式　本系统由高增益差动式直流放大器和衰减器组成。由此系统输入的微弱信号，经放大后加于垂直偏转板上，使电子束按被测信号的变化规律做上下运动。灵敏度调节旋钮的作用是调整被测信号在荧光屏上的幅度，共分16档。可根据被测信号的大小，拨到适当位置。例如，心肌细胞的跨膜动作电位约为120mV，如微电极放大器的增益为1，则示波器灵敏度可置于20mV/cm，此时荧光屏上可出现6cm高度的波形。

输入方式分为单端输入和双端输入。单端输入：信号由A端或B端输入，输入选择旋钮置于相应的A或B的位置。双端输入：信号由A、B两端输入，此时输入旋钮应置于A～B位置。

本机输入端为差动形式，输入方式可分为AC（交流）与DC（直流）两种，以供选择。此输入方式的选择，需根据被测信号的特性而定。在一般的生理实验中，可选用AC方式；而缓慢的电变化，如膜电位、体表胃肠电图、皮肤电等，则应用DC输入方式。

直流平衡调节：直流平衡旋钮用来调节放大器变换时的直流电位，使灵敏度在任一档次时光点均不会漂移出荧光屏。调节方法：先将扫描调至连续，灵敏度旋钮拨至20V/cm，再将直流平衡与位移旋钮调至中间位置，后轻调直流平衡的暗调电位器，将扫描线调到荧光屏的中央位置。逐挡转动灵敏度旋钮，并随时调节暗调电位器，使扫描线位于荧光屏的中央位置，直至调到灵敏度最高档为止。以后直流平衡的暗调电位器即不需要再调节。如实验中需要移动基线，只要用位移旋钮调节即可。

（4）触发选择旋钮 为了清晰地观察和测量电信号的参数，这就需要将刺激信号输入触发扫描发生器，使电子束扫描受到刺激器控制，刺激器输出与扫描同步，这样刺激所引起的反应也与扫描同步，使图像在荧光屏同一位置上重复出现。触发方式有：①电源触发；②上线与下线（AC、DC）内触发；③外触发（AC、DC）。可根据实验的具体要求，选择不同的触发方式。

（二）二道生理记录仪

生理记录仪是常用的生理学实验的仪器之一。生物学信号或生理变化经过放大后可以通过它的记录笔直接描记在记录纸上。由于记录笔有较大的惰性和较小的频响，故通常用于记录频率小于 100 次/秒和持续时间大于 10ms 的信号变化而不用于快反应信号，如神经的动作电位。在生理学实验中，常常使用二道记录仪（图 1 – 22）。

在启动生理记录仪的电源开关前，应先把所有开关置于"断"的位置，控制走纸的琴键也置于"停"。然后接通市电，开启本机电源开关，指示灯即亮。放下抬笔架，将换能器插座与本机接通。机械－电换能器与 A1B1，血压换能器与 A2B2，分别组成放大系统。机器运转前必须调零。调零应分级进行，先调后级放大器（A1 或 A2），此时应将后级放大与前级放大断开，可用二芯导线插头插入后级输入插座，使之断路。然后将放大器开关置于通的位置，旋转调节旋钮使笔尖居于中线。此时也可检查时标与实验描记笔的反应。此级检验完毕后，拨去二芯输入短路，再检查前级放大器（B1 或 B2）功能。

在未拨通前置放大器的开关前，应先把放大器灵敏度置于最低档，若是调整 A1B1 放大系统，则将 B1 的时间常数旋钮置于交流（AC）任一档，旋钮 B1 的调零旋钮使笔尖居于中线，再将时间常数置于直流（DC）档。旋动灵敏度旋钮，从最低档到最高档逐一转换，描笔尖均应居中线不动，若有偏离可调"直流平衡"。在调整前置放大器时，一定不要使输入端短路。因此，先要接通换能器，或使电极与动物标本接触良好，以免描笔产生剧烈震动而折断，然后才能开启前置放大器的开关。开启后若描笔偏离中线，则调节换能器的"调零"，使之回到中线，以后就可以开始进行实验。

实验完毕，应断开前、后级放大器的输入、输出开关，将灵敏度置于最低档，抬起笔架，切断电源，拔下插头。

若作血压换能记录，其后级放大系统的调零与前述相同，在检查前置放大器时，应接好血压换能器的输出线，并将血压换能放大器的输入、测量开关均置于"断"位，灵敏度置于最低档，然后才能拨去在调整后级时插入的二芯断路插头，拨通血压换能器输入开关。若笔尖偏离中线，则调节放大器的"调零"使之居中，然后旋动灵敏度旋钮，从最低档到最高档，拨通每一档时笔尖应不离开中线；若离开，就应调"直流平衡"（调好后在实验时即不能再扭动，否则影响血压绝对值的观测）上述步骤进行完毕后才能拨通血压放大器的测量开关，此时若描笔偏离中线，可调换能器的"调平衡"，使描笔回到中线。一切完毕后才能打开通向换能器的血管导管，开始描记血压，进行实验。

（三）BL－420F 生物信号采集与分析系统介绍

BL－420F 生物信号采集与分析系统是新一代概念型生物功能实验系统，其性能指标和使用方便性远远超过目前市场上销售的国内外任何同类产品。比如，其可编辑波形的刺激器，目前国内还没有任何一家产品能够实现，其 4 通道扫描速度独立可调，系统自身集成的多种专用数据分析功能，目前国外还没有任何一家产品能够实现。

1. 系统硬件指标

（1）采用 USB2.0 全速传输方式。

（2）系统可内置（放入计算机机箱内）、可外置。

（3）单通道最高采样率达 1MHz，最低采样率 0.01Hz。

（4）使用 16 位精度的 A/D 采样芯。

（5）放大器具有宽输入动态范围：$\pm 1V \sim \pm 20\mu V$，相当于 $1 \sim 50000$ 倍的放大倍数。

（6）采用 5 阶贝塞尔滤波器，滤波范围为 1Hz ~ 30kHz。

（7）波形可编辑的光电隔离刺激器，刺激器的输出波形幅度高达 100V，可以输出三角波、方波、正负方波、正弦波或自己编辑的任意波形。

（8）内置 12 导联标准心电选择电路，1 通道可任意选择 12 导联标准心电波形。

（9）无需手动按钮就可直接进行多设备同步级联，扩展为 8 ~ 16 个采样通道的新设备。

2. 系统软件指标

（1）可任意拖动灵活改变窗口宽度的双视观察系统，在不停止实时实验观察的同时查看以前记录的数据，而且可实现不同状态下实验波形前后变化的对比。

（2）为了适应于实验教学工作，该系统预设计了 10 大类共计 55 个实验模块，为国内外同类产品中预制实验模块最多的产品。

（3）为了适应于科研工作，该系统设计了众多的实验数据分析功能，能够对原始波形或记录的波形进行实时地微分、积分、频率直方图以及频谱分析等数据处理工作。

（4）具有多种通用数据测量方式　包括单点测量、两点测量、区间测量、实时测量等，可测量出波形的最大、最小、平均值，斜率、时间、频率、均方差等参数。

（5）众多的专用数据测量功能　血流动力学实验参数的分析、心肌细胞动作电位参数的测量、苯海拉明的拮抗参数（PA_2、PD_2）的测定等测量功能，还可以按照 Bliss 法计算 LD_{50}、**** 值、计算 t 检验和半衰期值等。

（6）四个通道扫描速度独立可调，零扫描速度采样，通用程控刺激等功能更具有独特魅力。

（7）实时采样过程中，可以根据需要随时改变采样率。

（8）用户可以根据需要设定 1 ~ 16 个显示通道（5 ~ 16 通道可用于分析）。

3. BL－420F 实验模块

实验类型	具体实验项目名称			
	序号	实验名称	序号	实验名称
肌肉神经类	1	刺激强度与反应的关系	6	肌肉收缩－兴奋的时相关系
	2	刺激频率与反应的关系	7	痛觉实验
	3	神经干动作电位的引导	8	阈强度与动作电位关系
	4	神经干兴奋传导速度的测定	9	细胞放电
	5	神经干兴奋不应期测定	10	心肌不应期测定

续表

实验类型	序号	实验名称	序号	实验名称
循环系统	1	蛙心灌流	7	兔动脉血压调节
	2	期前收缩－代偿间歇	8	左心室内压与动脉血压
	3	全导联心电图	9	血流动力学模块
	4	心肌细胞动作电位	10	急性心肌梗死及药物治疗
	5	心肌细胞动作电位与心电图	11	阻抗测定
	6	兔减压神经放电		
呼吸系统	1	膈神经放电	3	呼吸相关参数的采集与处理
	2	呼吸运动调节	4	肺通气功能测定
消化系统	1	消化道平滑肌电活动	3	消化道平滑肌活动
	2	消化道平滑肌的生理特性	4	苯海拉明拮抗参数的测定
感觉器官	1	肌梭放电	3	视觉诱发电位
	2	耳蜗生物电活动	4	脑干听觉诱发电位
中枢神经系统	1	大脑皮层诱发电位	4	诱发脑电
	2	中枢神经元单位放电	5	脑电睡眠分析
	3	脑电图		
泌尿系统	1	影响尿生成的因素		
药理学	1	PA_2 值的测定	6	药物对实验性心律失常的影响
	2	药物的镇痛作用	7	药物对麻醉大鼠的利尿作用
	3	尼可刹米对吗啡呼吸抑制解救作用	8	垂体后叶素对小白鼠离体子宫的作用
	4	药物对离体肠肌的作用	9	电惊厥实验
	5	传出神经系统药物对麻醉大鼠血压的影响		
病理生理学	1	大白鼠实验性肺水肿	4	急性右心衰
	2	急性失血性休克	5	急性高钾血症
	3	急性左心衰合并肺水肿		

（丁启龙　卢娜）

General Introduction

Section Ⅰ   Purposes, Demands and Rules of Physiological Experiment Courses

Purposes and demands

Physiological experiment is one of the important links for developing students' skill. It's purpose is to make students master the basic experimental technologies initially, understand scientific methods of how to acquire knowledge of physiology, examine and solidify basic theory of physiology by doing some representative experiments; to cultivate serious attitude toward science, rigid request, accurate working method and seek the truth from facts of working style in experiments; to cultivate student's ability of observing and comparing things objectively, ability of analyzing and synthesizing and ability of independent thinking.

Ⅰ. Preparations

1. Read the experimental instructions carefully to understand the purpose, demand, steps and procedure of the experiment.

2. Review the correlating theories in order to fully understand and foresee the due results of each step.

3. Be familiar with the instruments and basic operating methods.

4. Pay attention to and estimate the possible errors occurring in the experiment.

Ⅱ. Precautions

1. Keep equipment and supplies in a tidy, clean and orderly way.

2. Operate the experiment with a serious attitude following as the steps. Don't alter anything at your will. Don't do anything with no relation to the experiment. Be careful to protect the animals and specimens, save materials and drugs.

3. Observe the phenomenon carefully and patiently during the experiment, record it and think it over: ①What has happened? ②Why did it happen? ③What is the physiological significance of it?

Ⅲ. Arrangement

1. Wash and clean everything. Report to the instructor immediately if something was damaged.

2. Arrange the experimental record, draw a conclusion and write the experimental report.

Results process

Results observed in the experiment should be changed into measurable indexes in order that the changing regularities can be studied, so it's necessary to analyze and arrange the results from the experiment.

Measurable results, including length, height, velocity and weight, should be given correct unit and numeric value.

Generally, results that have curve record should be recorded in curve as possible as you can. Directions should be marked on the curves, such as stimulating symbols and time signs.

In order to be conveniently analyzed and compared, some experimental results can be recorded in the form of table or diagram. When tabulating, within the table you can list observing items on the left and changing numeric values of results on the right in sequence. A brief direction can also be attached to the table if it's necessary. The following should be noticed when tabulating:

1. List numeric value table of experimental results just beside the diagram.

2. Abscissa represents stimulating conditions and ordinate represents reactions that have happened.

3. Annotate the coordinate axis appropriately, including dose unit.

4. Choose scale of suitable size for mapping, decide the length of the coordinate axis according to the dimension of the diagram.

5. Draw curve or bending line that pass through each point smoothly. If it isn't continuous variation it can also be shown in cylinder shape.

6. Mark experimental conditions under the diagram.

Data acquired in the experiment needs statistical disposal (appendix III), getting means, standard deviation and differential significant test so that experimental results can be evaluated.

Requests on writing report

I. Everyone should write a report on demonstrating experiment or experiment that has been done by his own. And the report must be finished on time.

II. The report should be written seriously according to specific requests of the experiment. The report must be written concisely, fluently and clearly. And punctuation mark should be used correctly. The following are the requests:

1. List your name, class, team, date, room temperature and air pressure.

2. Give the number and the title of the experiment.

3. Express the purpose of the experiment

4. It is unnecessary to describe the method of the experiment. You can explain it concisely if instrument and method altered temporarily or your operating technique influenced the credibility of the result.

5. Results is a very important part of the experiment, during the experiment you should record the phenomena actually and correctly as well as record whatever you observed in the experiment in time. You should fill your report according to your record instead of your memory, or else there would be errors and omissions when that experiment finished. Results processing has been described in the former item.

6. Discussion and conclusion: Discussion is to explain and analyze the results on the basis of the former theories. The possible causes should be considered and analyzed when the results are not the expected, and the physiological significance of the results should be pointed out. Experimental conclusion is a general and summary judgment drawn from the results, in other word, it's a summari-

zation of concepts, principles and theories that the experiment could examine. In the discussion, theoretic analysis that has not been tested sufficiently should not be written in your conclusion.

Writing the discussion and drawing the conclusion are creating works. You shouldn't copy the book blindly but write the report seriously. The references should be marked on.

[Appendix] The normal pattern of the report

Report on physiological experiment

Name _____ Class _____ Team _____ Date _____ Room temperature _____ Air pressure _____

Number and title _____

Purpose _____

Method _____

Results _____

Discussion and conclusion _____

Laboratory rules

1. Arrive the lab on time, obey the disciplines, and wear white – gown in the lab.

2. Do the experiment attentively. Don't do anything with no relation to the experiment.

3. Keep quiet in the laboratory. Don't make noises.

4. Form a good habit. Be sure to keep environment and instruments orderly and clean. Parts of animal body, fragments and residues should be put in the appointed places.

5. Return public equipments and supplies and drugs to their original places after using.

6. Exchange instrument with other teams is not allowed. Report to the director or superintendent immediately if the instrument is damaged or disordered.

7. Take good care of the public properties, such as instruments, furniture and test animals. Save water and electricity, drugs, cotton, distilled water and solutions. If there is something that should not have been damaged or has been consumed excessively, it should be compensated by the team or the individual according to the situation.

8. Put everything in order and keep everything clean after the experiment toform a good habit.

9. Students who are on duty for the day should clean the laboratory, tackle the dead body of animals and keep everything in a proper way, turn off electricity and water, and close windows and doors.

Section Ⅱ Biopsy

Physiological experiment uses living animal or human body as observing objection and experimental material. Biopsy technology is critical to the success of the experiment. During the experiment, student should put emphasis on learning and mastering these operating technologies in order to improve their operating skills.

Generally there are two kinds of physiological experiment methods, in vitro and in vivo, the latter includes chronic and acute experiments. Acute in vivo experiment is to operate on an animal to exposure the specific organ in order that its functions and changing regularities could be studied on condition that the animal has been anesthetized or it's brain or spinal cord has been destroyed, such as observing in vivo heart activity or studying kidney urinary function. Acute ex vivo experiment is to take organs or tissues needed out of animal body that is alive or just has been put to death and place them in near – normal physiological artificial environments to observe their physiological functions, for example, ex vivo cardiac perfusion, activity of ex vivo intestine, studying neuromuscular physiological functions by using sciatic nerve – gastrocnemius muscle specimen. Acute experiment cannot last long. Observations and studies can only be carried out in definite period and animals cannot survive the experiment. Chronic experiment is a kind of experimental method that use integral and conscious animals as objections in specific terms. Using this method you can observe certain physiological functions of the animal continuously and repeatedly in a longer period. It needs to perform some sterile surgical operations on the animal body, such as gastrointestinal fistula operation, concealing electrode in certain part of the organic or cutting an organ. Experiment can only becarried out after the animal recovery. It takes a long time for this methods. So during the experiment, animals need special nursing.

Commonly used surgical instruments and their uses

Commonly used surgical instruments include operating scalpel, surgical scissors, surgical forceps, needles used to destroy frog's spinal cord and glass dissecting needle during the physiological experiment.

Ⅰ. **Operating scalpel**　It is mainly used to cut and dissect tissues. Its bladeis replaceable according to the operating site and property. There are four ways of holding a scalpel.

1. Holding a scalpel like holding a bow It is the most commonly way of holding a scalpel.

And it is used to cut skins of abdomen, cervical part or thigh (Fig. 1 – 1).

2. Holding a scalpel like holding a pen It is often used to cut small and short incision gently and accurately. Such as dissecting blood vessels and nerves, cutting peritoneum incisions (Fig. 1 – 2).

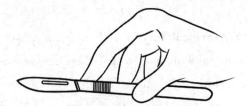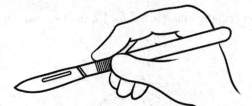

Fig. 1 – 1 　Holding a forceps like
holding a bow
　　　　　Fig. 1 – 2 　Holding a forceps like
holding a pen

3. Grasping a scalpel It is often used to cut incision which has a wide range or is hard to cut. Such as amputation and long skin incision.

4. Holding a scalpel with its blade upward It is often used to cut tissues upward in case of damaging deep tissues, such as cutting abscess.

Ⅱ. **Surgical scissors**　It is mainly used to shear coarse and soft tissues, such as skin or muscle. It can also be used to separate tissues, with its pointed end inserting in the interspaces to separate connective tissue that has no big vessels. Surgical scissors are found in the curved or straight va-

21

riety, with a sharp or blunt nose. Moreover, eye scissors is another small surgical scissors, which is used to shear soft tissues, including blood vessels and nerves. Eye scissors is also found in the curved or straight variety. Correct way of holding a surgical scissors is to hold the scissors with thumb and fourth finger, and put index finger above the scissors (Fig. 1 – 3).

III. Hemostatic forceps It is mainly used to stop bleeding by clamping vessels or hemorrhagic spots, to separate tissues, to pull sutured lines, to clip and pull surgical needles. The correct way of holding a hemostatic forceps is similar to that of the surgical scissors (Fig. 1 – 4). The way of opening a hemostatic forceps is: First utilizing thumb and fourth finger of right hand to press the forceps, then opening the forceps with a screwing action.

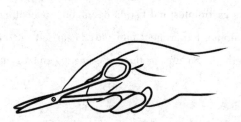

Fig. 1 – 3 Correct way of holding
a surgical scissors

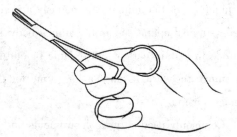

Fig. 1 – 4 Correct way of holding
a vascular forceps

According to operating needs, vascular forceps are found in the curved or straight, toothed or long lug, atraumatic, long or short variety. For example, straight kind serves in shallow part of operating field or subcutaneous part to stop bleeding. Curved kind serves in deep part to stop bleeding. Mosquito forceps serves in refinedhemostasia or separating tissues.

IV. Needle holder It is used to hold needles while suturing all kinds of tissues. The needle should be hold by the pointed end of the needle holder. The clamped site of the needle is one – third borderline between its end and its middle part. The correct way of holding a needle holder is similar to that of a surgical scissors. In order to be convenient, thumb and fourth finger should not have to be put into the annulus but hold near the proximal lug (Fig. 1 – 5).

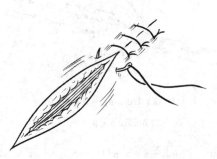

Fig. 1 – 5 Correct way of
holding a needle holder

V. Surgical forceps It is mainly used to clamp or raise tissues so that they can be easily striped, sheared or sutured. Surgical forceps are divided into two kinds: toothed or smooth forceps. Toothed forceps is used to clamp tough and firm tissues, such as skin, fascia or muscle tendon. Smooth forceps is used to clamp fragile tissues, such as vessel, nerve or mucosa. The correct way of holding a surgical forceps is given in Fig. 1 – 6, clamping tissues with you thumb, index finger and middle finger properly, slightly and steadily.

VI. Bone forceps It is used to cut bone tissue. Such as opening cranial cavity or opening medullary cavity of bone. Bone forceps are found in scissors or butterfly type (Fig. 1 – 7), the former is used to cut bone matrix, the latter is used to cut specula.

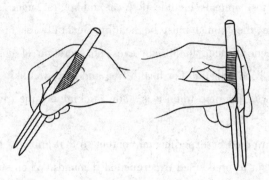
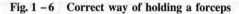

Fig. 1 – 6   Correct way of holding a forceps

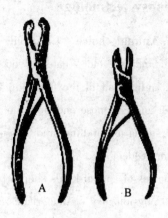

Fig. 1 – 7   Bone forceps

A. Butterfly type   B. Scissors type

Ⅶ. Cranial drill   It is mainly used to drill bouche when opening the cranium (Fig. 1 – 8).

Ⅷ. Needles used to destroy frog's spinal cord   It is used to destroy cerebral medulla and spinal cord. It has needle handle and needle body (Fig. 1 – 9A).

Ⅸ. Glass dissecting needle   It is specially used to separate nerve and vessel. The head can be found in the curved or straight variety, with round and smooth pointed end (Fig. 1 – 9B).

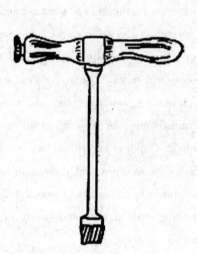

Fig. 1 – 8   Cranial drill

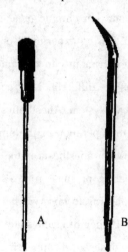

Fig. 1 – 9   Needle used to destroy frog's spinal cord (A) and glass dissecting needle (B)

Ⅹ. Surgical needle   It is mainly used to suture all kinds of tissues. They are designed in various styles and are available in different lengths, shapes. Including round needle, cutting needle, curved needle and straight needle. Round needle is used for transfixing soft tissues. Cutting needle is used for suturing tough tissues like skin. Curved needle is preferred in suturing within small, deep tissues.

Ⅺ. Artery clamp   It is mainly used to block artery bleeding in a short period, e. g. used in arterial cannula.

Biopsy technology

Ⅰ. **Animal choice**　Commonly used test animals include dog, cat, rabbit, rat, mice, guinea pig, toad and frog etc. Whatever you choose, the animal must be healthy. Generally, as to health mammal animal, all of the following are needed: sheen fur, bright eyes, no secretion of nose and eyes, wet and cool nose end, active reaction, good appetite. For health frog and toad, wet skin, liking activity, sitting on hindlimb and supporting with forelimb when it is static, sticking out the trunk, all these are needed.

Choices of animal kinds should be determined by experimental content so that animals' dissecting and physiological characteristics can adapt to predefined experimental demands. When studying the afferent impulse of aortic arch decompression nerve, rabbit is usually chosen as studying objection. Because rabbit's decompression nerve is concomitant with vagus nerve, forming a tract in cervical part and is easy to be found and separated. When studying electrical activity of cardiac specific conduction system, dog's Purkinje fiber or rabbit's sinoatrial node is usually chosen as experimental materials. Dog's Purkinje fiber is thick in cardiac ventricle and is easy to be dissected and separated. In physiology study, especially in basal theoretical study, choosing animal appropriately is usually critical to the success of the experiment. But higher animal is not always the better choice. Demands of the experiment should be taken into consideration.

Ⅱ. **Animal anesthesia**　In chronic or acute in vivo experiment, the animal must be anesthetized before the operation. During experiment or operation, anesthesia can relieve pain and keep the animal calm so that the experiment can be done successfully. There are many kinds of anesthetics but their acting principles are different. They can causephysiological function change except for anesthetizing the central nerve system. Anesthetics should be chosen cautiously according to the properties of the experiment, the operation or the animal kind. Animals must be properly anesthetized; it will cause adverse effect when anesthesia is too deep or too light. Depth of anesthesia can be judged from respiration, disappearing of some reflexes, tension degree of muscles and dimension of pupil. People often use simple way to observe the depth of anesthesia by stimulating corneal reflex or pinching muscle of thigh. Proper drugged state is that respiration is deep, slow and steady, corneal reflex and kinesthetic response are disappearing and muscles are relaxing.

1. **Kinds and uses of commonly used anesthetics**　Anesthetics can be divided into two kinds: local anesthetic and general anesthetic. Local anesthesia often use 0.5% ~ 1.0% procaine hydrochloride or 2% cocaine hydrochloride for skin or mucosa surface anesthesia. In physiological experiment, general anesthesia is usually adopted, such as volatile diethyl ether and non – volatile barbiturates, anhydroglucochloral.

(1) Diethyl ether　It is a kind of respiratory narcotic which is suitable to all kinds of test animals. When using diethyl ether to anesthetize cat, rabbit or rodents, the animal can be put in a special glass bell jar that contains ethyl absorbent cotton. The animal will be anesthetized after inhaling it for about 15 ~ 20 seconds. When anesthetizing dog, you can put mouth muffle on the mouth of the animal, and drip diethyl ether on the mouth muffle gradually and keep the animal quietly.

Diethyl ether stimulates the respiratory tract to secrete mucus. Atropine sulfate (0. 1 ~ 0. 3mg/kg weight) can be injected (intramuscular injection, i. m. or subcutaneous injection, sc.) to prevent the respiratory tract from being blocked.

Diethyl ether is safer and can be easily controlled. Its maintainable time is short. The animal can be easily awakened after anesthesia. Diethyl ether needs special management to prevent the animal from awakening early or being anesthetized excessively.

（2）Pentobarbital sodium　Pentobarbital is one of the most commonly used anesthetics, usually in 5% water solution form (intraperitoneal injection, i. p. or intravenous injection, i. v.). Its effect starts quickly and maintenance time is about 2 ~ 4hour after one dosage and needs no special management. If needed additional injection during the experiment, it can be injected through vein with 1/5 dosage, the maintenance time is 1 ~ 2hour. Serious inhibition of respiratory and circulatory system will occur when it is injected excessively, which is fatal to the animal.

（3）Ethyl carbamate　Another name of it is urethane. It is soluble in water, commonly used concentration is 20% ~ 25%. It is suitable to all kinds of animals, such as cat, dog, rabbit (i. v. or i. p.), for frog, it can be injected through subcutaneous lymphatic bladder.

Non – volatile anesthetic is convenient for use and its maintenance time is longer. Animal needs no special care during the experiment and depth of anesthesia can be easily controlled. Most laboratories adopt this kind of anesthesia. Its shortcoming is that the animal awakes slowly.

Dosage and usage of commonly used anaesthetic are given in the following table (Table 1 – 1)

2. Administration pathway and methods of anesthetics　Administration pathways of non – volatile anesthesia include intravenous injection, intraperitoneal injection, intramuscular injection, subcutaneous injection or lymphatic bladder injection.

Table 1 –1　Dosage and usage of commonly used anaesthetic

Anaesthetic	Animal kind	Administration Pathway	Drug Concentration	Dosage (mg/kg weight)	Maintenance Time (hour)	Remarks
Diethyl ether	All kinds of animals	Trachea inhalation	—	Suitable dose	Shorter	Stimulate the respiratory tract, can be prevented by injecting atropine(sc. or im.)
Pentobarbital sodium	Dog/cat/rabbit	Vein	3%	30	2 ~ 4	Steady anesthetization, using caffeine or phenylethylamine for saving.
	Dog/cat/rabbit	Abdominal cavity		35		
	Rodent	Abdominal cavity		40		
	Bird	Muscle		50 ~ 100		
Ethyl carbamate	Dog/ cat/ rabbit	Vein	20% ~ 25%	1000	2 ~ 4	Soluble in water. Affection on organ function is very small.
	Dog/cat/ rabbit	Abdominal cavity		1000		
	Rodent	Abdominal cavity		1000		
	Bird	Muscle		1250		
	Frog	Subcutaneous lymphatic bladder		2000		
Alphachloralose	Dog/ rabbit	Vein	1%	60 ~ 80	3 ~ 4	Low solubility. Can be heated but no boiled. Affections on respiration and vasomotor center are small.
	Cat	Abdominal cavity		60 ~ 80		
	Rodent	Abdominal cavity		80 ~ 100		

Anaesthetic	Animal kind	Administration Pathway	Drug Concentration	Dosage (mg/kg weight)	Maintenance Time (hour)	Remarks
Pentothal sodium	Dog cat Rabbit	Vein Vein	2.5% ~5%	15 ~25 10 ~20	0.5 ~1.5	Solution isn't stable, dispensing when using, not suitable for injection (sc. im.). Damages on cardiovascular and internal organs are small. Injecting slowly to prevent from anesthetizing excessively.
Phenobarbital sodium	Dog cat rabbit Dog cat rabbit Pigeon	Vein Abdominal cavity Muscle	10%	80 ~100 100 ~150 300	24 ~72	Anesthesia induction period is long and anesthesia depth can't be easily controlled. Not suitable for BP experiment. Using phenylethylamine and tetrachloromathane when anesthesia is exceeded.

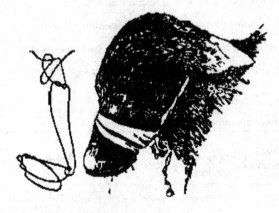

Fig. 1 – 10　Ways of binding a dog's nose and mouth

（1）Intravenous injection　It is usually used to anesthetize dog and rabbit. Dog must be tranquilized before being anesthetized, especially strange dog, to prevent it from hurting people. The dog's nose and mouth should be bound with coarse cotton band: winding from lower jaw to upper jaw to tie a knot, then winding to lower jaw to tie another knot, pulling the band to the back of the dog's head to tie the third knot and a slipknot (Fig. 1 – 10). The dog's cephalic vein that is in the medial part of forelimb and small saphenous vein which is in the lateral part of hindlimb are usually chosen for injection and blood collection. Before injection, you should cut coated hair of the injection site, hold and press the concentric tip of the vein with your hand to make the vessel become congestion and expansion. Along the vessel direction, you should prick the needle into subcutaneous part just beside the vessel, and then prick into the vessel. For the time being, you would see recurrent blood. Thereafter, you can fix the needle with one hand and inject slowly with another hand (Fig. 1 – 11).

The commonly used injection site of rabbit is marginal vein of its ear. The external vessel of rabbit ear is vein and the central vessel is artery. Before injection, you'd better fix the animal in rabbit box, expose it's head outside the box to prevent it from struggling. Firstly, you should cut coated hair of the injection site; clamp the concentric tip of marginal vein with index finger and middle finger of left hand to make it become congestion, and fix the ear with thumb and ring fin ger, then hold injection syringe with right hand and prick it into the vein along the vessel direction. After pricking, you should move index finger and middle finger of left hand to the head of the needle, combining with the thumb to fix the needle in the vein. Thereafter, you can inject slowly with another hand (Fig. 1 – 12). It illustrates that the needle doesn't go into the vein if injection resistance is maximum or the injection site is swelling. You should pull the needle out and prick once more. First injection should start from axifugal tip of the vein in order that it could be injected repeatedly.

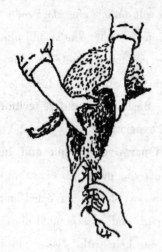

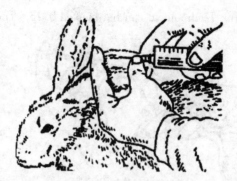

Fig. 1 – 11　Injection of small saphenous vein of dog's hindlimb　　　**Fig. 1 – 12　Injection of marginal vein of rabbit's ear**

（2）Intraperitoneal injection It is usually used to anesthetize cat and rodent. When anesthetizing cat, you should grasp its skin plica of nuchal region tightly, prick needle into enterocoelia quickly and pull the needle out instantly after injection. Cat may get angry frequently and it's claw and tooth may hurt people. For play it safe, you should put cat in a cloth bag and inject after sealed. When anesthetizing rodent, safety is also important. You can inject a mouse in a handhold way (Fig. 1 – 13). You should clamp its tail with little finger and ring finger of left hand, grasp ear and skin of cervical part quickly with the other three finger, with its abdomen upward, prick needle into lateral part of linea alba abdominis on hypogastric region with your right hand, with needle and skin forming a 45° angle. If resistance disappears after the needle passing through abdominal

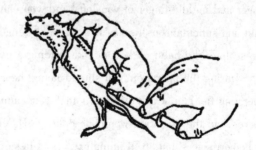

Fig. 1 – 13　Injection of enterocoelia of mouse

muscle, keeping the needle in still and drawing back slightly, if there are no intestinal contents, urine and blood being drawn out, you could inject anesthetic gently.

（3）Intramuscular Injection　Animal's two sides of buttock or thigh are usually chosen as injection part, including monkey, dog, cat and rabbit. First you should fix the animal, then hold injection syringe with your right hand, there would have a 60° angle between needle and muscle, prick needle into the muscle and massage the injection part to help the drug absorption.

（4）Subcutaneous injection　It is not commonly used in injecting anesthesia. Subcutaneous injection part of mouse is usually on its back. You can pull its skin and prick needle into subcutaneous part. Swaying the needle slightly, if the needle can be swayed easily it means that the needle has been pricked into subcutaneous part. Then the drug can be injected. When pulling the needle out, you'd better pinch injection part slightly with your finger to prevent drug solution from leaking out. As to rat, guinea pig, rabbit and cat, their back, medial surface of thigh or buttock are often chosen as injection part because at which subcutaneous fat is little.

（5）Lymphatic bladder injection   It is usually used to anesthetize frog or toad. Because frog's skin is thinner and its elasticity is very poor, drug solution will outflow after the needle being pulled out, it is suitable to choose pectoral lymphatic bladder as injection site. You should prick the needle into oral mucosa, entering subcutaneous lymphatic bladder through myometrium of lower jaw, then inject drug. Each animal can be injected 0. 25 ~ 1ml solution at a time (Fig. 1 – 14).

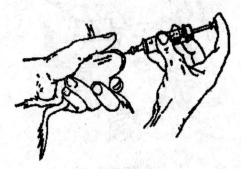

Fig. 1 – 14   Lymphatic bladder injection of frog

Ⅲ. Basic manipulative technique of acute animal experiment

1. Operative incision and hemostasis

Before carrying out skin incision on mammal animal body, you should cut coated hair of the incisional part and area around the incision. You should cut hair with scissors, avoiding raising hair, to prevent skin from being injured and put hair in a glass beaker that contains water, to prevent hair from flying up to pollute the environment. Before operation, you should take notice of dimension and dissection structure of the incision; obeying principles that cut less vessels and nerves. At the same time, you should take the coincidence of incision and direction of layers of tissues fiber into consideration as possible as you can. Incision dimension should be appropriate and not too large. After fixing the skin of two sides of superior extremity of the incision with thumb, index finger and middle finger of you left hand, you can hold operating scalpel with your right hand to cut skin and subcutaneous tissues with proper strength and directly reaching myometrium. You can hold the scalpel like holing a bow or like holding a pen.

During the operation, you should notice hemostasis at any time to avoid badly mutilated in the operating field in which condition that you cannot tell the differences between blood vessels and nerves, and the operation would be delayed. Different hemostatic methods can be adopted according to hemorrhage situation. If miniature vessel hemorrhaging, you can press it by using lukewarm saline gauze to stop bleeding. When major vessel hemorrhaging, you should find the petechia first and clamp it with hemostatic forceps, then ligature it with a thread. If large vessel is damaged, you should stop bleeding accurately and quickly, or else the experiment will be affected if losing blood too much. During the experiment you should close the wound temporarily or cover the wound with lukewarm saline gauze to prevent the tissue from becoming dehydration.

2. Operative knot   It is not only a important technique in surgical operation, but also a basal technique in acute animal experiment. There are many kinds of operative knots. Quadrate knot is the most commonly used in physiological experiment. There are one – handed tied knot, bimanual tied knot and holding forceps tied knot. One – handed tied knot is most convenient but the ligature must be remained longer. Holding forceps tied knot is used in conditions that ligature is too short or ligature site is too deep.

3. Operation on neck

（1）Tracheal separation　You should fix the animal in supine position, shear coated hair of its abdominal part of neck, and cut skin along cervical midline adjacent to inferior part of throat with operating scalpel. Length of incisions: rabbit or cat is about 5 ~ 7cm, dog is about 10cm; rat or guinea pig is about 4cm. In mid – abdominal part of trachea, separating the subcutaneous connect tissues layer by layer with your hand or hemostatic forceps, you will see sternohyoid muscle which is covering the abdominal part of trachea. Separating sternohyoid muscle in the midline with hemostatic forceps, then the trachea will be exposed.

（2）External jugular vein separation　External jugular vein of mammal is thick, its wall is thin and its distribution is superficial. It lies in subcutaneous part of neck, lateral margin of sternal mastoid. While you separating the vein, you can pinch unilateral skin of the incision with your thumb and index finger of left hand, and then turn it over outward; you will turn the dark purple thick vein on your index finger. Separating connective tissue with glass dissecting needle or exquisite hemostatic forceps along lateral part of the vein, then the external jugular vein can be separated, crossing a thread under it for availability.

（3）Common carotid artery separation　It lies in the lateral part of trachea. Its abdominal part is covered by sternohyoid muscle and sternothyroid muscle. When separating, you can pinch sternal muscle of unilateral part of separated trachea, turn it over outward and you can turn common carotid artery and nerve tract on your index finger, separate connect tissue in the lateral part of the artery with glass dissecting needle or hemostatic forceps, then you will separate the common carotid artery, cross a thread for availability. Paying attention to the neurovascular tract which is formed by connect tissue encysted cervical nerve and common carotid artery. When separating the artery, you should notice the position and ambulation of the nerve and not injury the concomitant nerve.

（4）Nerve separation　On the basis of the common carotid artery separation, raising the artery and you can see nerves of different caliber. Separate connect tissue around the nerves carefully with glass dissecting needle, separating 2cm of which you can cross a thread for availability. Nerve distribution of cervical part is different according to the differences of animal kind. The following is characteristics of cervical nerves of common used test animals. There are three nerves in the neurovascular tract in cervical part of rabbit, in the lateral part of which is vagus nerve that is thickest and of white color; sympathetic nerve lies in the middle part and it is grey and thinner; decompression nerve lies between vagus nerve and sympathetic nerve, it is thinnest and belongs to afferent verve. Cat's vagus nerve and sympathetic nerve is concurrent, sympathetic nerve is thinner than vagus nerve, decompression nerve is combined with vagus nerve. In dog's later odorsal part of common carotid artery there is a thick vagus – sympathetic nerve stem. Knot ganglion of vagus nerve is adjacent to anterior cervical ganglion of sympathetic nerve. From below the first cervical vertebra vagus nerve enters the cervical part and it is concomitant with sympathetic nerve stem. They are encysted by dermal root sheath to form a vagus – sympathetic stem. After entering the thoracic cavity the two nerves are separated and migrated.

4. Operation on abdominal region   In animal experiment, linea alba abdominis is the most commonly used site for abdominal incisions. It is a white aponeurosis line where nerve and vessel distribution is scarce, beginning from sternal xiphoid eminence to pubic symphysis. Linea alba abdominis incisions will not injury muscles, nerves and vessels, damages that it causes to the animal is very light and hemorrhagic tendency is small. Lengths of linea alba abdominis incisions are different according to the differences of experimental demands and animal kinds. For example, when observing motor activity of stomach and small intestine of rabbit, you need to cut an incision of 8 ~ 10cm under the sternal xiphoid eminence so that the stomach and small intestine can be exposed sufficiently. In rabbit's urine formation regulatory experiment, you need to cut an incision of 2 ~ 3cm upward from pubic symphysis, then the bladder can be exposed.

5. Operation on thigh   Femoral vessels and nerves are also usually used in animal experiment. Such as inserting cardiac catheter, measuring blood pressure, injection and blood collection. Vessels and nerves of thigh are usually passing through femoral triangle that is commonly used for femoral operation. Femoral triangle is a triangular region formed between pectineal muscle and posterior margin of the back of sartorius muscle. In femoral triangle there are femoral artery, femoral vein and femoral nerve.

Separation of blood vessel and nerve: you should fix the animal in supine position, touch artery pulsation with your finger in medial root part of thigh, cut coated hair, cut a 4 ~ 5cm incision with a surgical scalpel parallel to vessel direction; separate subcutaneous connection tissue with hemostatic forceps, then separate sartorius muscle and pectineus at their point of intersection and pull the back of sartorius muscle outward, below which you will see neurovascular bundle which is encysted by fascia (Fig. 1 – 15); separate the connective tissue membrane of neurovascular bundle with mosquito forceps carefully and the nerve and the vessel can be separated, then cross a thread for availability. The natural position of neurovascular is that femoral vein lies in medial part; femoral nerve lies in lateral part and femoral artery lies between them.

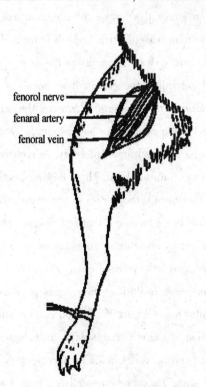

fenorol nerve
fenaral artery
fenoral vein

Fig. 1 – 15   Femoral neurovascular tract of rabbit

Ⅳ. Blood collection technology   Because we use different kinds of animals, have different requests of experiments and need different quantity of blood, we choose different methods to collect blood. The following are commonly used methods of blood collection:

1. Rabbit and guinea pig

(1) Heart blood collection   You should fix the animal in supine position, cut coated hair of left thoracic part where is corresponding to heart site, sterilize skin with iodine tincture or alcohol, choose a site where heartbeat is most obvious for puncture. Generally, for rabbit, it should be punctured into the third intercostal

space where is 3mm apart from the left border of breastbone; for guinea pig, punctured into the fourth to sixth intercostal space. You'd better palpate heartbeat with your left hand when puncturing. When the needle is approaching to heart you may feel the heartbeat. For the time being, you should prick the needle inward into the ventricle. Blood will flow into the syringe because of the heartbeat. If the needle has been prick into the heart and there is no blood that can be drawn out, you can move the needle inward or outward slightly. After $6 \sim 7$ days of blood collection, the procedure can be repeated. Each time you can draw $20 \sim 25$ml blood from rabbit, and $6 \sim 7$ml from guinea pig.

(2) Central artery blood collection of rabbit ear   You should put rabbit in rabbit box, inuncte rabbit ear with alcohol cotton to make it congested. There is a central artery in the center of rabbit ear that is longitudinal, thick and bright red. Fixingrabbit ear with your left hand and holding syringe with your right hand, at the end of central artery you can prick the needle into it in centripetal direction. Drawing slightly and you will see the blood flows into the syringe. Each time you can draw 15ml blood (paying attention to hemostasis). Choosing No. 6 needle for blood collection. Because central artery is easy to get spasmodic contraction, congestion of rabbit ear is necessary before blood collection. Blood collection can be carried out when the artery is expanding and has not have spasmodic contraction, when time lasts long the artery may contrast permanently and blood collection can't be carried out.

In addition, for rabbit and guinea pig, blood can also be drawn from their femoral vein, cervical vein, femoral artery and common carotid artery. Generally blood collection can be carried out after the separation of artery and vein.

2. Mouse and rat

(1) Caudal vein blood collection   you should put the rat in a fixed cylinder and leave its tail outside. Massage the tail with you hand or warm it with warm water ($45 \sim 50℃$), or you can smear the tail with dimethylbenzene to make the caudal vein congested. Shear the caudal endpoint (mouse is about $1 \sim 2$mm; rat is about $5 \sim 10$mm) and blood may flow out. Crush the tail gently from root to tip for several times and you can collect a few drops of blood.

If the experiment needs blood collection repeatedly at regular intervals, you can shear a short segment of the tail at each time. Pressing the wound with cotton ball to stop bleeding after blood collection, and smearing the wound instantly with 6% liquid collodion to form a pellicle to protect it.

(2) Post – orbital venous plexus blood collection   First, you should make hard glass capillary which is about $7 \sim 10$cm in length, 0.6mm in caliber of one end and 0.3mm in wall thickness. The blood collection site is post – orbital venous plexus that lies between eyeball and orbital posterior part. When collecting blood, you should catch the animal from its back with your left hand and hold its cervical part with your index finger and thumb, utilizing the light pressure you laying on the cervical part to make blood regurgitation of head vein become difficult and make eyeball become evaginated sufficiently. You should hold the sterilized capillary with your right hand, insert its pointed end into the animal's medial eyeend, and push it slightly toward throat direction for about $4 \sim 5$mm running parallel with nasal orbital wall, then it will reach the post – orbital venous plexus. Hold the glass capillary in horizontal position and attracted slightly, blood will flow into the capillary. You can

use 1% heparin solution moistening the medial wall of the capillary before blood collection to prevent blood from coagulating. You should draw the capillary out after blood collecting and release your left hand at the same time to stop bleeding. Using this method, each time you can draw 0.2ml blood from mouse and 0.5ml from rat. Generally, post – operative hemorrhage of puncture hole or other combined symptoms will not occur. You can draw blood repeatedly from the same puncture hole after a few minutes according to experimental demands. Guinea pig and rabbit can also be drawn blood from their post – orbital venous plexus except mouse and rat (Fig. 1 – 16).

3. Dog and cat   For these animals, blood can be drawn from their subcutaneous vein of forelimb and hindlimb. The basic method is similar to that of intravenous injection. Be carefully to draw blood slowly in case that the pinhole may attach to the wall of the vessel. In this way you can draw 10 ~ 20ml blood. Moreover, Blood can also be drawn from cervical vein, cervical artery and femoral artery, the basic methods are similar to that of operation on neck and operation on thigh. If the experiment needs a large quantity of blood, you can draw blood from the heart. The method is similar to that of rabbit.

Ⅴ. Methods of putting to death

1. Dislocation of vertebra   Holding back of the head of the mice with your thumb and index finger of left hand, pressing it downwards, holding the tail with your right hand, pulling it backwards and upwards, in this way, its vertebra will dislocate and the animal will die instantly (Fig. 1 – 17).

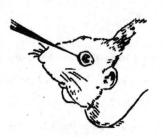 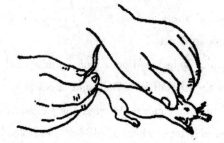

Fig. 1 – 16   Post – orbital venous plexus blood collection   Fig. 1 – 17   Dislocation of vertebra of mouse

2. Air embolism   Animal will die of embolism if you inject air into its vein. Cat, dog and guinea pig can be put to death in this way. Rabbit can be injected through its marginal vein, dog can be injected through its subcutaneous vein of forelimb and hindlimb. Animals can be put to death by injecting air into their vein, rabbit and cat need 20 ~ 40ml air and dog needs 80 ~ 150ml air.

(Wang Qiujuan)

Section Ⅲ   The common apparatus in physiological experiments

The physiological apparatus are constituted of four parts, namely stimulating system, probe system, regulating signal system and recording and monitoring system generally.

For exciting the body, isolated organs or cell, the stimuli need to be given. The common stimuli equipment is electronic stimulator. When the physiological phenomenon is electric signal, the probe system may be an introductory electrode, including the tiny glass electrode to record the unicellular electric activity and the crassitude metal electrode to record the electric activity of a cluster of cells. When the physiological phenomenon is another energy form, such as the mechanical constriction, the pressure, sound and so on, the probe system may be a transducer. Because the physiological electric signal is weak, only $10\mu V \sim 100mV$, it must be amplified by a amplifier, and then be recorded in the recorder or showed on the oscillograph. The recording system usually is an oscillograph or a pen type recorder. Fig. 1 – 18 shows the installing scheme of these instruments.

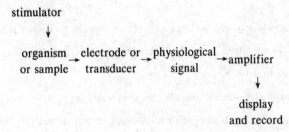

Fig. 1 – 18   The installing scheme of physiological instruments

1. Stimulating system   Various stimuli factors, such as the light, sound, electricity, temperature, machine and chemical factors can stimulate the excitable tissue to produce the physiological reaction. But in physiological experiments, the electrical stimulator is used in common. Because the stimulating parameters are easy to be controlled in this kind of stimulator, and the tissue is less hurt or not hurt at all. In the common stimuli system, we primarily introduce the electrical stimulator and kinds of stimuli electrodes.

A. Electronic stimulator   An electronic stimulator is an apparatus that can produce electric stimuli which have the certain form of waves (Fig. 1 – 19). The waves are mostly square wave, sine wave and dissymmetry wave (such as telepathy electric wave). Because the square wave is simple and it is easy to be produced and controlled strictly, and its current in the front craggedness edge is effective, and the stimulating intensity is calculated easily, the square wave is often adopted.

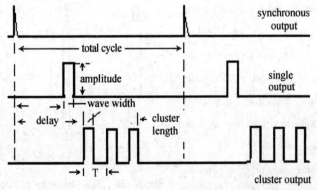

Fig. 1 – 19   The wave form and parameters in electronic stimuli

The stimuli strength, namely the height of the square wave, may be expressed as voltage or current strength. The current strength is general from several μA to several ten mA. The voltage is below

200V. If the strength is too weak, the stimuli can't lower the cell rest potential (the absoluteness value) to the threshold potential and cannot cause the cell stimuli. If the strength is too high, the stimuli may cause the electrolysis and hot effect inside the tissue, and it will harm or destroy the tissue. So in experiments, the excessive strong or weak stimuli should be avoided.

Stimuli time is the continuous time of the square wave, namely the wave width. The stimuli continuous time is generally from several ten μs to several seconds. While adopting the stimuli of a single direction square wave, the stimuli time should not be very long; otherwise the harmful effect will be produced. In order to decrease the electrolysis and hot effect inside the tissue, the stimuli time should be shortened and the stimuli square wave with plus/minus double directions should be adopted as far as possible. Moreover, usage of the best stimuli time and the stimuli strength is closely related. Generally speaking, while using a double direction square wave of 1ms wave width, the square wave amplitude of 10 V is regarded as good. If the wave width is lowered to 0. 5 ms, the amplitude often need to be enlarged to 40 ~ 50V.

When using the continuous stimuli, the stimuli frequency may be adjusted. The stimuli frequency is the repetitive frequency of the stimuli square wave, generally less than 1000 times/second. If the frequency is too high, a part of the stimuli may fall into the refractory period of the tissue, and the tissue has no response, which leads to asynchronous of the stimuli and physiological effect. The stimuli frequency may be chosen according to the different tissue. In physiological experiments, the stimuli frequency with 60 ~ 100 times/second is good. When a continuous stimulus is applied, the "cluster length" can still be regulated according to the experiment. The "cluster length" is the continuous time of square wave with repeating frequency, namely the time of producing several square waves.

Other functions are provided in electronic stimulator besides the adjustable stimuli parameters above. Total cycle is the cycle of the synchronous pulse. The synchronous pulse expresses an initial time point of stimuli. The synchronous pulse, imported to the whole experimental system, causes a common initial time point in every instrument in order to keep the time synchronous. The time from the synchronous pulse to appearance of the square wave is called "time delay". While regulating the "time delay", the physiological response caused by the square wave or a square wave stimulus is showed in the middle of the fluorescence screen in oscillograph in order to observe and record expediently.

B. Stimulating electrode Stimulating electrodes, made by metals, can be divided into the common electrode, the protective electrode and the non - polarizable electrode etc. according to their functions (Fig. 1 - 20A and B). This text introduces the former two kinds of electrodes.

The common electrode and the protective electrode are made of silver wire or stainless steel wire. Generally two metal wires are embedded into the organic glass or the

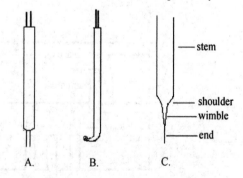

Fig. 1 - 20   The structure of stimulating electrodes

A. Common electrode B. protective electrode

C. the glass tiny electrode

bakelite frame, and the stimuli end is bare. They are used as stimulating electrode outside of cells. Since the stimuli end of its insulating frame is curled into a hook shape and two metal wires are embedded into the hook with only nudity in the hook, the protective electrode can protect its surrounding tissue from being stimulated.

2. Probe system

A. The tiny glass electrode A tiny electrode, as a part of the probe system in the physiological instrument, is applied extensively to measure the unicellular electric activity. The tiny electrodes include the tiny metal electrode (can be made of the stainless steel wire, tungsten wire, platinum wire etc.) and the tiny glass electrode (Fig. 1 – 20C). There are many methods of making the tiny glass electrode, please refer to the relevant articles.

B. Transducer A transducer is a device by which a kind of energy can be transformed into another one. As a part of the probe system, it may transform the non – electric physiological phenomenon such as the mechanical energy, sound, light, magnetism and temperature etc. into electric signals. Then the electric signals, after being amplified by a prepositive amplifier, are showed on an oscillograph or recorded on a recorder. There are many kinds of transducers, such as tension – electricity transducer, pressure – electricity transducer, light – electricity transducer, sound – electricity transducer and temperature – electricity transducer etc. This text introduces the former three kinds of transducers.

(1) Tension – electricity transducer (tension transducer) and pressure – electricity transducer (pressure transducer)　This two transducers extensively applied in the physiological research. Tension transducer can measure contraction and diastolization of the tissue or organs in vitro or in vivo. Pressure transducer, can measure every kind of pressure (such as blood pressure, the pressure inside chest, the pressure inside lung, the pressure inside ventricle and the pressure inside gastrointestinal tract etc.). The basic principle is that a physiological phenomenon with non – electric characteristic is transformed into an electric signal by a strain patch. The strain patch includes a resistance wire strain patch and a semiconductor strain patch. They are usually installed in an electric road of Wheatstone bridge.

(2) Light – electricity transducer　The transducer is primarily constituted of photosensitivity element – photoelectric cell or light battery. The basic principle is that the light with strong or weak changes is transformed into a current change. This current is transformed into a potential, and then the potential can be directly introduced in an oscillograph or a recorder. This transducer can be used to measure the change of the pressure or the displacement, and even sphygmus or spontaneous motion of small animals etc. It includes the pressure transducer and the pull transducer made of a light battery.

3. The regulating signal system

After receiving a stimuli, the tissue excitation in a animal can be observed on an oscillograph. Because the bioelectricity is often very weak and the amplification in the oscillograph is still not enough, a bioelectric signal must be amplified by a prepositive amplifier and then its variational waves can be just showed on an oscillograph or a recorder. The function of a prepositive amplifier is amplifying the weak bioelectricity at first before a main amplifier enlarges it.

There are many kinds of amplifiers. According to the purpose, they can be divided into the voltage, the current and power amplifier. According to the frequency, they can be divided into the direct current (breath, pulse etc.), low frequency (action potential etc.), high frequency and video frequency amplifier. According to the coupling method, they can be divided into the direct current coupling, the resistance/capacitance coupling and transformer – coupling amplifier etc. In the following unit, the relevant function and index of an amplifier are introduced in brief.

(1) The Frequency Response   An amplifier has different amplificatory multiples on signals with different frequencies, namely amplifying the same multiple on signals in a certain scope of frequency. The frequency scope between the upper limit frequency and lower limit frequency is the frequency response scope, namely the amplifier transmission bands. When an amplifier is chosen, its frequency response must be suited for the frequency response scope of the physiological signal being enlarged. Generally, the frequency response scope of a bio – amplifier is $10 \sim 15 Hz$ in an AC amplifier and $0 \sim 10$ kHz in a DC amplifier.

(2) Time Constant   It is very importance whether the time constant is appropriate on the graph definition, accuracy and no distortion. In an electric physiological experiment, in order to record rightly every quick change or the slow potential, a choice circuit of time constant (namely high and low frequency compensation or attenuation) is placed in the input end of a prepositive amplifier or between the prepositive and the postpositive amplifier. When recording a quick potential, choose a small time constant (such as $0.001s$); but when recording a slow potential, choose a big time constant (generally for 2 seconds). When recording the electric activity in the central nervous system, the time constant is not less than $0.1s$. Please refer to the table 1 – 1 for choosing the time constant.

(3) The Amplificatory Multiple   The amplifier multiple is the amplifying ability of an amplifier, and shows its sensitivity. A prepositive amplifier mainly amplifies the voltage. Ku is expressed as an amplificatory multiple of a voltage amplifier.

$$Ku(\text{voltage gain}) = \frac{\text{output voltage}}{\text{input voltage}}$$

Therefore the voltage amplificatory multiple, namely the ratio of the output voltage and the input voltage in the amplifier, can be calculated by the values of the output voltage and the input voltage measured. In electrical physiological experiments, the amplificatory multiple of the amplifier should be chosen according to the intensity of the bioelectrical signal. For example, when recording the trans – membrane potential in nerve or myocardial fiber, the sensitivity is adjusted to $5 \sim 10 mV/cm$. When recording electrical activity of nerve in vivo, the sensitivity is adjusted to $50 \sim 100 \mu V/cm$. To choose the sensitivity in recording every bioelectrical signal, please refer to the table 1 – 1.

(4) Signal – to – Noise   Besides amplifying bioelectrical signals, each amplifier may amplify the irregular voltage or current at the same time. These disorderly and irregular voltage or current are called the amplifier noise. In the electronics, the ratio of signal and noise (signal to noise) is thought as the amplifier function when amplifying a weak signal.

$$Signal - to - Noise = \frac{\text{signal power}}{\text{noise power}}$$

Therefore, only when the signal – to – noise is more than 1, the weak signal may be amplified effectively. Otherwise, because the signal and the noise are amplified with same multiple, it is useless no matter how high the multiple is. For example, the brain electricity in human is dozens of μV, if the noise of the electroencephalogram (EEG) machine equals to that of the importing end and the latter voltage is over 100 μV, then EEG waves will be drowned in the noise and can't be distinguished. Therefore the signal − to − noise is also the important function index of the amplifier. So in a good amplifier, both of the signal − to − noise and the amplificatory multiple must be high.

The noise of an amplifier is divided into the endogenous noise and the exterior noise. The amplifier or auxiliary facilities produce the endogenous noise. For example, the transistor and resistance produce the noise because of electron hot sport. The exterior noise comes from the AC or DC magnetic field or electromagnetic radialization in the surroundings, generally named this noise as interference. The method of distinguishing the amplifier noise and interference is that the noise potential remained on the oscillograph is the amplifier noise, and the dissolving noise is the exterior in terference signal after the input end connected to the ground.

In electric equipments, the effective steps of repressing the noise and eliminating the interference are the shield and the ground connecting. For example, the interference can be expelled availably by shielding the interference source and the experiment instruments especially the experimental object. Generally, the electrical physiological experiment had better be done in a shield room or a shield box, and all instruments used should have metal machine hull, each conjunctive line among instruments should be a shield line. Especially, the input line of the amplifier and the line between the prepositive and postpositional amplifier should be well shielded, and the bareness on the joint should be reduced as far as possible. The ground connecting is that a point and an equipotential point or an equipotential surface are linked by a low resistance in order to constitute a circuit and a benchmark potential of the system. It is the reason why the potential is called the earth potential. In electrical physiological experiments, a point of paralleling connection should be adopted to connect the ground system.

(5) Input Impedance and Output Impedance The impedance matching plays a very important role during amplifying, and also is a main index of an amplifier for successfully searching, amplifying and showing the signal from the signal source.

Generally, for a system of multi − class amplifiers, especially bioelectric amplifiers, the higher input impedance is required (more than 1 $M\Omega$). At this rate, it can lighten the burden of the signal source and decrease the loss of the biologic signal. In the research work of the microelectrode, because the microelectrode point is fine (generally $0.5 \sim 1\mu m$) and the inside resistance is very high (generally $10 \sim 20$ $M\Omega$ or higher), this will require the microelectrode amplifier to have specially high input resistance (generally 10,000 $M\Omega$ or higher). Otherwise, the input voltage of the amplifier would be very small because the inside resistance of the signal source is high and the output voltage of the weak biological signal is mostly consumed on this resistance. Therefore the impedance transformation must be made so that the input impedance could exceed that of the microelectrode.

4. The recording and monitoring system

A. Oscillograph

Oscillograph is an electronic instrument for observing the change of the voltage or current and measuring its values. Each electric signal or non – electric signal that can be transformed to the voltage or the current may be showed on an oscillograph.

The core of an oscillograph is an electronic oscillotron. Besides there is a scan signal generator, an amplifier and a power supply.

(1) The electronic oscillotron   The oscillotron is constituted of an electronic gun, a deflexion system and a fluorescence screen (Fig. 1 – 21).

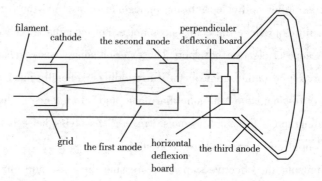

Fig. 1 – 21   The structure of the electronic oscillotron

a. Electronic gun: it is a special device that can produce the electron beam and then focus. It is constituted of filament, cathode, control grid, three anodes and so on.

The function of the filament and the cathode is to shoot electron, and the control grid can control the strength of the electron ray, sequentially can control the brightness of the light point on the fluorescence screen. The first anode and the second anode, loaded with certain voltages respectively, can be combined to become an electron lens, and then focus the electron beam to a point on the fluorescence screen. Therefore the first anode is the focus anode. The knob of "focus" on the panel exerts the focusing function by regulating the voltage loaded in the first anode. The third anode is accelerating anode, and can accelerate the electron movement, and it also can absorb the secondary electron shot from the screen.

b. The Deflexion System: It includes two pairs of mutual perpendicular deflexion boards, namely a pair of perpendicular deflexion board (the y – axis deflexion board) and a pair of horizontal deflexion board (x – axis deflexion board). When changing the voltage on the perpendicular deflexion board, the electron beam can move up and down. The horizontal deflexion board can control the movement of the electronbeam left and right, and form a scan base line. The knobs of the "horizontal shift" and the "perpendicular shift" on the panel of the oscillograph may change the position of the light point by regulating the voltage on the two pairs of deflexion board. In an electric physiological experiment, the biological signal is inputted to the y – axis and the x – axis represents time, then the light point can move in straight lines on the fluorescence screen following the time.

c. The Fluorescence Screen: The fluorescence screen is a glass screen on the bottom of the oscillotron. There is a layer of fluorescence material on the wall of the screen. When the electron beam with a high speed beats a point on the screen, this point gives out light. The more the number of the electron beating on the screen in time unit is, the brighter the light sent out by the screen is. The electron beam beats the fluorescence material to give out light, but the irradiance is still kept in a period after the electron beam has stopped, and this period is named the remaining brightness time. Generally, when observing the high frequency signal, it is proper to choose an oscillotron with a short remaining brightness; but when observing the signal with the low frequency and the slow variety, it is proper to use an oscillotron with a long remaining brightness.

(2) Proper usage of the SBR – 1 model oscillograph

a. General notice

a) When turn on the machine, each knob on the panel is generally placed in the following position; Brightness Degree; middle position; Trigger Potential; automatism or consecution; x – axis function; Normal; Sensitivity; 20 V/cm; Perpendicular Position; center position.

b) After the power supply is turned on, the cooling fan begins to work. After warming up 30 minutes, its function becomes stabilization, and then can be used. The instrument can continue working 8 hours.

c) If the heat dispersion is in bad condition or the machine is malfunction inside, and the temperature in the machine attains 55 ℃, the oscillograph will automatically stop working. The reason should be found out and the malfunction be expelled before use it again.

d) During the usage or maintenance, if the power supply is cut off, it could be switched on at least 3 minute later, otherwise it may be damaged.

b. Brightness degree and focus; the brightness degree knob can be used to regulate the brightness. When turning it clockwise, the light point gradually becomes bright. During the experiment, the light point should not be too bright, generally convenience for the observation.

The regulation of the focus should be done at slow scan. The reason is that the light point is clear and easy to be recognized. It is OK to regulate the light point to the roundest and the most minimum.

The knob of scale brightness can be used to control the brightness of the floodlight on the front – panel in the fluorescence screen. The brighter it is, the clearer the scale is. The abscissa on the scale may be used to measure the time of the signal, and the ordinate on the scale may be used to measure the voltage of the signal.

c. The perpendicular amplificatory system and the input fashion

This system is constituted of a differential DC amplifier with high gain and an attenuator. The weak signal imported by the system is imputed to the perpendicular deflexion board after being amplified, and drives the electron beam to move following its variational regularity. The function of the sensitivity knob is to adjust the signal amplitude in the fluorescence screen. The knob can be placed in suitable position according to the intensity of the signal. For example, the action potential in myocardial cell is about 120 mV, and if the gain of the microelectrode amplifier is 1, the sensitivity of the oscillography should be placed in 20 mV/cm, the height of the wave on the fluorescence screen is 6cm.

The input fashion is divided into the single end input and the double end input. The signal is imported from the A end or the B end, or imported from the A and B ends at the same time.

According to its characteristic, the input fashion of the signal is divided into AC (exchange current) and DC (direct current). In a general physiological experiment, the AC fashion is used. But for the slow electric change, such as the membrane potential, the gastrointestinal potential on the surface of the body and the skin potential etc, the DC input fashion should be chosen.

The regulation of the direct current equilibrium: The equilibrium knob is used to regulate the direct current potential when the amplificatory multiple is changed, in order that the light point can't drift out of the fluorescence screen. Regulate the sensitivity knob, the DC equilibrium knob, the displacement knob and the hidden resistor to make the scan line locate in the central position on the fluorescence screen all the time.

d. The trigger choice knob: For clearly observing and measuring the parameter of the electric signal, the stimulating signal should be imported to the trigger scan generator. Then the stimulator controls the scan of the electron beam. After the input and the scan are synchronized, the wave will appear repeatedly in the same position of the fluorescence screen.

The trigger fashion includes ① the power supply trigger; ② the inside trigger of upper line and bottom line (AC, DC); and ③ the outside trigger (AC, DC). Choose different trigger fashions according to the specific request of the experiment.

B. Two channels physiological recorder

The recorder is one of the common instruments. Its pen can directly record the biological signal or the physiological change that has been amplified on the record paper. Because the pen has very big sloth and its frequency respond is small, the changes with the frequency below 100 times/ second or with the continuance larger than 10 ms may be recorded, but it is not used in recording the changes with quick variety, such as the active potential of nerve. In physiological experiments, twochannels physiological recorder is often used (Fig. 1 – 22).

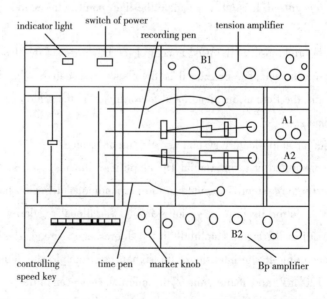

Fig. 1 – 22   The front – panel diagram of the two channels physiological recorder

Before turning on the power switch of the physiological recorder, all switches should be placed first in the "break" position, and the control key of the paper is also placed in the "stop". Then turn on the power supply switch, and the indicator light brightens at once. Lay down the uplifting pen rack, and then connect the transducer with this machine. The mechanism – electricity transducer and A1B1, the blood pressure transducer and A2B2 constitute to an amplificatory system respectively.

Before the machine working, the base line should be set to zero. The zero setting should be done step – by – step, first regulating the prepositive amplifier (A1 or A2), and then regulating the postpositive amplifier. At this time, the connection between the prepositive and the postpositive amplifier should be interrupted by inserting a plug of a line with two cores into the jack of the postpositive input. Then place the switch of the amplifier in the "turn – on" position, and set the pen nib in the centerline by regulating the zero setting knob. After completing the zero setting, draw out the two cores line in the input short – circuit, and check the function of the prepositive amplifier (B1 or B2) again.

Before turning on the prepositive amplifier, place the sensitivity of the amplifier at the lowest level. If adjusting the amplificatory system of A1B1, place the time constant knob of B1 at any level (AC), and circumvolve the zero setting knob of B1 to place the pen nib in the centerline. Then again set the time constant at the direct current (DC) level. Before adjustment of the prepositive amplifier, ensure that the input end is not in the short circuit. Therefore, first connect the transducer to the machine, or connect the electrode to the sample of the animal, and then turn on the prepositive amplifier in order to prevent the violent vibration that may break the pen. If the pen nip is in the centerline, the experiment may be started.

After the experiment being completed, shut the input and output switches in the prepositive and the postpositive amplifier, then place the sensitivity switch at the lowest level, uplift the pen rack, turn off the power supply and pull out the plug.

When recording the blood pressure, the zero setting of the postpositive amplifier is the same as above. When checking the prepositive amplifier, the first step is connecting the pressure transducer to the machine, placing the input switch of the transducer and the measuring switch in "break" position, and the sensitivity knob at the lowest level, then pulling out the plug with a two cores line and turning on the input switch of the blood pressure. If the pen nip deviates from the centerline, the "zero setting" knob of the amplifier should be regulated to bring it to the centerline. After the above steps being completed, turn on the measuring switch of blood pressure amplifier. If the pen deviates from the centerline, the "adjust equilibrium" should be adjusted to return the pen to the centerline. After all adjustments are completed, the vessel cannula leading to the transducer can beopened to begin recording the blood pressure.

C. Introduction to BL – 420F biological signal acquisition and analysis system

BL – 420F biological signal acquisition and analysis system is a new generation of conceptual biological function experiment system, the performance index and convenience are far better than any products sold in the market at home and abroad. For example, the stimulator can edit the waveform while no other domestic product can achieve it at present, the scanning speeds of the four channels are adjustable independently, and the system integrates a variety of special data analysis functions, until now, there is no other foreign product able to achieve them.

1. System hardware indexes

(1) Use USB 2. 0 full speed transmission.

（2）The system can be built inside（put in the computer case）or outside.

（3）The maximum sampling rate of single channel is 1 MHz, and the minimum sampling rate is 0.01 Hz.

（4）Use A/D sampling core with 16 - bit accuracy.

（5）The amplifier has a wide dynamic input range: $\pm 1V \sim \pm 20 \mu V$, equivalent to an amplification multiple of 1 - 50000.

（6）The 5 - order Bessel filter is adopted, and the filtering range is 1 Hz ~ 30 kHz.

（7）The waveform can be edited by photoelectric isolation stimulator, the output waveform range of the stimulator is up to 100 V, you can output triangular waves, square waves, positive and negative square waves, sine waves, or any waveform you can edit yourself.

（8）It is equipped with 12 lead standard ECG selection circuit; 12 - lead standard ECG waveform can be arbitrarily selected in 1 channel.

（9）Multi - device synchronization cascade can be carried out directly without manual button, which is extended to new devices with 8 ~ 16 sampling channels.

2. System software indexes

（1）The double - view observation system, which can be dragged freely and flexibly change the window width, can view the previously recorded data without stopping the real - time experimental observation, and can realize the comparison of the changes before and after the experimental waveform in different states.

（2）In order to adapt to the experimental teaching work, they pre - designed a total of 55 experimental modules in 10 categories, which is the largest number of prefabricated experimental modules among similar products at home and abroad.

（3）In order to adapt to scientific research, they designed a number of experimental data analysis functions: real - time differentiation, integration, frequency histogram and spectrum analysis of the original waveform or recorded waveform.

（4）It has a variety of general data measurement methods, including single - point measurement, two - point measurement, interval measurement, real - time measurement, etc. It can measure the maximum, minimum, average value, slope, time, frequency, mean square deviation and other parameters of the waveform.

（5）Many special data measurement functions: analysis of hemodynamic experimental parameters, measurement of myocardial cell action potential parameters, determination of diphenhydramine antagonistic parameters（PA_2, PD_2）and other measurement functions. LD_{50}, **** value, t test and half - life value can also be calculated according to Bliss method.

（6）The scanning speed of four channels is adjustable independently, zero scanning speed sampling, universal program - controlled stimulus and other functions have unique charm.

（7）During real - time sampling, the sampling rate can be changed at any time as required.

（8）Users can set 1 ~ 16 display channels according to their needs（5 ~ 16 channels can be used for analysis）.

3. Experimental modules

The Experimental Type	Specific experimental projects			
	No.	Name	No.	Name
Muscle & Nerve	1	Relationship between stimulus intensity and response	6	The relationship between muscle contraction and excitation
	2	The relationship between stimulus frequency and response	7	Pain experiment
	3	The guidance of nerve stem action potential	8	Relationship between threshold intensity and action potential
	4	Determination of nerve trunk conduction velocity	9	Cell discharge
	5	Determination of excitatory refractory period of nerve trunk	10	Determination of myocardial refractory period
Circulation system	1	Frog heart perfusion	7	Arterial blood pressure regulation in rabbits
	2	Preterm shrinkage – compensation intervals	8	Left ventricular and arterial pressure
	3	Full – lead electrocardiogram	9	Hemodynamic module
	4	Cardiomyocyte action potential	10	Acute myocardial infarction and drug therapy
	5	Cardiomyocyte action potential and electrocardiogram	11	The impedance measurement
	6	Rabbit decompression nerve discharge		
Respiratory system	1	Phrenic nerve discharge	3	Collection and processing of respiratory parameters
	2	Respiratory motor regulation	4	Measurement of pulmonary ventilation function
Digestive system	1	Electrical activity of digestive tract smooth muscle	3	Digestive tract smooth muscle activity
	2	Physiological characteristics of digestive tract smooth muscle	4	Determination of antagonistic parameters of diphenhydramine
Sensory Organ	1	Muscle spindle discharge	3	Visual evoked potential
	2	Cochlea bioelectrical activity	4	Brainstem auditory evoked potential
Centralnervous system	1	Cortical evoked potential	4	Evoked EEG
	2	Central neuron unit firing	5	EEG sleep analysis
	3	Electroencephalogram (EEG)		
Urinary system	1	Factors that influence urine production		
Pharmacology	1	Measurement of PA_2 value	6	Effects of drugs on experimental arrhythmias
	2	The analgesic effect of drugs	7	Diuretic effect of drugs on anesthetized rats
	3	The rescue effect of nikethamide on morphine respiratory depression	8	Effect of pituitrin on mouse uterus in vitro
	4	Effects of drugs on intestinal muscles in vitro	9	Electroconvulsive Experiment
	5	Effects of efferent nervous system drugs on blood pressure in anesthetized rats		
Pathophysiology	1	Experimental pulmonary edema in rats	4	Acute right heart failure
	2	Acute hemorrhagic shock	5	Acute hyperkalemia
	3	Acute left heart failure with pulmonary edema		

(Ding qilong　Lu Na)

第二章 神经与肌肉

Nerve and muscle

实验一 组织兴奋性的观察

扫码"学一学"

【实验目的】

利用蟾蜍坐骨神经－腓肠肌标本，观察电刺激神经引起肌肉的反应，进而印证神经肌肉组织的生理特性。

【实验原理】

肌肉、神经、腺体称为可兴奋组织，它们有较大的兴奋性。不同组织、细胞的兴奋性表现（兴奋）各不相同，神经组织的兴奋性表现为动作电位，肌肉组织的兴奋性主要表现为收缩活动。因此，观察肌肉是否收缩可以判断它是否产生了兴奋。一个刺激是否能使组织发生兴奋，不仅与刺激形式有关，还与刺激时间、刺激强度、强度－时间变化率三要素有关，用矩形脉冲电刺激组织，则组织兴奋只与刺激强度、刺激时间有关。用矩形电脉冲刺激组织，在一定的刺激时间（波宽）下，刚能引起组织发生兴奋的刺激称为阈刺激，所达到的刺激强度称为阈强度；能引起组织发生最大兴奋的最小刺激，称为最大刺激或顶刺激，相应的刺激强度叫最大刺激强度或顶强度；介于阈刺激和顶刺激间的刺激称为阈上刺激，相应的刺激强度称阈上刺激强度。某些药物（如普鲁卡因）可降低组织的兴奋性，使刺激阈强度大大增大，甚至使组织完全失去兴奋性（阈强度变为无穷大）。

刺激神经使神经产生兴奋，并沿神经纤维传导，兴奋通过神经肌接头的化学传递，使终板膜上产生终板电位，终板电位可引起肌肉也产生兴奋（AP），传遍整个肌纤维，再通过兴奋－收缩耦联使肌纤维中粗细肌丝产生相对滑动——宏观上表现为肌肉收缩。肌肉收缩的形式，不仅与刺激本身有关，而且还与刺激频率有关。当刺激频率较小，使刺激间隔大于一次肌肉收缩舒张的持续时间，则肌肉收缩表现为一连串的单收缩；增大刺激频率，使刺激间隔大于一次肌肉收缩的收缩时间、小于一次肌肉收缩舒张的持续时间，则肌肉产生不完全强直收缩；继续增加刺激频率，使刺激间隔小于一次肌肉收缩的收缩时间，则肌肉产生完全强直收缩。本实验利用蟾蜍坐骨神经－腓肠肌标本，观察矩形脉冲电刺激坐骨神经引起腓肠肌收缩的情况。

【实验材料】

1. 器材 BL－420F 生物信号采集与分析系统（或二道生理记录仪，电子刺激器），蛙手术器械一套，肌板，双凹夹，小烧杯（50ml 或 100ml），滴管，蛙板，棉花，线少许，图

44

钉，滑轮。

2. 药品 任氏液，1%普鲁卡因。

3. 对象 蟾蜍。

【实验方法】

1. 蟾蜍坐骨神经-腓肠肌标本制备

（1）破坏脑和脊髓 取蟾蜍一只，左手握住，用食指压住头部前端，拇指按压背部，使头前俯。右手持探针由头前端沿中线向尾方划触，触及凹陷处即枕骨大孔，其位置在两鼓膜连线中点将探针由此垂直刺入，再将探针尖端向头方向插入颅腔，左右搅动，捣毁脑组织。而后，将探针退出再由枕骨大孔向后刺入脊椎管捣毁脊髓。待四肢紧张性完全消失，即表示脑和脊髓完全破坏。

（2）剪除躯干上部及内脏（五剪法）并剥皮（图2-1） 第一、二剪：用手术剪从上肢下缘开始，沿两侧将腹部侧面肌肉及皮剪开，直至下肢上部；第三剪：沿上肢下缘将皮剪一环口，使上部皮和下部皮分开，并且自腹面将内脏器官全部剪下，再用镊子将腹腔内脏及腹部皮肤全部向下剥下。第四剪：自下肢上部腹侧将已剥下的内脏及皮全部剪去；第五剪：剪去肛周一圈皮肤。

用镊子夹住上肢下缘背侧环口下的皮，左手握住蟾蜍头部，将蟾蜍下部皮肤全部剥下，自上肢下缘将脊柱剪断以除去上肢及其以上部分。将标本放在蛙板上并滴上任氏液，再将手及用过的器械洗净。

（3）游离坐骨神经 将标本背位并用图钉固定于蛙板上，沿脊柱两侧用玻璃针分离坐骨神经，于根部穿线结扎并剪断。轻轻提起扎线，逐一剪去神经分支，游离坐骨神经后将它团在趾骨联合内侧。将标本腹位放于蛙板上，用图钉将脊柱和下趾尖端固定，用玻璃针划开梨状肌及其附近的结缔组织，沿坐骨神经沟找出坐骨神经大腿部分，用眼科镊子将腹部的坐骨神经小心夹出（夹住扎线），手执结扎神经的线，剪断坐骨神经所有分支，一直游离至膝关节。

（4）制成坐骨神经-腓肠肌标本 将分离干净的坐骨神经搭于腓肠肌上，在膝关节周围剪断全部大腿肌肉，并用粗剪刀将股骨刮干净，在股骨的上部剪断（保留2/3股骨）。再在跟腱处以线结扎，剪断并游离腓肠肌至膝关节处，在膝关节以下将其小腿其余部分全部剪断，而得到坐骨神经-腓肠肌标本（图2-2）。将标本放入任氏液中浸泡10分钟左右，待其兴奋性稳定后再进行实验。

2. 坐骨神经-腓肠肌标本固定及仪器连接

（1）坐骨神经-腓肠肌标本的股骨固定于肌板上电极旁的小孔内，并使腓肠肌在股骨上方，肌腱扎线与换能器（选用100克换能头）头端小钩相连，坐骨神经置于刺激电极上（若记录仪是记纹鼓则如图2-3连接）。

（2）电子刺激器输出与肌板上的刺激电极相连（负极靠近腓肠肌）。

3. 观察项目

（1）阈强度、顶强度的测定 将电子刺激器上的工作方式置于"单脉冲"，触发方式置于"外"，强度粗调×1V，强度细调为0；波宽2～5ms。开启电源后，调节强度细调钮，由0逐渐增大，分别按手动单次钮刺激神经，用生理记录仪（或记纹鼓）记录肌肉收缩曲线，根据收缩曲线确定阈刺激，阈上刺激及最大刺激强度（顶强度）。记录仪

扫码"看一看"

走纸速度 5～10mm/s，灵敏度根据收缩大小置于 5mV/cm 左右，时间常数为 DC 或 2s，滤波为 30Hz。

（2）腓肠肌单收缩、不完全强直收缩、完全强直收缩记录　将刺激器上的工作方式置于"单脉冲"，触发方式置于"内"用最大刺激强度，串个数为 1，波宽 2～5ms，选择主间隔分别为 1000ms、500ms、200ms、100ms、50ms（即选择不同刺激频率 $F = 1/t$）。开启电源后，以不同主间隔分别刺激神经，每次刺激持续约 2s，然后把触发方式置于"外"，刺激即停止（每次调换主间隔时间时一定要没有刺激输出）。观察并记录单收缩、不完全强直收缩及完全强直收缩曲线，其刺激频率分别为多少？

（3）普鲁卡因麻醉坐骨神经结果观察　用 1% 普鲁卡因棉花条包裹于神经中段，1～2分钟后，用上述同样刺激观察肌肉收缩反应。待肌肉收缩反应消失后，用电极直接刺激肌肉，观察其收缩反应。去掉棉花条，将标本取下用任氏液浸泡 3～5 分钟后，观察恢复情况。

【实验指导】

1. 预习要求
（1）兴奋性、兴奋的概念。
（2）神经肌接头化学传递的机制。
（3）骨骼肌的收缩原理。
（4）肌肉收缩的外部表现和力学分析。

2. 操作要点
（1）熟练地调试仪器　将仪器如图 2-4 所示装置好，接通电源并进行调试，注意刺激器主间隔（T_1）、延迟（T_2）、波宽（T_3）、串间隔（T_4）均不能为 0，且要求 $T_1 > T_2 + T_3$，记录仪要接地良好，消除干扰并且灵敏度适当。

（2）掌握坐骨神经-腓肠肌标本的制备方法　注意不要损伤坐骨神经及腓肠肌，尤其是坐骨神经与腓肠肌连接处。分离标本时只用玻璃分针，不可用手和金属器械触摸；分离神经时避免过度牵拉，避免所有不良刺激及损伤。

（3）实验应在尽可能短的时间内完成，否则神经肌接头处容易疲劳，进而影响实验结果。

（4）蟾酥对人皮肤无甚损害，若不慎溅入眼内，可立即用生理盐水冲洗，在制作标本时，可先用布盖住耳后腺稍加挤压，以促使其排尽。

3. 注意事项
（1）不能用器械尖端或粗糙物碰触神经肌肉。
（2）要经常用任氏液湿润标本，以免干燥死亡。
（3）调换电子刺激器刺激参数时，应保证刺激器一定没有刺激输出。
（4）仪器均必须接地良好，否则会影响实验。

4. 报告要点
（1）获得清晰的实验结果曲线。
（2）讨论刺激强度、频率与肌肉收缩的关系及刺激神经引起肌肉收缩的原理。
（3）讨论普鲁卡因对神经的作用原理。

5. 思考题

（1）为什么要将制备好的坐骨神经 – 腓肠肌标本先放在任氏液中浸泡一段时间？

（2）本实验中肌肉收缩的潜伏期、收缩期和舒张期是如何划分的？

（3）说明骨骼肌产生不完全强直收缩及完全强直收缩的发生机制（从细胞分子水平）。

（傅继华）

1　Observation on the tissue excitation

PURPOSE

To observe the reaction of sciatic nerve – fibula muscle with the electric stimulation and prove the physiological reaction of nerve – muscle tissue.

PRINCIPLE

Muscle, nerve and gland are called excitable tissue, which are more excitable than other tissue. Different sort of tissue and cell shows different excitability. Nerve excitability represents as active potential (AP) and muscle represents as contraction. So we can judge the muscle's excitation by observing it's contraction. Whether a stimulus could lead to excite is not only decided on the way of stimulus, but also decided on duration, strength and ratio of strength – duration, which called three essentials. When stimulus is in a rectangle pulse, the excitability of tissue only depends on duration and strength. After a proper stimulus duration with a rectangle pulse, the lowest stimulus leading to tissue excitability is called threshold stimulus, the strength is called threshold intensity. The lowest stimulus that could lead to the highest excitability of tissue is called max stimulus or top stimulus, and the intensity is called max stimulus intensity or top intensity. That called up – threshold stimulus between threshold stimulus and top stimulus, the intensity called up – threshold intensity. Some drugs (such as procaine) can reduce the excitability of tissue, enlarge the threshold, or disannul it's excitability.

Nerve can be excite when it is stimulated. That can be conducted through the nerve fiber and chemical transmission through neuromuscular junction, which cause the end – plate potential on the end plate. The end – plated potential will cause an muscle's AP, which would conduct through all the muscle fiber, cause sliding of the actin filaments into the channels between the myosin filaments through excitation – contraction coupling, that is muscle contraction. The form of contraction is not only decided on the stimulus, but also decided on stimulus frequency. When the internal of stimulation is longer than the period of single muscle contraction and relaxation period, the contraction is called single twitch. Enlarging the stimulus frequency, which is longer than the period of contraction but shorter than the period of relaxation, cause a incomplete tenustion. Enlarging the frequency continuously, which is shorter than the period of contraction, cause a complete tetanus. In this experiment, we will observe muscle contraction with toad's sciatic nerve – fibula muscle sample through electric stimulus.

MATERIALS

1. Equipments BL – 420F biological signal acquisition and analysis system（or two – channel recorder，stimulator），operating table for frog，frog board，beaker（50ml or 100ml），dropper，cotton ball，drawing pins，pulley.

2. Solutions Ringer's solution，1% procaine.

3. Object Toad.

METHODS

1. Preparation of sciatic nerve – fibula muscle sample

（1）Destroy brain and spinal cord Hold a toad with left hand，press the front of it's head and back with forefinger. Hold probe with right hand，touch it's skin from the middle line to the end，prick the skin vertically at the hole of occipital bone，then insert the head of probe into the brain and destroy it. Then take out of the probe，insert it into the back of occipital and destroy it. It shows that brain and spiral cord has been destoried when the movement of toad's four limb disappear.

（2）Cut away the upper part of it's body and internal organs，shell it's skin（Fig. 2 – 1） First and second clip：from the lower edge of upper limbs，cut the skin on the two sides of abdomen，to the upper of the lower limbs；Third clip：cut the skin horizontally and separate the lower skin and upper skin，and cut all the internal organs. Forth clip：cut away all separated organs and skin；Fifth clip：cut away a circled skin around anus.

Tweeze the skin at lower edge of upper limb，which is at the beginning of the first clip，hold it's head with left hand，shell all the skin，cut away all of the upper part of the body at the lower edge of upper limb，put the sample on the frog board and drip Ringer's solution to the toad，clean all the used tools and your hands，and make a good preparation for the next phrase.

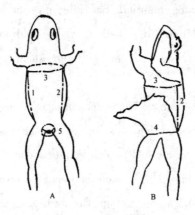

Fig. 2 – 1 Shearing the viscus of toad with five – scissoring method.

A. planform B. side elevation 1st，2nd，3rd，4th，
5th clip express as 1，2，3，4，5

Fig. 2 – 2 Preparation of the sciatic nerve – fibula muscle specimen

（3）Separate sciatic nerve Fix the back of sample on the frog board with pins，separate the sciatic nerve along the spiral cord，tie the end of it and cut away. Put the ligation thread and cut the branch of nerve. Fix the sample with pins. Cut the muscle and tissue with glass needle，separate the sciatic nerve from the sciatic nerve ditch, cut out it carefully andtie it with a ligation thread, hold the thread, cut all the branches to the knee joint.

(4) Get the sample Put the sciatic nerve on the fibula muscle, cut all the muscle at knee joint, scrape the thighbone with a big scissors, cut the upper thighbone (remain 2/3 of it). Ligate it at Achille's tendon, cut away the fibula muscle and separate it, and cut away the other part below the knee joint. Then we get the sample. Dip the sample in Ringer's solution for about 10 minutes.

2. fixation of the sample and connection of the equipment

(1) Fix the thighbone of the sample in a hole near the electrode, put the fibula muscle above the thighbone, connect ligation thread with a hook on the head of transdncer, and put the sciatic nerve on the electrode (Fig. 2 – 3).

(2) Join up the output of electronic stimulator and electrode.

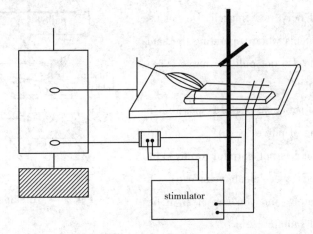

Fig. 2 – 3 Equipment for recording muscle contractions when it is stimulated

3. Observation items

(1) Threshold intensity and upper intensity. Put the button of wave on "single wave" of the stimulator, put the button of way on "out", put the button of intensity on " × 1v"; set the width of wave on "2 ~ 5ms". Turn on the electric power, adjust it's intensity, and then stimulate the nerve with pushing hand control button, record the muscle – shrink – curve, work out the threshold stimulating, up stimulating and upper intensity.

(2) The recording of single contraction, incomplete tetanus and complete tetanus Put the button of wave on "single wave", put the button way button on "in" with the highest intensity wave width of 2 ~ 5ms, choose internals and set it at 1000,500,200,100,50ms. Turn on the stimulate the nerve with different internals, and make each stimulation last for 2 seconds. Then put the way button on "out", the work will be paused. Observe and record the response of the single contraction, incomplete tetanus and work out it's stimulating frequency.

(3) Observe the response of put procaine on sciatic nerve Wrap the middle of the nerve with cotton dipped with 1% procaine for about 2 minutes, observe the response of the sample that is mentioned on the above. Then, stimulate the sample directly with electricity, record it's response. Through away the cotton, put the sample in Ringer solution for 3 ~ 5 minutes, observe the result.

GUIDANCE

1. Preview

（1）Mastevs the concept of excitability.

（2）Mastevs the mechanism of the chemical transmitter at nerve – muscle joint.

（3）Understand the principle of contraction.

（4）Understand the response of contraction and analysis its mechanism.

2. Manipulation

（1）Adjust the equipment（Fig. 2 – 4） connect the equipment, turn on the power, pay attention to T_1, T_2, T_3, T_4 of stimulator, do not put away one of it on "0", and you must set $T_1 \geqslant T_2 + T_3$.

（2）Master the method of preparation of sciatic nerve – fibula muscle. Do not destory the sample, especially of the joint of nerve and muscle. Do not use hand and other metal tools when separating the sample except glass needle; Do not pull the nerve excessively when seperating.

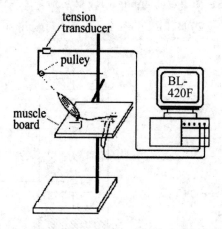

Fig. 2 – 4   Linking equipments

（3）Finish the practice as soon as possible in order to avoid fatiguing of nerve

（4）The toad – cake is not harmful to our skin, if it was spattered your eyes, clean your eyes with normal saline immediately, and you can clean it before the preparation of sample

3. Notices

（1）Do not touch nerve and muscle with the top of tools and coarse object.

（2）Wet the sample with Ringer solution, in order to keep it good at work.

（3）Make sure there isn't any sign output from stimulator, when changing the parameter.

（4）Make sure that all the equipment were connected well, or it would affect the result.

4. Reports

（1）Get the clear curve of the result

（2）Discuss the relationship between intensity frequency and contraction, and work out the principle of contraction

（3）Discuss the principle of procaine's effect on nerve

5. Questions

（1）Why must we dip a sample of sciatic nerve – fibula muscle into Ringer solution for a while?

（2）How to divide incubation period, contraction period and diastole period of muscle contraction?

（3）Illustrate the mechanism of incomplete tetanus and complete tetanus?

（Fu Jihua）

实验二　神经干动作电位观察

扫码"学一学"

【实验目的】

用示波器观察蛙类坐骨神经干的单相、双相动作电位基本波形，并了解其产生原理。通过操作实践，学习电生理实验仪器的使用方法。

【实验原理】

在有效刺激作用下（常用电刺激），神经纤维膜内外产生去极化，当其去极化达到阈电位时，能诱发膜产生一次在神经纤维上可传导的快速电位反转，此即为动作电位（AP）。神经干动作电位是神经兴奋的客观标志，处于兴奋状态的部位对静止部位而言，膜外电位呈负电性质，当神经冲动通过以后，膜外电位又恢复到静息时水平。

如果两个引导电极置于正常完整的神经干表面，兴奋波先后通过两个电极处，便引导出两个方向相反的电位偏转，称为双相动作电位。如果两个引导电极之间神经组织有损伤，兴奋波只通过第一个引导电极，不能传至第二个引导电极，则只能引导出一个方向的电位偏转波形，称为单相动作电位。

神经干由许多神经纤维组成，故神经干动作电位与单根神经纤维的动作电位不同，它是由许多神经纤维动作电位综合成的综合性电位变化。所以神经干动作电位幅度在一定范围内可随刺激强度的变化而变化。

【实验材料】

1. 仪器　BL-420F生物信号采集与分析系统（或示波器，电子刺激器），神经标本屏蔽盒，蛙板，小烧杯，滴管，瓷板，蛙手术器械一套。

2. 药品　任氏液。

3. 对象　蟾蜍。

【实验方法】

1. 蛙坐骨神经干标本制备　标本制备方法基本同坐骨神经-腓肠肌标本制备法，只是为了获得尽量长的神经干标本，在分离到腓肠肌后再继续沿神经一分支（胫神经）一直分离至踝关节附近，末端结扎并剪断。

2. 仪器连接和调试

（1）将示波器、刺激器、神经屏蔽盒等接好，用刺激器触发示波器，使扫描同步（图2-5）。

（2）将神经屏蔽盒内所有电极用浸有任氏液的棉球擦净。

（3）用镊子夹住已制备好的神经标本的一端，将其放置于电极上，用滤纸片吸去标本上过多的任氏液。

（4）示波器 y 轴灵敏度用5mV/cm或2mV/cm，x 轴扫描速度用0.5~0.1ms/cm，刺激器刺激波宽0.1~1.0ms，刺激频率适当，刺激强度在1.0V左右，调节刺激器的延迟旋钮，使动作电位波形正好出现在荧光屏的适中位置。

3. 观察项目

（1）双相动作电位的观察 计算双相动作电位时程及上升相、下降相宽度及幅值，计算自伪迹起点至动作电位起点所需的时间。

（2）调节刺激强度求出在相应刺激波宽下动作电位产生的阈强度和顶强度。

（3）单相动作电位的观察 用镊子将两个记录电极之间的神经夹伤，此时示波器上呈现单相动作电位，观察其形状并计算时程、幅值及伪迹至单相动作电位起点所需的时间。

【实验指导】

1. 预习要求

（1）复习动作电位、静息电位产生的原理。

（2）复习动作电位在神经纤维上的传导机制。

（3）复习刺激器、示波器的使用方法及注意事项。

2. 操作要点

（1）熟练地应用与调试刺激器和示波器，掌握仪器使用注意事项，正确使用仪器，注意仪器接地是否良好。

（2）坐骨神经标本制备时应特别小心，防止损伤神经，手术操作应规范化。

（3）本实验可以将计算机连接起来使用，具体连接如（图2-6），刺激器同步输出可同时触发示波器扫描和计算机采样，生物电信号必须首先放大，然后一方面用示波器观察，另一方面输入计算机之 A/D 卡由计算机采样、贮存，计算机可将采样结果显示于荧光屏，并按要求处理结果及从打印机打印图形及处理结果，软件可采用 BL－420F 生物信号采集与分析系统。

3. 注意事项

（1）制备坐骨神经标本时应谨慎，避免损伤神经，切勿用利器或手指触及神经，分离的神经标本应尽量长些。

（2）神经的两端不能碰在屏蔽盒上，也不要把神经两端折叠在电极上，以免影响动作电位的大小和波形。

（3）开始时刺激不要过强，应由弱刺激逐步加至适宜强度，以免过强刺激伤害神经标本。

4. 报告要点

（1）画出双相动作电位和单相动作电位图形，并求出时程、幅值等结果；测量某一刺激波宽下的动作电位刺激阈强度、顶强度。

（2）讨论双相及单相动作电位产生原理，神经冲动传导机制。

（3）说明伪迹产生原因。

5. 思考题

（1）为什么双相动作电位上升相和下降相宽度和幅度不一样，且第一相（上升相）幅值大于第二相（下降相），但宽度小于第二相？试问是否有可能达到上升相和下降相方向相反而幅度和宽度相同？

（2）神经干动作电位的幅度在一定范围内随着刺激强度的变化而变化，这是否与神经纤维动作电位的"全或无"性质相矛盾？

（傅继华）

2 Observation on the action potential of nerve trunk

PURPOSE

To observe the basic monophasic, biphasic AP wave forms by oscillograph, and understand the principle. To study the use of electric physiological instruments in practice.

PRINCIPLE

Under the effective stimulation (most using electric stimulation), inside and outside of the nervous fiber membrane produces depolarization. When the polarization rises to threshold potential, it will causes a rapid potential reverse that can transmitting on the nervous fiber, which is called action potential (AP). The AP of nerve trunk is the objective symbol when nerve is exciting. It's negative that outside membrane potential of area which is in exciting condition, compared with the restingcondition. When the nerve impulse has traversed, the outside membrane potential returns to the resting level.

If two lead electrodes are placed on the surface of the normal intact nerve trunk, when a excitative wave traverses two electrodes in turn, the electrodes will lead two reverse potential deflections, called biphasic AP. If the nerve tissues are damaged between two lead electrodes, the excitative wave will only traverse the first lead electrode, other than second lead electrode, resulting in leading unidirectional potential deflective wave – form, called monophasic AP.

Nerve trunk is composed of many nervous fibers, so the AP of nerve trunk is different to the AP of single nervous fiber, which is a synthetical potential change composed of much AP of nervous fibers. Therefore, the AP range of nerve trunk changes with the stimulation intensity to a certain extent.

MATERIALS

1. Equipments BL – 420F biological signal acquisition and analysis system (or Oscillograph, electric – stimulator), shield – box for nerve specimen, operating table for frog, beaker, burette, china board, a set of operating tools for frog.

2. Solution Ringer's solution.

3. Object Toad.

METHODS

1. Preparation for sciatic nerve trunk sample of toad Take a toad and damage its brain and spinal cord, cut out the top of body and viscus, shell its skin, and then dissociate sciatic nerve carefully by hand along two sides of spine, ligate it at the root and cut it out. Clamp it out from belly with minute tweezers, ligate the nerve at ankle and cut it out. Before the trial, nerve specimen should be immersed in Ringer's solution for about then minutes until irritability issteady.

2. Connection and adjustment of eguipment

（1）Connect oscillograph、stimulator and nerre shield – box. Start up oscillograph with stimulator to ensure synchronous scan (Fig. 2 – 5).

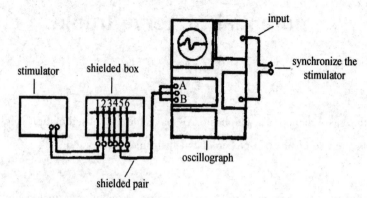

Fig. 2 – 5 Link equipments to lead AP of nerve trunk

（2）Scrub all electrodes in the shield – box by cotton swab with Ringer's solntion.

（3）Clamp one end of the simple and put it on the electrode, suck excessive Ringer's solution of the specimen with filter paper

（4）Adjusting: oscilloscope sensitivity 5mV/cm or 2mV/cm as y axis

scan – velocity 0. 5 ~ 0. 1ms/cm as x axis

stimulating – wave width 0. 1 ~ 1. 0ms

stimulating intensity 1. 0V

frequency should be proper when the wave of action potential appears on the suitable place of monitor.

3. Observation items

（1）observe the biphasic AP: calculate the biphasic AP period, the width and range of rise phase and decrease phase calculate the time from pseudo – track starting – point to AP starting – point.

（2）adjust the stimulation intensity: calculate the threshold intensity and top in tensity which are produced by AP at relevant stimulation wave – width.

（3）observe the monophasic AP: clip to harm the nerve between two record electrodes by tweezers, then AP will appear on the oscillograph. Observe its shape and calculate its period, range and time from pseudo – track starting – point to AP starting – point.

GUIDANCE

1. Preview

（1）review the principle of AP and resting potential occurrence.

（2）review the mechanism of AP conducting on nervous fiber.

（3）review the methods and attentions of stimulator and oscilloscope.

2. Manipulation

（1）Operate and adjust the stimulator and oscillograph skillful, master points for attention of apparatuses and use them correctly, notice whether or not the ground connections of apparatuses are well.

(2) Prepare the sciatic nerve simple carefully The operation should be standard.

(3) This experiment can link the computer to use, concrete linking as follows (fig. 2 - 6). Stimulator synchronous output can trigger the oscilloscope scanning and computer sampling at the same time. The bioelectric signals need to be enlarged first, then on one hand observe by oscilloscope, and on the other hand input the signals to the computer A/D card for sampling and saving. The computer can display the sampling outcome in screen, handle the outcome according to request and print thefigure and outcome. The software can use the EBS general bioelectric signal sampling and operating system which is invented by FuJihua.

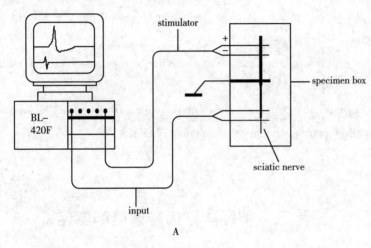

A

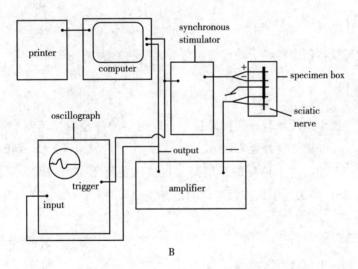

B

Fig. 2 - 6　Linking equipments

A. Using D - 95　B. common method

3. Notices

(1) Preparation for the specimen should be cautious, you must not touch the nerve with sharp things and fingers, and separate the specimen as long as possible.

(2) The ends of nerve shouldn't touch the shield box and fold the ends of nerve on electrodes, avoid influencing the size and shape of AP.

(3) Stimulation shouldn't be too strong at first, and then increase gradually weak stimulation to

suitable intensity. Avoid damaging the specimen under over – stimulation.

4. Reports

（1）Draw the biphasic and monophasic AP figures, calculate the period, range etc. ; measure the AP threshold intensity and top intensity in some stimulation wave – width.

（2）discuss the principle of biphasic and monophasic AP occurrence, the conduct mechanism of nerve impulse.

（3）explain the reason of pseudo – track occurrence.

5. Questions

（1）Why the width and range of biphasic AP rise phase and descent phase are different. why the range of first phase（rise phase）is larger than that of second phase（descent phase）, but the width is smaller than second phase?

Whether or not it is possible that the width and range of rise and descent phase are equal when their directions are opposite.

（2）The AP range of nerve trunk changes with the stimulation intensity to a certain extent, does it contradictory to all or none phenomenon of nervous fiber AP?

（Fu Jihua）

实验三　神经冲动传导速度的测定

【实验目的】

学会用电生理仪器测定神经干动作电位传导速度的方法并了解其原理。

【实验原理】

动作电位在神经干上传导有一定的速度。不同类型的神经传导速度不同，神经纤维越粗则传导速度越快。蛙类坐骨神经干以 Aα 类纤维为主，传导速度为 35～40m/s。

测定神经冲动在神经干上传导的距离与通过这段距离所需的时间，可根据距离（s）、时间（t）、速度（v）的关系求出神经冲动的传导速度，即 $v = s/t$。

【实验材料】

同"神经干动作电位观察"实验。

【实验方法】

1. 蟾蜍坐骨神经标本制备　同"神经干动作电位观察"实验。

2. 仪器连接和调试　同"神经干动作电位观察"实验。

3. 观察项目

（1）如图 2 – 7 所示，将坐骨神经标本的粗端放于刺激电极 A、B 上，细端放于记录电极 D、E 上，拉直神经标本，使 A 电极接正极，B 电极接负极，C 电极联 D、E 两记录电极的屏蔽线外壳，并与示波器接地相连。刺激强度适当（小于顶强度），此时可在示波器上见到一双相动作电位，测出伪迹起点至动作电位起点的时间 t_1，并测出两记录电极间距离 s_1。

（2）E 电极不动，改变 D 电极位置，测出 DE 间距离 s_2，这时用同样刺激强度可观察到一双相动作电位，测出伪迹起点至动作电位起点时间 t_2。

（3）神经冲动传导速度 $v = (s_1 - s_2)/(t_2 - t_1)$。

【实验指导】

1. 预习要求 预习神经冲动产生及传导原理。

2. 操作要点 同"神经干动作电位观察"实验。

本实验也可以将计算机连接起来使用，连接方法同"神经干动作电位观察"实验所述，t_1、t_2 可由计算机自动求出，还可求得神经冲动传导速度 v。

3. 注意事项

（1）神经干一定要粗端放于刺激电极一侧，并且刺激电极正、负极必须如以上所述连接。

（2）$|s_1 - s_2|$ 必须达到一定值，若太小则 $|t_1 - t_2|$ 将很小，v 的计算结果将会有较大误差。

4. 报告要点 正确记录实验结果，计算神经干冲动传导速度，并分析本实验所测得的神经冲动传导速度是其中哪类纤维的速度。

5. 思考题

（1）神经冲动传导速度是否可以用以下方法测定：测出刺激电极负极至第一记录电极间距离 s，测出刺激伪极起点至动作电位起点时间 t，则 $v = s/t$，为什么？

（2）通过实验能否分别测出蛙坐骨神经中三类神经纤维的传导速度？

（傅继华）

3　Measurement of conduction velocity of nerve impulse

PURPOSE

To study the method of measuring conduction velocity of action potential by electric – physiological equipments and its principle.

PRINCIPLE

Action potential has a regular velocity. Commonly, the more thick the nerve is, the more quick the velocity conducts. Fiber – A a is the main to the frog, its velocity is about $35 \sim 40 \text{m/s}$. By measuring the distance and time of nerve, conduction velocity can be calculated from the equation $v = s/t$.

MATERIALS

1. Equipments BL – 420F biological signal acquisition and analysis system (or oscillograph, electric – stimulator), shield – box for nerve specimen, operating table for frog, beaker, burette, china board, a set of operating tools.

2. Solution   Ringer's solution.

3. Object   Toad.

METHOD

1. Preparation for sciatic nerve sample of toad   Take a toad and damage its brain and spinal cord, cut out the top of body and viscus, shell its skin, and then dissociate sciatic nerve carefully by minute hand along two sides of spine, ligate it at the root and cut it out. clamp it out from belly with minute tweezers, ligate the nerve at ankle and cut it out. Before the trial, nerve specimen should be immerse in Ringer's solution for about then minutes until irritability is steady.

2. Connection and adjustment of eguipment

（1）Connect oscillograph. stimulator and nerve shield – box. Start up oscillograph with stimulator to ensure synchronous scan.

（2）Scrub all electrodes in the shield box by cotton swab with Ringer's solution

（3）Clamp one end of the sample and put it on the electrode, suck excessive Ringer's solution of the specimen with filter paper.

（4）Adjusting: oscilloscope sensitivity 5mV/cm or 2mV/cm as y axis

scan – velocity $0.5 \sim 0.1$ms/cm as x axis

stimulating – wave width $0.1 \sim 1.0$ms

stimulating intensity 1.0V

frequency should be proper when the wave of action potential appears on the suitable place of monitor.

3. Observation items

（1）As the following diagram, put the thick end of nerve specimen on stimulating – electrode A and B, and put the other end on recording – electrode D and E. Pull the sample straight and then connect A with anode, B with negative pole, C with D and E which link oscilloscope. As a bi – direction action potential appears on the oscilloscope, the time t from the starting point of pseudo – electrode to that of action potential can be measured and so does the distance s_1 between D and E.

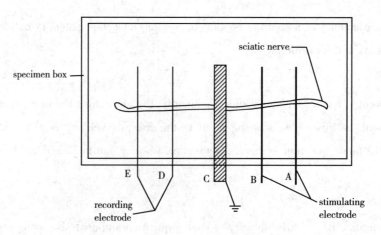

Fig. 2 – 7   **Specimen box for stimulating**

（2）Change the site of D, measure again. When distance s_2 of a bi – direction impulse can be observed by the same intensity stimulating, time t_2 will be gained.

（3）Equation: $v = (s_1 - s_2)/(t_2 - t_1)$.

GUIDANCE

1. Preview   Preview the occurrence and conduction principle of nerve impulse.

2. Manipulation

（1）Master the use of apparatuses.

（2）Operating should be standard.

（3）Computer may be used.

3. Notices

（1）The thick end of nerve muscle should be put on the stimulating – electrode.

（2）If $(s_1 - s_2)$ is too small, the result will be error.

4. Report   Record the results correctly and calculate conduction velocity of nerve impulse carefully.

5. Questions

（1）If s is from negative pole of stimulating – electrode to the fist recording – one, and t is from the starting point of pseudo – electrode to that of action potential, is the equation $v = s/t$ right?

（2）Can the three types of conduction velocities of nervous fibers in frog's sciatic be measured respectively?

（Fu Jihua）

实验四　蟾蜍坐骨神经不应期的测定

【实验目的】

测定蟾蜍坐骨神经的绝对不应期和相对不应期，并了解其测定原理。

【实验原理】

用一台电子刺激器输出两个电脉冲，通过调节两刺激脉冲间隔，可测得坐骨神经的绝对不应期和相对不应期。将两刺激脉冲间隔由最小逐渐增大时，开始只有第一个刺激脉冲产生 AP，第二个刺激脉冲不产生 AP，当两刺激脉冲间隔达到一定值时，此时第二个刺激脉冲刚好能引起一极小的 AP，这时两刺激脉冲间隔即为绝对不应期。继续增大刺激脉冲间隔，这时由第二个刺激脉冲产生的 AP 逐渐增大，当两刺激脉冲间隔达到某一值时，此时由第二个刺激脉冲产生的 AP，其大小刚好和第一个刺激产生的 AP 相同，这时两刺激脉冲间隔即为相对不应期。继续增大刺激间隔，此时由两刺激脉冲产生的 AP 将始终保持完全一致。

【实验材料】

同"神经干动作电位观察"实验。

【实验方法】

1. 蟾蜍坐骨神经标本制备 同"神经干动作电位观察"实验。

2. 仪器连接和调试基本 同"神经干动作电位观察"实验，只是刺激器输出需用串脉冲，串个数为2，两刺激脉冲间隔通过串间隔调节。

3. 观察项目

（1）顶强度的测定 用单脉冲刺激坐骨神经，刺激频率适当，刺激波宽用0.2～0.5ms，刺激强度由0逐渐增大，找出该坐骨神经的刺激顶强度。

（2）坐骨神经绝对不应期的测定 用两个串脉冲刺激坐骨神经，刺激强度用顶强度，刺激波宽同1，串间隔由0.6ms开始逐渐增大。当串间隔达到一定值时，第二个刺激脉冲也开始引起一微弱的动作电位，此时的串间隔即为绝对不应期。

（3）坐骨神经相对不应期的测定 在观察项目（2）的基础上进一步增大串间隔，这时由第二个动作电位幅值刚好达到第一个动作电位幅值大小时，此时的串间隔即为相对不应期。

（4）重复以上实验，在相对不应期内增大测试刺激的强度时，缩小的第二个动作电位幅度可达到第一个的水平。但如果在绝对不应期内，虽然增大刺激强度，却不能引起神经的第二次兴奋。

【实验指导】

1. 预习要求

（1）复习神经兴奋性产生的原理及其变化规律。

（2）复习神经绝对不应期、相对不应期的产生原理。

2. 操作要点

（1）同"神经干动作电位观察"实验。

（2）本实验可与计算机连接起来使用，将生物电信号和刺激脉冲分别输入计算机之A/D卡，计算机可自动描记生物电图形及刺激脉冲波，并自动求出绝对不应期及相对不应期。

3. 注意事项 同"神经干动作电位观察"实验。

4. 报告要点

（1）描记神经干动作电位图形，并描记处于绝对不应期及相对不应期时，由2个串脉冲引起的动作电位图形。

（2）记录顶强度、绝对不应期、相对不应期的大小。

（3）结合实验结果，讨论神经在一次兴奋后兴奋性变化的规律及原理。

5. 思考题

（1）本实验为什么要用顶强度刺激，用不同刺激强度刺激测得的绝对不应期和相对不应期会一致吗？

（2）试分析神经纤维绝对不应期、相对不应期和神经干绝对不应期、相对不应期的生理意义，它们有什么异同？

（傅继华）

4　Measurement of refractory period on toad sciatic nerve

PURPOSE

To measure absolute and relative refractory period one on toad sciatic nerveand study the principle of measurement.

PRINCIPLE

Make an electric – stimulator output two pulses, adjust the interval of pulses to get the absolute and relative refractory period on toad sciatic nerve. As adjusting the pulse interval that increases gradually, only the first pulse yields AP at the beginning, while the other not. To the extent that the second pulse causes a minimum AP, the pulse interval is called absolute refractory period. Continue increasing the interval until the AP is as large as that from the first pulse, this pulse interval is called relative refractory period. After that, the two APs are not changed.

MATERIALS

1. Equipments　BL – 420F biological signal acquisition and analysis system (or Oscillograph, electric – stimulator), shield – box for nerve specimen, operating table for frog, beaker, burette, china board, a set of operating tools.

2. Solution　Ringer's solution.

3. Object　Toad.

METHOD

1. Preparation for sciatic nerve sample of toad　Take a toad and damage its brain and spinal cord, cut out the top of body and viscus, shell its skin, and then dissociate sciatic nerve carefully by minute hand along two sides of spine, ligate it at the root and cut it out. clamp it out from belly with minute tweezers, ligate the nerve at ankle and cut it out. Before the trial, nerve specimen should be immersed in Ringer's solution for about ten minutes until irritability is steady.

2. Connection and adjustment of eguipment

(1) Connect oscillograph stimulator and nerve shield – box. start up oscillograph with stimulator to ensure synchronous scan.

(2) Scrub all electrodes in the shield box by cotton swab with Ringer's solution.

(3) Clamp one end of the sample and put it on the electrode, suck excessive Ringer's solution of the specimen with filter paper.

(4) Adjusting: oscilloscope sensitivity 5mV/cm or 2mV/cm as y axis

scan – velocity $0.5 \sim 0.1$ ms/cm as x axis

outputting two cluster pulses and stimulating – wave width $0.2 \sim 0.5$ ms

stimulating intensity 1.0V

frequency should be proper when the wave of action potential appears on the suitable place of monitor.

3. Observation items

（1）Measurement of top – intensity

Make single pulse stimulate sciatic nerve by stimulus – intensity increasing gradually from zero, the top – intensity can be found.

（2）Measurement of absolute refractory period

Make the two cluster pulses stimulate sciatic nerve, use top – intensity as stimulus – intensity, adjust wave width to 0. 2 ~ 0. 5ms and cluster interval increasingly from 0. 6ms when an weak action potential caused by the second pulse is appearing, the cluster interval is called absolute refractory period.

（3）Measurement of relative refractory period

From the above（2）, continue the interval increasing. When the range of the second action potential is the same with the first one, the cluster interval is called relative refractory period.

（4）If enlarge stimulus – intensity while reduce the second action potential range in relative refractory period, the first level will also be gained. But if in absolute period, the sample will do not get the second stimulation.

GUIDANCE

1. Preview

（1）Review the principle of nerve irritability occurrence and its changing regulation

（2）Review the principle of nerve absolute and relative refractory period.

2. Manipulation

（1）Master the use of apparatuses.

（2）Operating should be standard.

（3）Computer may be used.

3. Notices

（1）The thick end of verve muscle should be put on the stimulating – electrode.

（2）If $(s_1 - s_2)$ is too small, the result will have errors.

4. Reports

（1）Trace the wave form.

（2）Record the roof – intensity, absolute and relative periods.

（3）Discuss the regulation and principle of nervous irritability change after one stimuli.

5. Questions

（1）Why to use roof – intensity stimulating while not stimulus – intensity for measuring absolute and relative periods? Is that the similar?

（2）Try to analysis the differences of nerve fiber's absolute and relative period and state its significance?

（Fu Jihua）

实验五　脊髓反射

扫码"学一学"

【目的要求】

观察几种常见的脊髓反射（屈肌反射、搔抓反射等），学习测定反射时的方法，了解反射弧的组成并探讨反射弧的完整性与反射活动的关系。

【实验原理】

在中枢神经参与下，机体对刺激所起的反应过程称为反射。较复杂的反射需要较高级中枢部位的整合，而一些较简单的反射，只需通过中枢神经系统的低级部位就能完成。将动物的高位中枢切除，仅保留脊髓的动物称为脊动物，此时动物产生的各种反射活动为单纯的脊髓反射。由于脊髓已失去高级中枢的正常调节作用，故利于观察和分析研究反射过程的某些特征。

任何反射活动均需通过一定的反射弧才能完成。反射弧由感受器、传入神经、反射中枢、传出神经和效应器五部分组成。反射通过反射弧各组成部分所需的时间称为反射时，即由刺激作用于感受器开始，到效应器出现反射活动所经过的时间。反射时的长短与反射弧在中枢交换神经元的多少及是否有中枢抑制存在等有密切关系。反射时也与刺激强度有关，在一定的条件下与一定的刺激强度范围内，刺激愈强，反射时愈短。反射活动的完成依赖于反射弧的完整性。如果一反射弧中任一环节被中断，反射活动都将不能进行。

【实验材料】

1. 器材　蛙手术器械，蛙板，肌夹，表面皿，小烧杯，秒表，铁架台，滤纸片，棉花，纱布。

2. 溶液　0.5% 及 2% 硫酸溶液。

3. 对象　蟾蜍。

【实验步骤】

1. 制备脊蟾蜍　取蟾蜍 1 只，用剪刀横向伸入口腔，沿两侧鼓膜后缘保留其下腭，将其颅脑部剪去制成脊蟾蜍。用棉球压迫创口止血。用肌夹夹住下腭，将脊蟾蜍挂在铁站架上，等候片刻再行实验。

此外，也可用探针由枕骨大孔刺入颅腔，捣毁脑组织以制备脊蟾蜍。

2. 观察脊髓反射

（1）屈肌反射　以盛有少量 0.5% 硫酸的表面皿接触蟾蜍后肢趾尖皮肤，观察反应。

（2）搔抓反射　用一小片滤纸浸以 2% 硫酸粘贴在蟾蜍腹部皮肤上，观察反应。

3. 测定反射时　于表面皿内盛少量 0.5% 硫酸。分别先后将左右两后肢的最长趾浸入其中（浸入 2～3mm 为宜，浸入时间不要超过 10s），同时按秒表。记录足趾浸入硫酸至腿部开始屈曲收缩所需的时间（以秒计算）。观察后立即将该足趾浸入盛有清水的烧杯中洗净，然后用纱布抹干。按上法重复一次，求两次的平均值，此即用酸刺激足趾部皮肤引起下肢屈肌反射的反射时。

4. 反射弧分析

（1）上述测定反射时的实验，是利用正常脊髓反射活动。

（2）将测过反射时的脊蟾蜍一侧小腿的皮肤做一环形切口，再由此切口将其下肢的皮肤剥掉（不可留有任何小的皮肤附着在肌肉上），稍停片刻，待蟾蜍静止下来，再以0.5%的硫酸浸此无皮肤包围的趾端，记录其反射情况有无变化。再用2%的硫酸浸过的棉花涂擦腹部，观察两下肢有无反应。

（3）取下蟾蜍将正常腿（未剥掉皮肤腿）侧的背部脊椎旁皮肤剪开，找到由脊髓发出通往下腿的神经，将通往正常腿侧的神经——剪断，再重复用0.5%硫酸刺激正常下腿趾，观察有无反应。再以2%硫酸浸过的棉花涂擦腹部，观察左、右两腿反应情况。

（4）以金属探针捣毁脊髓后再以2%硫酸浸过的棉花涂擦腹部，观察下肢有无反应。

【实验指导】

1. 预习要求　复习反射、反射弧组成、反射中枢及反射中枢活动的一般规律等内容。

2. 操作要点　脊蟾蜍制备法及寻找由脊髓发出通往下腿神经的方法。

3. 注意事项

（1）剪去颅脑的部位应适当，太高则部分脑组织保留，可能会出现自主活动；太低则伤及上部脊髓，可能使上肢的反射消失。

（2）实验时每次浸入硫酸的足趾及其范围应该相同，以保持刺激强度一致。

（3）刺激后要立即洗去硫酸以免损伤皮肤。洗后应擦干蟾蜍趾上的水渍，防止硫酸被稀释。

4. 报告要点　列表记录各实验结果并加以解释；根据结果讨论反射与反射弧的关系。

5. 思考题

（1）决定和影响反射时长短的体内、体外因素主要有哪些？

（2）反射弧实验中利用了几种反射？其反射途径如何？

（3）除屈肌反射和搔抓反射外，你还可举出哪些脊髓反射？

（郭青龙）

5　Spinal reflex

PURPOSE

To observe several spinal reflexes (flexor reflex and scratch reflex) and learn the measurement of reflex time in order to understand the conformation of reflex arc and the relationship between the integrity of reflex arc and the reflex activity.

PRINCIPLE

The response process of the organism for stimulation is named reflex in the participation of central nervous system. Complex reflex needs the conformity of superior centrum, while some simple reflexes only need the participation of inferior centrum. The animals, which superior centrums are cut and spinal cord is remained only, are called spinal animals. Their various reflex activities are pure spinal reflex. Since the normal modulation of superior centrum cannot regulate spinal cord, spinal animals are advantageous for observing and analyzing the character of some reflexes.

Every reflex activity needs a certain reflex arc. A reflex arc consists of sensor, afferent nerve, reflex centrum, efferent nerve and effector. The time spent during the reflex going through every part of the reflex arc is called reflex time, that is, the time from the sensor receiving stimulation to the effector showing reflex activity. The length of reflex time has a close relation with the number of exchange neuron and the central inhibition in centrum. The reflex time is also associated with stimulus intensity. In some conditions and in a range of stimulus intensity, the more stronger the stimulus is, the more shorter the reflex time is. The completion of a reflex activity relies on the integrity of the reflex arc. The reflex would be interrupted if any part of the reflex arc was broken.

MATERIALS

1. Equipments　Frog operating instruments, frog board, muscle clamp, watch – glass, little beaker, stopwatch, iron stand, filter paper, cotton, gauze.

2. Solutions　0. 5% and 2% sulphuric acid.

3. Object　Toad.

METHODS

1. Preparation of spinal toad　Put a scissor into the buccal cavity of the toad horizontally. Cut down its cranio – brain along posterior border of drum membrane on two sides but remain its submaxilary. Stress the wound with cotton balls for hemostasia. Clamp its submaxilary with a muscle clamp and hang the toad on the stand. Start the experiment after a while.

In addition, spinal toad can be prepared by a probe sticking into cranial cavity from great occipital foramen to destroy brain tissue.

2. Observing spinal reflex

(1) Flexor reflex Dip the skin of the toe top of the toad hindlimb in 0. 5% sulphuric acid on a watch – glass. Then observe the response of the toad.

(2) Scratch reflex Paste a piece of filter paper with 2% sulfuric acid on the skin of the toad abdomen. Observe the response of the toad.

3. Measurement of the reflex time　Put some 0. 5% sulfuric acid on the watch – glass. Immerse the longest toe on the left and right hind limb in the watch glass respectively (2 ~ 3mm depth, not longer than 10 seconds) and start the stopwatch at the same time. Write down the time from the toe putting into sulfuric acid to the leg beginning flexion (expressed with seconds). Immerse the toes into water in beaker to wash up and rub them to dry with a piece of gauze. Repeat the above and then calculate the average time. It is the time of the lower limb flexor reflex induced by the acid as a stimulator.

4. Analyses of the reflex arc

(1) The above experiment that the reflex times were measured is a normal spinal reflex.

(2) After the determination of reflex time, cut a circular nick on the skin of one side shank in the spinal toad. Strip its skin of lower limb from the nick (do not remain any little skin on muscles). When the toad calms down after a while, dip the top of the toe not surrounding with skin in

0.5% sulfuric acid and record its response. Rub the abdomen skin with cotton dipped by 2% sulfuric acid and observe the response of lower limbs.

（3）Cut the skin of back vertebra on the normal leg side（surrounding with skin）and open to look for the nerves that are from spinal cord to the normal lower leg. Cut off the nerves one by one and stimulate the normal toe with 0.5% sulfuric acid again and observe the response of the toad. Rub the abdomen skin with cotton dipped by 2% sulfuric acid and then observe the response of lower limbs.

（4）Destroy the spinal cord with metal probe and then rub the abdomen skin with cotton dipped by 2% sulfuric acid, then observe the response of lower limbs.

GUIDANCE

1. Preview　Review reflex, reflex arc, reflex centrum and the general rules about the activity of reflex centrum.

2. Manipulation　Manipulation requirements are the methods of preparing the spinal toad and finding the nerves from spinal cord to lower limbs.

3. Notices

（1）The place where the cranio – brain will be cut should be chosen properly. If it is too high some brain tissues may be remained and independent activity may appear. If it is too low the upper spinal cord may be injured and the reflex of upper limb may be disappeared.

（2）The depth dipped in 0.5% sulfuric acid should be same in order to maintain the same stimulus intensity.

（3）After stimulation sulfuric acid should be washed up immediately with water to prevent skin injury. And then wipe the water on the toe of the toad to prevent diluting sulfuric acid.

4. Report　Write down the results of the experiment in the table and then give explanation. Discuss the relationship between reflex and reflex arc according to the results and relative theory.

5. Questions

（1）What are the main factors in vivo and in vitro of determining and affecting the length of reflex time?

（2）How many kinds of reflex are utilized in the experiment of reflex arc? What are their pathways?

（3）What other spinal reflex can you list except flexor reflex and scratch reflex?

（Guo Qinglong）

实验六　血－脑屏障

【目的要求】

血液中某些物质不易透入脑组织或脑脊液。本实验证实血－脑屏障的存在。

【实验原理】

在毛细血管与脑组织周围间隙和脑脊液之间，存在着一种对物质交换的屏障，称为"脑屏障"，它能选择性地让某些物质透过，而另一些物质却不易透过。根据物质通过血管与脑之间界面的弥散速度和物质在脑组织中的含量等，进一步将脑屏障分成三部分：血－脑屏障；血－脑脊液屏障及脑脊液－脑屏障。实验证明，碱性染料（正电荷）易于通过血－脑屏障；而酸性染料（负电荷）则易于通过血－脑脊液屏障。血－脑屏障有重要的生理意义。

造成脑屏障的原因主要有以下几点：脑组织毛细血管的内皮细胞无窗孔，且内皮细胞之间有紧密连接，紧密连接被认为是血－脑屏障的结构基础；大多数脑组织毛细血管的外侧被一层神经胶质细胞伸出的"脚板"（血管周足）所包围，这些"脚板"也影响毛细血管的通透性，对血－脑屏障可能起辅助作用。毛细血管内皮外有一层厚约 200Å 的基膜。此外，脉络丛上皮细胞之间的闭锁小带被认为是血－脑脊液屏障的结构基础。

【实验材料】

1. **器材**　1ml 注射器，针头，剪刀，镊子，蛙板，大头针。
2. **溶液**　1% 台盼蓝溶液。
3. **对象**　小白鼠。

【实验步骤】

取小白鼠 1 只，皮下注入 1% 台盼蓝 0.5ml。30 分钟后将动物处死，做全身解剖，观察脑、脊髓与其他脏器的颜色有无区别，并与正常鼠相应器官进行比较。

【实验指导】

1. **预习要求**　复习教材中血－脑屏障有关内容。
2. **操作要点**　小白鼠捉持法及小鼠皮下注射方法。
3. **注意事项**　注入台盼蓝后，小白鼠肺脏与肝脏染成暗蓝色，一定要与正常小白鼠相应脏器比较才能得出正确结论。
4. **报告要点**　根据脑、脊髓与其他脏器的颜色不同，说明出现这一现象的原因。
5. **思考题**　何谓血－脑屏障？如何证明之？其生理意义如何？

（郭青龙）

6　Blood – brain barrier

PURPOSE

Some substances in blood are difficult in entering cerebral tissues and/or cerebrospinal fluid. This experiment is to verify the existence of blood brain barrier.

PRINCIPLE

There is a substance exchange barrier called "blood brain barrier" between blood capillary and the spaces surrounding brain tissues and cerebrospinal fluid. It can select some substance to go through easily and the other substances to go through difficult. According to the diffusion rate between blood and brain and the contents of some substances in brain tissues, the blood brain barrier can be divided into three parts further: blood – brain barrier, blood – cerebrospinal fluid barrier and cerebrospinal fluidbrain barrier. Experiments have verified that the basic dye is easily to pass blood-brain barrier and the acid dye is easily to pass blood – cerebrospinal fluid barrier. The blood brain barrier has an important physiological significance.

There are several causes in forming blood brain barrier. Firstly, there is no window in blood capillary endothelial cells in brain and there is tight junction among endothelial cells, which is considered as the structural basic of blood brain barrier. Secondly, the outer laterals of most of blood capillaries are surrounded by feet plate (perivascular feet) of neuroglial cells, which can affect the permeability of blood capillaries and have assistant functions to blood brain barrier. Thirdly there is a layer of basal membrane about 200A in out of the blood capillary endothelium. Lastly the occludens zonula among choroid plexus epithelial cells are considered as the structural basis of blood cerebrospinal fluid barrier.

MATERIALS

1. **Equipments**   1ml syringe, injection needle, scissor, forceps, frog board, pins.

2. **Solution**   1% trypan blue.

3. **Objects**   Mouse.

METHOD

Take a mouse and inject 1% trypan blue 0.5ml subcutaneously. Kill the mouse after 30 mins and dissect the whole body. Observe whether the colors of brain and spinal cord are different from those of other organs and compare them with corresponding organs in normal mice.

GUIDANCE

1. **Preview**   Review the associated contents of blood brain barrier.

2. **Manipulation**   Pay attention to the method of holding a mouse and subcutaneous injection in mouse.

3. **Notice**   The lung and liver of a mouse would be dyed into dark blue after injection oftrypan blue solution. Correct conclusion can be gained only by comparing these organs with corresponding organs in normal mice.

4. **Report**   Explain the cause of the difference in colors of brain and spinal cord from other organs.

5. **Questions**   What is the blood brain barrier? How to verify it? What is the physiological significance?

(Guo Qinglong)

实验七　脑内乙酰胆碱的定性测定

扫码"学一学"

【目的要求】

证明脑内含有乙酰胆碱（乙酰胆碱为中枢神经系统递质）并了解其测定方法。

【实验原理】

乙酰胆碱可作用于 N_2 型受体，使腹直肌产生收缩反应，随后乙酰胆碱被胆碱酯酶水解为胆碱和乙酸。毒扁豆碱等胆碱酯酶抑制剂可抑制胆碱酯酶活性而使乙酰胆碱堆积。本实验通过脑提取液与外源性乙酰胆碱对腹直肌作用的比较，以证明脑内可能含有乙酰胆碱。

已知脑内许多部位存在乙酰胆碱递质系统。乙酰胆碱主要分布于以下部位：①脊髓前角运动神经元支配骨骼肌接头处的神经递质，其分支与闰绍细胞形成突触联系的递质；②丘脑外侧核的神经元与大脑皮层感觉区之间的突触传递递质；③脑干网状结构中的某些神经元之间，边缘系统的海马以及大脑皮层内部等处。

乙酰胆碱主要是在胆碱能神经末梢内，由胆碱乙酰化酶和乙酰辅酶 A 在胞质液中促进胆碱乙酰化而形成。乙酰胆碱形成后即贮存在囊泡中。当神经冲动到达时，乙酰胆碱量子式释放入突触间隙，作用于突触后膜上 M 胆碱受体而发挥生理作用，随后很快被神经末梢部位的胆碱酯酶（ChE）水解而失效。体内的 ChE 分两种，一种叫真性 ChE，又叫乙酰胆碱酯酶（AChE），主要存在于胆碱能神经突触后膜上，水解 ACh 比水解其他胆碱酯类更快，一般指的胆碱酯酶即指真性胆碱酯酶。另一种叫丁酰胆碱酯酶（BU－ChE），主要存在于各型胶质细胞、血浆及肝脏中，水解苯甲酰胆碱及丁酰胆碱等。毒扁豆碱（依色林）属易逆性抗胆碱酯酶药，用药后可使组织内 ACh 蓄积。

【实验材料】

1. 器材　BL－420F 生物信号采集与分析系统，张力换能器，蛙手术器械，浴管，温度计，心杠杆，滴管，烧杯（250ml），铁站架，注射器（1ml、10ml），玻棒，试管，缝衣针，线。

2. 溶液　任氏液，10^{-5} mol/L 乙酰胆碱溶液，10^{-3} mol/L 毒扁豆碱任氏液，10^{-5} mol/L 毒扁豆碱任氏液。

3. 对象　蟾蜍，小白鼠。

【实验步骤】

1. 制备腹直肌标本　用探针毁坏蟾蜍脑脊髓后，剪开腹壁皮肤即可看到腹直肌。在腹正中线自耻骨端至剑突将两条腹直肌分开，并与两侧腹斜肌分离，在每条腹直肌的两端各以线结扎，剪断后取下（图 2－8），将此标本装于浴管中并加入 10^{-5} mol/L 毒扁豆碱任氏液，浸腹直肌 30 分钟以上。实验装置见图 2－9。

2. 制备脑提取液

（1）取一试管加任氏液 5ml，放于水中加热至沸。

扫码"看一看"

（2）取小白鼠1只，腹腔注射10^{-3}mol/L毒扁豆碱任氏液0.2ml，出现抽痉时立即取脑并快速用滤纸吸去脑上血液，放入上述试管中继续加热2分钟，用玻棒捣碎脑后静置20分钟，待冷却至室温后吸取上清液备用。

3. 测定

（1）放掉浴管中的溶液换以任氏液，滴加10^{-5}mol/L乙酰胆碱5～10滴，用记纹鼓记录（手拨转法）腹直肌的收缩曲线高度（1～2分钟内应出现反应）。

（2）标本用任氏液洗三次，使基线回至原来水平，换以备用脑提取液，按上法记录收缩高度后，回收脑提取液，标本用任氏液洗三次。

（3）在上述脑提取液中加鼠血10滴，37℃水浴中保温10分钟，待冷却后加入浴管中观察腹直肌有无收缩。

（4）用任氏液洗标本三次后重复第1项，再加任氏液洗三次。

（5）取一试管加入任氏液5ml，并滴加10^{-5}mol/L乙酰胆碱5～10滴，再加鼠血10滴，混匀后在37℃水浴中保温10分钟。待冷却后，加入浴管中观察腹直肌有无收缩。

【实验指导】

1. 预习要求　复习神经递质章节，了解乙酰胆碱的分布、化学结构、合成、释放、失活及作用原理。

2. 操作要点　制备腹直肌标本和脑提取液的方法。

3. 注意事项

（1）每次用药后，标本均需用任氏液洗三次，换洗时描笔应离开记纹鼓，以免曲线受影响。

（2）浴管内的任氏液，一定要超过标本，并在实验过程中保持同一高度。

（3）加热小鼠脑组织的时间不可过长。

（4）实验步骤测定项中，（3）（5）两项水浴保温最好同时做，这样可平行对照，也可节省时间。但测定时仍按实验讲义所述进行。

4. 报告要点　用配有文字说明的记录曲线表达实验结果，并测量每条曲线的高度，根据结果进行讨论。

5. 思考题　中枢神经系统内的递质主要有哪些？ACh是兴奋性还是抑制性递质？

（郭青龙）

7　Qualitative determination of ACh in brain

PURPOSE

To verify the existence of acetylcholine (ACh, a transmitter in central nervous system) in brain and get to know its measurement method.

PRINCIPLE

ACh can act on N_2 receptor to make abdominis rectus muscle contract. After that ACh is hydrolyzed into choline and acetic acid by choline esterase. The cholinesterase inhibitors, such as physostigmine, can inhibit the activity of choline esterase and then pile ACh up. The experiment proves that ACh may be existent in brain by comparing extract fluid from brain with extraneous ACh.

It is realized that many sites in brain have ACh transmitter system. ACh, as a transmitter, is distributed in following sites: ① nerve – muscle connection and the synapses. Motorial neurons in anterior horn of spinal cord are cholinergic neuron, which axon and cells of skeletal muscle constituted nerve – muscle connection or and Renshaw's cell in the horn constituted synapses; ②the synapse between thalamo lateral neurons and sensory area of cerebral cortex; ③the synapses between some neurons of reticular formation of brain stem, hippocampi of limbic system and interior of cerebral cortex.

$$CH_3CO - CoA + HO-CH_2-CH_2-N^+\overset{CH_3}{\underset{CH_3}{-}}CH_3 \xrightarrow{\text{choline acetylase}} CH_3C\overset{O}{-}O-CH_2-CH_2-N^+\overset{CH_3}{\underset{CH_3}{-}}CH_3$$

Acetylcholine, mainly in cholinergic nerve ending, is synthesized by choline acetylase and acetyl coenzyme A in cytoplasm of the ending, and then is stored in vesicle. Achs are released in quantal manner to synaptic cleft and act on M cholinoceptor that will show physiological action when nerve impulses are coming. After that, ACh will be hydrolyzed quickly by choline esterase (ChE) and become inactivity in nerve ending. ChE *in vivo* is divided into two kinds: One is called true ChE, which is also named as acetylcholinesterase (AChE) as we all refer usually. It can be seen mainly on postsynaptic membrane of cholinergic nerve and can hydrolysis ACh fast than other choline esters. Another is called butylcholinesterase (BU – ChE) that is existed in glial cells, plasm and liver and can hydrolyze benzoyl choline and butylcholine. Calabarine (Eserine) that causes accumulation of ACh in tissue after administration belongs to a reversible anticholinesterase drug.

MATERIALS

1. Equipments BL – 420F biological signal acquisition and analysis system, tension transducer, operating instruments for frog, bath tube, thermometer, heart lever, drip tube, beaker (250ml), iron stand, syringe (1ml, 10ml), glass needle for separation, test tube, needles and thread.

2. Solutions Renshi's solution, ACh solution (10^{-5} mol/L), calabarine in Renshi's solution (10^{-3} mol/L), calabarine in Renshi's solution (10^{-5} mol/L).

3. Objects Toad, mouse.

METHODS

1. Preparations of rectus abdominis muscle sample Destroy brain and spinal cord of a toad with a metal probe, shear skin of along the midline of abdominal wall. Then rectus abdominis muscle can be seen. Separate rectus abdominis muscle to two parts from the pubic symphysis to the xiphoid at midline of abdomen. Separate with a forfex rectus abdominis muscle from obliquus abdominis muscle. Ligate both ends of each rectus abdominis muscle with thread, cut each end and get a rectus abdominis muscle sample (Fig. 2 – 8). Put the sample to the bath tube and add calabarine Renshi's solution (10^{-5} mol/L) for 30minutes. Experimental devices are arranged as showed in Fig. 2 – 9.

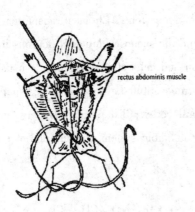

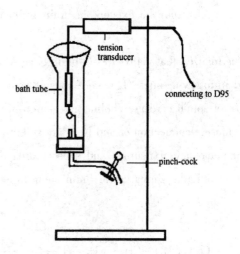

Fig. 2 - 8　The preparation of rectus abdominis muscle sample

Fig. 2 - 9　The experimental instrument

2. Preparation of cerebral extract

(1) Add 5ml Renshi's fluid to a test tube and heat it to boil.

(2) 0. 2ml calabarine Renshi's solution (10^{-3} mol/L) was injected into abdominal cavity of a mouse. After convulsion of the mouse was happened, snap the neck of the mouse firstly, open the cranial cavity and take out the brain, and then suck blood on the surface of the brain with filter papers. Put the brain into above – prepared test tube and heat it for 2 minutes. Pound the brain to fragments with a glass stick (or pestle) and lay the tube at the room temperature for 20minutes. Take the supernate for use.

3. Measurement

(1) Drop out the solution in bath tube and exchange Renshi's solution. Add ACh (10^{-5} mol/L) 5 ~ 10 drops, and then record the height of contract of the muscle (the response should be observed in 1 ~ 2minutes). The record paper in BL – 420F should be stopped.

(2) Wash the sample with Renshi's solution for three times to insure the base line reach the original level. Add cerebral extract to the bath tube and record as the above. Retrieve cerebral extract in a test tube and wash the sample with Renshi's solution for three times.

(3) Add 10 drops blood of mouse to the extract tube and keep the tube warm for 10minutes at 37℃ in water bath after full mixed. After waiting for cooling, add it to the bath tube and observe contraction of rectus abdominis muscle.

(4) Redo the first item after the sample was washed with Renshi's solution for three times. Clean it with Renshi's solution for three times after observation.

(5) Add Renshi's solution 5ml and ACh (10^{-5} mol/L) 5 ~ 10 drops to a test tube, then put blood of mouse 10 drops into it. Keep the tube warm for 10minutes at 37℃ in water bath after full mixed. Then put them into the bath tube and observe if rectus abdominis muscle would contract.

GUIDANCE

1. Preview　Review neurotransmitter and be familiar with distribution, chemical structure, release, inactivation and mechanism of ACh.

2. Manipulation　Prepare rightly rectus abdominis muscle sample and cerebral extract.

3. Notice

（1）Clean sample for three times with Renshi's solution after the effect of drug was seen.

（2）Renshi's solution in bath tube must be higher than sample and controlled at the same height during the experiment.

（3）The time that cerebral tissue of mouse was heated should not be too long.

（4）Keeping the test tubes warm in water bath in the third and the fifth item in the experiment may be done at the same time in order to compare with each other and save time. But the measurement should be done as above steps.

4. Report　Describe the experimental result with recording curves that have letter interpretation. Measure the height of each curve and discuss basis of the result.

5. Questions　What transmitters are there in central nervous system? What is ACh, excitatory or inhibitory transmitter?

（Guo Qinglong）

实验八　刺激兔大脑皮层引起的躯体运动

扫码"学一学"

【实验目的】

在不开颅的前提下，利用家兔颅骨上的骨性标志安放刺激电极，进行家兔大脑皮层功能定位。

【实验原理】

大脑皮层运动区控制着躯体的运动。直接电刺激大脑皮层某些区域，可引起动物躯体某一局部的运动。在人类，中央前回是第一运动区，刺激其不同部位可引起躯体不同肌肉收缩，具体有下列特点：①对躯体运动的调节支配具有交叉性质，即一侧皮层主要支配对侧躯体肌肉，但对头面部多数肌肉，支配是双侧性的；②具有精细的功能定位，即刺激皮层一定部位，引起一定的肌肉收缩，从运动区的上下分布来看，其定位安排是躯体的倒影；③功能代表区的大小与运动的精细复杂程度有关，与肌肉大小无关，运动愈精细复杂的肌肉，其代表区也相对愈大；④刺激所得的肌肉运动反应单纯，主要为少数个别肌肉收缩，不发生肌肉群的协同性收缩。不同种类的动物，躯体不同部位运动在皮层表面代表区的精细度不一样，动物愈高级，代表区的精细程度愈高，反之则比较粗糙。本实验即以电刺激方法观察家兔大脑皮层对躯体运动的控制及特点。

【实验材料】

1. 仪器　普通大头针，钢尺，铅笔，手术剪，镊子，旧止血钳，手术刀，小榔头，注射器5ml，注射针头，YSD－4型多用仪（或DCQ－3型电子刺激器），棉花，胶泥。

2. 药品　30%过氧化氢，1%普鲁卡因，生理盐水。

3. 对象　家兔。

【实验方法】

1. 固定 将兔固定于兔箱，剪去头顶部毛，用1%普鲁卡因约5ml注入兔头顶部皮下组织内，进行局部麻醉。用手术刀在兔头顶部做一长约4cm切口，用止血钳分离组织并用过氧化氢溶液破坏周围组织，然后用生理盐水洗净以暴露颅骨。

2. 确定刺激点 测量和刺激点是本实验的关键，规定七条标志线（图2-10）。

（1）矢状线 与矢状缝重合的直线。

（2）旁矢状线 眶后切迹内侧线，与矢状线平行，左右各一条。

（3）切迹连线 双侧眶后切迹前缘连线。

（4）冠状线 冠状缝的重叠划线。

（5）顶冠间线 顶间前线与冠状线之间的平分线。

（6）顶间前线 通过人字缝顶点与冠状线的平行线。

3. 安放电极 垂直打入大头针，电极深度为4～5mm，左右对称，各一枚。

（1）1号电极 头部运动矢状线旁2mm与切迹连线后1mm会合处。

（2）2号电极 咀嚼运动，旁矢状线外2mm与冠状线前1mm会合处。

（3）3号电极 前肢运动，矢状线旁2mm与冠状线后2mm会合处。

（4）4号电极 竖耳运动，顶冠间线后2mm与旁矢状线内不到1mm会合处。

（5）5号电极 竖尾运动，顶间前线前4～5mm与矢状线旁1～2mm会合处。

（6）无关电极的安放 在切迹连线前10～20mm处。

4. 刺激强度 规定刺激频率64Hz，波宽6ms的恒压矩形脉冲刺激，无全身电感应时为最佳，从阈下强度开始以0.5V/次梯度上升并记录最佳刺激强度。

5. 观察 按要求分别电刺激1、2、3、4、5号电极，观察动物的反应并记录结果。

【实验指导】

1. 预习要求

（1）复习锥体系和锥体外系的组成及其功能。

（2）复习大脑皮层对躯体运动调节的特点和原理。

2. 操作要点

（1）熟练掌握用普鲁卡因局部麻醉动物的方法，注意要麻醉好，否则手术时动物会挣扎。

（2）暴露颅骨时要尽量做到少出血，不要弄破颅骨，正确寻找矢状缝、人字缝和冠状缝。

（3）正确确定七条标志线，正确定位五个刺激电极位置。

3. 注意事项

（1）电刺激家兔大脑皮层各点时，动物不要固定于兔箱中，以便正确观察各项指标。

（2）刺激大脑皮层引起骨骼肌收缩的潜伏期较长，故每次刺激应持续5～10s才能确定有无反应。

4. 报告要点

（1）正确记录刺激每个电极时动物所产生的运动反应，并记录最佳刺激强度。

（2）根据实验现象，说明大脑皮层对躯体运动控制的特点，讨论锥体系及锥体外系的组成及功能。

5. 思考题

（1）兔大脑皮层表面是否也如人大脑皮层中央前回一样，存在着支配躯体运动的精细定位区，为什么？

（2）用什么方法可以确定体表某个部位的浅感觉在大脑皮层上的定位区？

（傅继华）

8 Somatic movements elicited by stimulation of rabbit cerebral cortex

PURPOSE

To locate the function of cerebral cortex by putting stimulus – electrode on the bone – mark of rabbit's cranium without open skull.

PRINCIPLE

Cerebral cortex motor area controls bodies movements. In human beings, precentralgyrus is the first motor area which can cause contraction of different body muscles with stimulating, as is followed：①Crossing character；one side cerebral cortex dominates the opposite side body muscles except for the bi – side controlling on head. ②Delicate function localization；the function localization appears an inverted image at the motor area. ③The side of function area is related to how the movement is complicated The more refine the movement is, the larger the function area is. ④No muscle nest cooperativity contraction. In addition, high – ranking animals have more delicate function area than low – ranking ones.

MATERIALS

1. Equipments Pins, steel rule, pencil, surgical scissors, tweezers, hemostat, scalpel, small hammer, 5ml syringe, needle, stimulator, cotton, glue.

2. Solutions 30% hydrogen peroxid solution, 1% procaine, normal saline solution.

3. Object Rabbit.

METHODS

1. Fix Fix the rabbit in the box and cut out the fur on its head roof, inject about 5ml of 1% procaine about 5ml by subcutaneous injection, and make a nicking about 4cm long. Isolate it with hemostat and destroy with hydrogen peroxide solution, until the exposure of skull, after that, wash it tissures with saline solution.

2. Stimulating sites Refer to the following illustration for location seven mark lines on skull.

3. Putting electrodes Strike pins into skull

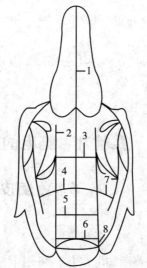

1. sagittal line
2. par a–sagittal line
3. interin cisure line
4. coronal line
5. interparietocor onal line
6. anter or interparietal line
7. coronal suture
8. lam bdoid suture

Fig. 2 – 10 Planform of the surface of rabbit's skull

vertically as electrodes. The depth is about 4~5mm, the right is symmetrical with the left.

(1) Electrode 1: The crossing of line 1 and line 3 as caput movement area.

(2) Electrode 2: The crossing of line 2 and line 4 as chewing movement area.

(3) Electrode 3: The crossing of line 1 and line 4 as forelimb movement area.

(4) Electrode 4: The crossing of line 2 and line 5 as uprighting ear movement area.

(5) Electrode 5: The crossing of line 1 and line 6 as uprighting tail movementarea.

4. Stimulating intensity   Require: stimulus – frequency is 64Hz, the wave width of rectangular constant pulse is 6ms, latent period < 10s, it's the best when without electric – induction on body, increasing the intensity from sub – threshold by interval of 0.5V and record the best stimulus – intensity.

5. Observation items   Stimulate electrode 1,2,3,4,5 each other according to request, observe the movement of rabbit and record.

GUIDANCE

1. Preview

(1) Review the composition of pyramidal system and extrapyramidal systems and their functions.

(2) Review the characteristic and principle of cerebral cortex controlling body movement.

2. Manipulation

(1) Master local anesthesia with Procaine.

(2) In operation, do your best for less bleeding and don't intact skull.

(3) Locate the seven lines and five position of stimulation accurately.

3. Notices

(1) When stimulating, Don't fix the rabbit in box for right observation.

(2) It should be lasting 5~10s to confirm response.

4. Reports

(1) Record the reaction and the best stimulus – intensity.

(2) According to the response, state the characteristic of cerebral cortex controlling body movement, discuss the composition of pyramidal and extrapyramidal systems and their functions.

5. Questions

(1) Dose the rabbit's cerebral cortex have the delicate localization which controls body movement? Why?

(2) How can we locate the cerebral area that deputes superficial sense of some part of body?

(Fu Jihua)

实验九　脑电的观察（示教）

A.　兔脑皮层电图

【目的要求】

大脑皮层存在持续不断的电变化，可用电极经多道生理记录仪引出的皮层电图来显示大脑电活动的情况。

【实验原理】

在人类和其他脊椎动物的皮层表面放两个电极，或将一个电极放在皮层表面，另一个无关电极放在远处，这时在两个电极之间可记录到连续的电位波动，称皮层电图。已知皮层电活动可分为 3 种，即单个神经细胞的电活动、自发性的脑电活动以及由特定刺激所引起的诱发电位。后两种电变化是大量神经细胞活动时的总和表现。而大脑皮层内神经细胞上发生的电现象不外 3 种，即神经冲动（发生在脑体或轴突上）、兴奋性突触后电位和抑制性突触后电位。现已证明两点：皮层电图主要反映的是皮层神经元的突触活动；自发脑电活动和皮层诱发电位主要与突触活动有关，而与神经冲动无关。因此在环境安静时，皮层电图记录的是大脑皮层自发脑电活动（由突触后电位变化形成，发生在胞体和树突上。当皮层的浅层结构出现兴奋性突触后电位或是皮层的深层结构出现抑制性突触后电位时，皮层表面都产生负的电位波动。反之，如果上述层次出现相反的突触活动，则产生正的电位波动。上述电活动与丘脑功能有关，并受网状结构功能的影响）；而动物受刺激时，则皮层某一局限区域也能记录到皮层诱发电位，它是感觉器官、感觉神经或感觉传导途径上任何一点受刺激时，在中枢神经系统所引出的电位变化，是在自发脑电波的背景上出现的。本实验所记录的皮层电图主要反映自发脑电活动。皮层电图的频率和波幅主要取决于动物种类、记录部位和觉醒的程度。

【实验材料】

1. 器材 BL-420F 生物信号采集与分析系统（或多道生理记录仪），引导电极，兔固定箱，手术刀，止血钳，中式剪，注射器（5ml、1ml），小镊子，纱布块，小锤。

2. 药品 1% 普鲁卡因，30% H_2O_2，磷酸锌粘固粉，牙托水，生理盐水，碘酒、酒精棉球。

3. 对象 兔。

【实验步骤】

1. 手术 取兔一只称重，固定于兔箱中。将头顶部毛剪去，用 1% 普鲁卡因 5ml 注入兔头顶部皮下组织内，进行局部麻醉，然后消毒头部皮肤，用手术刀在兔头顶部做一长约 3cm 的切口，用止血钳分离组织并用 30% H_2O_2 破坏周围组织，然后用生理盐水洗净以暴露颅骨。

2. 电极安放 将两个引导电极穿过颅骨分别放置在脑皮层的额叶与顶叶，再在其前方数厘米处的正中颅骨上放置一无关电极，然后将磷酸锌粘固粉与牙托水拌匀用以固定各电极。两个引导电极与无关电极输入到 BL-420F。

3. 记录 BL-420F 中，记录脑皮层电图的参数如下：采样周期 5~50ms，压缩比 1:1，增益 5000，滤波 0.1~0.01，时间常数 0.1~0.01s。记录时，调节记录纸的移动速度，以获得清晰的脑皮层电图记录。

【实验指导】

1. 预习要求 复习教材中自发脑电活动、脑皮层电图和皮层诱发电位等内容。

2. 操作要点 兔头顶部局部麻醉方法，引导电极的安放与固定。

3. 注意事项

（1）该实验最好在屏蔽室内进行或把动物用钢丝网屏蔽起来，以防止干扰。

（2）在更换引导部位时动作要轻，防止损伤皮层。

4. 报告要点　根据记录讨论兔清醒时的皮层电图，并说明其特点。

5. 思考题　皮层自发电位是如何产生的？

B. 人体脑电图

【目的要求】

观察正常人清醒时的脑电图，并初步分析其波形。

【实验原理】

把引导电极放在头皮上，通过与放大器相连的示波器（或脑电图仪），可以记录出大脑皮层的自发电活动，称为脑电图。引导的条件基本上与皮层电图相同。产生机制可参考皮层电图。由于其记录电极（引导电极）离开皮层较远、颅骨的电阻很大，所以与皮层电图相比，脑电图的振幅较小。此外，诱发电位的幅度一般较小，加之它是夹杂在自发性的脑电活动中，并要克服脑表面与电极间组织的电阻，故从脑电图上很难观察到诱发电位，这是脑电图与皮层电图的区别之一。脑电图的引导可以是双极的，即从两个放在颅顶上的电极之间引出；也可以是单极的，一个特异性电极放在头皮上，另一个无关电极放在远处（如耳垂）。脑电图波形按其频率和振幅的不同，可分为四类：α 波（8 ~ 13 次/秒，20 ~ 100μV），β 波（14 ~ 30 次/秒，5 ~ 20μV），θ 波（4 ~ 7 次/秒，100 ~ 150μV），δ 波（1 ~ 3.5 次/秒，20 ~ 200μV）。α 波是脑电图的基本节律，主要出现于大脑半球后半部，特别是枕叶部位，在安静闭目时即出现，持续 1 ~ 2 秒，而在睁眼、思考问题或突然听到声响时消失，此称"α 波阻断"。对脑电图的评定首先是注意它的频率、振幅、波形、分布和出现频率。

【实验材料】

1. 器材　BL – 420F 生物信号采集与分析系统（或前置放大器与示波器，或脑电图仪，或多道生理记录仪），脑电极，耳电极，导电胶，75% 酒精棉球。

2. 对象　人。

【实验步骤】

1. 安放电极　让受试者静坐椅上，姿势自如。用 75% 酒精棉球擦净耳垂及枕部皮肤各一小块，并分别将电极固定其上，再分别与脑电极导线、耳电极导线相连，各导线输入到 BL – 420F 或与脑电图机相连。电极与皮肤间涂有导电胶。

2. 仪器调试　打开 BL – 420F 脑电记录界面，设置相应参数。脑电图机接通电源前，控制面板上的各个旋钮放在应处的位置，然后通电，20 分钟后定标。

3. 记录

（1）定标后开动走纸记录一段脑电变化后，嘱受试者闭目，观察有无 α 波出现。

（2）受试者在闭目安静情况下，接受一声音刺激，观察 α 波是否减弱或消失。

（3）停止声音刺激，α 波重新呈现后，再嘱受试者睁眼 3 ~ 5 秒后闭目 10 ~ 15 秒，反复三次，观察有无"α 波阻断"现象出现。

【实验指导】

1. 预习要求　复习自发脑电活动和脑电图等内容，预习所使用生理仪器的操作方法。

2. 操作要点　引导电极的安置方法和脑电图机的使用方法。

3. 注意事项

（1）实验需在屏蔽室内进行，以防外界干扰。

（2）如有肌电干扰，嘱受试者均匀呼吸，放松肌肉，停止眨眼、咀嚼或吞咽等动作。

（3）更换导联时，应先将记录笔关闭，避免损坏记录笔。

（4）如用脑电图仪等，则可同时观察和记录大脑皮层多处的脑电活动。

4. 报告要点　根据实验记录讨论人清醒时的脑电图主要波形，并说明其特点。

5. 思考题

（1）试述脑电图产生的一般原理。

（2）如何识别 α 节律与 α 波阻断？

（郭青龙）

9　Observation on electroencephalogram （demonstration）

A. Electrocarticogram in rabbits

PURPOSE

Unceasing electrical activity is present in cerebral cortex, so electrocarticogram (ECOG) which was inducted by electrodes into a polygraph physiological recorder or BL – 420F can show the electrical activity in brain.

PRINCIPLE

ECOG is the continuous potential fluctuation between two electrodes that was put both on surface of cortex or one on surface of cortex and another indifferent electrode in distant place in human or other vertebrates. Potential activity in cortex can be divided into three kinds that are electrical activity of single nerve cell, spontaneous brain electrical activity and evoked potential (EP) induced by definite stimulation. The latter two activities are total electrical variation of a great quantity of nerve cells. Electric phenomenon of nerve cell in cerebral cortex has three types: nerve impulse (occurrence in cerebral body or axon), excitatory post – synaptic potential (EPSP) and inhibitory postsynaptic potential (IPSP). Two points have been certificated: (1) ECOG mainly reflects synaptic activity of nerve cell in cortex; (2) Spontaneous electric activity in brain and evoked cortex potential is related to synaptic activity but not to nerve impulse. So ECOG is the record of spontaneous electrical activity in cerebral cortex when animals are calm (occurred in cell body or dendrite and is induced by post – potential change. When EPSP was happened in superficial structure of cortex or IPSP was happened in deep structure of cortex, negative potential fluctuation was merged on surface of cortex. On the contrary, if adverse synaptic activity was happened in superficial lamella and deep structure, positive potential fluctuation was formed on surface of cortex. These electrical activities are related to function of thalamus and affected by function of reticular formation.); When animals were stimulated, EP on certain limited region ofcortex can be recorded and is potential variation in central nervous system based on spontaneous brain electric wave when sensory organs、sensory nerves or pathway of sensory conduction were stimulated. ECOG recorded in the experiment mainly reflex the spontaneous electrical activity in brain. Frequency and amplitude of waves in ECOG are dependent on animals' species、record site and the degree of awakening.

MATERIALS

1. Equipments   BL – 420F biological signal acquisition and analysis system, introductory electrode, fixing box for rabbit, scalpel, hemostat, scissors, syringe (5ml and 1ml), forceps, gauze, and little hammer.

2. Solutions   1% procaine, 30% H_2O_2, zinc phosphate cement, dental base acrylic resin liquid, 0.9% NaCl, iodine and 75% alcohol cotton balls.

3. Object   Rabbit.

METHODS

1. Anesthesia and operation   Weigh one rabbit, and fix it into the box. Shear hair of vertex. Inject 1% procaine 5ml into subcutaneous tissue of vertex in order to local anesthesia. Then sterilize skin of head with iodine and 75% alcohol. Cut an incision with a scalpel for 3cm at vertex of rabbit. After separating tissue with hemostat and destructing milieu – tissue with 30% H_2O_2, expose skull after washed clear with 0.9% NaCl.

2. Emplacement of electrodes   Put two introductory electrodes on the frontal lobe and parietal lobe of cortex in brain through cranium, respectively, several centimeters in front of which a reference electrode is put on the middle of cranium. Fix these electrodes with the mixture of zinc phosphate cement and dental base acrylic resin liquid. Connect two introductory electrodes and a reference electrode to BL – 420F.

3. Record   Parameters for recording ECOG in BL – 420F are sampling cycle 5 ~ 50ms, compression 1 : 1, gain 5000, filter 0.1 ~ 0.01, time constant 0.1 ~ 0.01s. When record was beginning, adjust properly the speed of recorder paper in order to trace the electrocarticogram clearly.

GUIDANCE

1. Preview   Review the theory about spontaneous brain electrical activity, electrocarticogram and cerebral cortex evoked potential.

2. Manipulation   Manipulative keys are the method of local anesthesia on the head of rabbit and the placement and fixation of introductory electrodes.

3. Notice

(1) It is recommended that the experiment be carried out in a shielded room, or that the animals be shielded with steel network to prevent the interference of the city electricity.

(2) Change gently the place of electrode to prevent injuring cerebral cortex.

4. Report   Discuss the electrocarticogram of conscious rabbit according to the record and write its character out.

5. Question　How does the spontaneous cerebral cortex potential produce?

B. Electroence pha logram of human

PURPOSE

To observe the electroence phalogram of normal conscious human and analyze its waveform initially.

PRINCIPLE

Electroencephalogram (EEG) is spontaneous electrical activity in brain that can be recorded by BL – 420F (or oscilloscope which was connected with amplifier) with introductory electrodes on scalp. The sites of two electrodes are the same as ECOG on the whole. The mechanism can reference ECOG. Amplitude of EEG's wave is small because recording electrode (introductory electrode) is far away from cortex and resistance of skull is big. In addition, the amplitude of evoked potential is small and it is mixed with spontaneous electrical activity in brain. Moreover, it should overcome resistance of tissue between cerebral surface and electrode. Therefore, it is difficult to observe EP in EEG that is different to ECOG. Introduction of EEG may be bipolar, which are from two electrodes on the parietal region, or monopolar, which a specific electrode set on scalp and another indifferent electrode in distant place (e. g. earlap). The waves of EEG can be divided into four kinds according to frequency and amplitude: a wave (8 ~ 13times/s, 20 ~ 100μV), β wave (14 ~ 30times/s, 5 ~ 20μV), θ wave (4 ~ 7times/s, 100 ~ 150μV), δ wave (1 ~ 3. 5times/s, 20 ~ 200μV)。 α wave is basic rhythm in EEG that is from post – section of cerebral hemisphere, especially from occipital lobe. It can be seen during calm and closed eyes and can last for 1 ~ 2 seconds. It disappears when opening eyes, thinking or hearing a sudden sound, which is called "α wave block". Evaluation of EEG is done according to frequency, amplitude, waveform, distribution and generant frequency.

MATERIALS

1. Equipments　BL – 420F biological signal acquisition and analysis system (or EEG, preamplification and oscilloscope, polygraph), cerebral electrode, ear electrode, conductive glue, 75% alcohol cotton ball

2. Object　Human.

METHODS

1. Emplacement of electrodes　Let quizzee sit on a chair silently and casually. Clean two parts of skin on an earlap and the occipital region with 75% alcohol cotton ball, on which two electrodes, connected with cerebral electrode and ear electrode, were fixed respectively. Every wire was linked to BL – 420F or EEG machine. There is conductive glue between electrodes and skin.

2. Adjustment of instrument　Open BL – 420F and select parameters. Every button in control panel should be set properly before the EEG machine is powered on. Calibration is done at 20 minutes after the power is on.

3. Record

(1) Record a period of electroencephalogram after calibration. Tell the quizzee to close his/her eyes and observe if a wave occurs.

（2）Observe if a wave goes weak or disappears when the eye – closed quiet quizzee is given a sound stimulation.

（3）a wave should occur again after the sound was stopped. Tell the quizzee to keep his eyes open for 3 ~ 5 seconds and then close for 10 ~ 15 seconds. Repeat for 3 times and observe if the phenomenon of "a wave block" occurs.

GUIDANCE

1. Preview   Review the associated contents with spontaneous brain – electric activity andelectrocorticogram. Preview the operation method of instruments.

2. Manipulation   Pay attention to the emplacement of introductory electrode and the usage of EEG machine.

3. Notices

（1）It is recommended that the experiment should be carried out in shielded room to prevent the interference.

（2）Tell the quizze to breathe steadily, relax muscles, stop nictitating, chew or swallow if interference of muscle electricity occurs.

（3）Recording pen should be closed at first when leads are changed lest the pen would be damaged.

（4）The electric activity in several places of brain can be observed and recorded with EEG machine in same time.

4. Report   Discusses the electrocorticography of conscious human according to the record result. Write its character out.

5. Questions

（1）Explain the general principle of EEG.

（2）How to recognize a rhythm and a wave block？

（Guo Qinglong）

扫码"学一学"

实验十　去大脑僵直

【目的要求】

观察去大脑僵直这一现象，以理解中枢对肌紧张的调节作用原理。

【实验原理】

正常机体即使在安静时，其骨骼肌也存在一定的肌紧张。肌紧张来源于脊髓的牵张反射，而脊髓的牵张反射受高位中枢控制（图 2 – 12）。高位中枢对于肌紧张的调节具有两重性，即有些部位对肌紧张起易化作用，使肌紧张加强，称为易化区，主要包括前庭核、小脑前叶两侧部和网状结构易化区；另一些部位则起抑制作用，使肌紧张减弱，称为抑制区，主要包括大脑皮层抑制区（4S 区等）、纹状体、小脑前叶蚓部和延髓网状结构抑制区。在正常情况下，抑制区与易化区的作用互相拮抗而取得相对平衡，使机体具有一定程度的肌紧张以维持姿势与平衡。如果在动物中枢的上、下丘之间横断脑干，则因抑制区被切掉较多，抑制区失去较高级中枢的兴奋作用，保留下来的抑制作用减弱，而易化作用相对增强，特别表现为伸肌紧张性亢进，此称去大脑僵直。实验可见动物四肢僵直，头向后仰，尾向上翘等现象。

【实验材料】

1. 器材　7 号注射针头，小锤，大头针，铅笔，直尺。

2. 对象　家兔。

【实验步骤】

1. 利用大脑皮层功能定位实验的兔，在颅骨的矢状缝与冠状缝交点至人字缝顶点，用笔划一直线（与矢状缝重合），将此线作三等分，前 2/3 与后 1/3 交点向左或向右旁开约 5mm 处为穿刺点。用大头针先在一侧穿刺点钻一小孔，将 7 号注射针头尖端自小孔垂直刺入至颅底，并向两侧作较大范围拨动，将脑干离断。取出针头，用胶泥封闭小孔止血即可进行观察。

2. 观察在上、下四叠体间离断脑干后，动物四肢肌、背部肌、颈肌紧张性有何变化。

【实验指导】

1. 预习要求　复习肌紧张调节机制。

2. 操作要点　掌握横切脑干的方法。

3. 注意事项

（1）切断脑干的部位不能偏低，以免伤及延髓呼吸中枢引起呼吸停止。

（2）如果切断部位偏高，则不出现去大脑僵直现象。此时可将针头稍向尾侧端倾斜再划几次。

（3）适度牵拉动物躯体和四肢，可加速出现或加强僵直现象。

（4）离断脑干过程中，动物强烈挣扎。应加以注意，以免损坏物品。

4. 报告要点　试述在上、下四叠体间离断脑干后，所观察到的现象的机制。

5. 思考题

（1）在中脑水平切断兔脑，其伸肌紧张性为何会发生变化？

（2）如在上述结果基础上分别切断延髓或切断脊髓背根，将对肌紧张产生什么影响？

（郭青龙）

10　Decerebrating rigidity

PURPOSE

To observe the phenomenon of decerebrating rigidity and understand how the nervous centrum modulates muscular tension.

PRINCIPLE

Skeletal muscles in normal bodies have muscular tension in some extent even ifbodies are calm. Muscular tension comes from stretch reflex of spinal cord, which is modulated by advanced centrum(Fig. 2 – 12). There are two parts in the modulation. One is the places called facilitative region which facilitate and strengthen muscular tension, including the vestibule nucleus, two sides of anterior lobe of cerebellum and reticular structure facilitative region; the other is called inhibitory region which inhibit and weaken muscular tension, including the inhibitory region of cerebral cortex (4S area etc.), striatum, vermis and reticular structure inhibitory region of medulla oblongata. Normally the inhibitory region and facilitative region are against each other and in relative balance, for which the body has muscular tension in some extent to maintain posture and balance. If the brain stem is transected between superior colliculus and inferior colliculus of the quadrigeminal body, the inhibitory region is cut a large part off and loses the excitation of high – level centrum. The inhibition becomes weak and the facilitation becomes relatively strong. It shows especially high tension of extensor and this phenomenon is called decerebrating rigidity. It can be seen in experiment that the limbs of animals is rigor, head raises backward and tail bends upward.

MATERIALS

1. Equipments   7# injection needle, little hammer, pin, pencil, ruler.

2. Object   Rabbit.

METHODS

1. From intersection between sagittal suture and coronal suture to top of lambdoid suture in rabbit skull (the rabbit has been used in function apposition of cerebral cortex), draw a straight line (overlapped with sagittal suture) with a pencil. The line was divided into three parts equally, and the puncture point is at 5mm from either side of the intersection of anterior 2/3 and posterior 1/3 of the line. Drill a pinhole with pin at the puncture point; penetrate vertically with 7# injection needle through the pinhole to base of skull. Turn the needle toward two sides to break brainstem. Pull out the needle and block pinhole with glue mud.

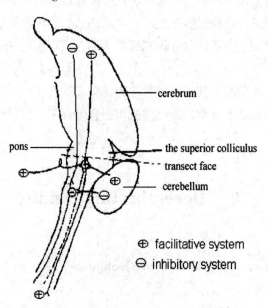

Fig. 2 – 12   The mechanism of decerebrate rigidity

2. Observe the tension changes of limbs muscles, back muscles and muscles of neck after the brain stem has been broken between the superior and the inferior colliculus of the quadrigeminal body.

GUIDANCE

1. Preview　Review the modulatory mechanism of muscle tension.

2. Manipulation　Pay attention to the method of intersection of a brain stem.

3. Notices

（1）Do not cut the brain stem too low in case of respiratory centrum injury in medulla oblongata which cause respiration.

（2）The decerebrating rigidity cannot be seen if the transect is too high. In this case, the needle should be inclined to the tail side and turn several times.

（3）Draging body and limbs of the rabbit properly can accelerate or strength rigor.

（4）Pay attention to avoiding damage of article because animal is struggling fiercely when its brain stem was break down.

4. Report　Explain mechanism of decerebrating rigidity induced by breaking brain stem between the superior and the inferior colliculus of the quadrigeminal body.

5. Questions

（1）Why did the extensor tension of rabbit change when rabbit's brain at midbrain was broken?

（2）If medulla oblongata or dorsal root of spinal cord is broken at the base of prior results, what will muscular tension happen?

（Guo Qinglong）

实验十一　豚鼠大脑皮层诱发电位

【实验目的】

了解大脑皮层感觉功能的定位及其电活动的表现形式，学习皮层诱发电位的记录方法。

【实验原理】

凡感觉器官、感觉神经或感觉传导途径上任何一点受刺激，在中枢神经系统引出的电位变化，称为诱发电位。如在皮层上某一局限区域引出的电位变化，称皮层诱发电位，这种方法可用于皮层感觉功能定位。本实验观察电刺激听神经或用声音刺激耳朵，在豚鼠颞叶皮层引出的诱发电位。

由于大脑皮层随时产生自发电活动，诱发电位经常是出现在自发脑电的背景上，前者振幅愈低，后者反应就愈清楚。因此实验时要用麻醉较深的动物，使自发脑电活动受到抑制，诱发电位才能清楚地显示出来。

【实验材料】

1. 器材　双线示波器，直流前置放大器，刺激器，耳机或喇叭，引导电极（可用不锈钢针或小号缝衣针），刺激电极（用直径小于0.3mm的不锈钢针，表面涂以绝缘物，尖端裸露），无关电极（用大头针等），10ml注射器，注射针头（6号），普通剪，止血钳，解剖刀，眼科镊子，玻璃分针，小三角尺，烧杯（500ml，400ml），滴管。

2. 药品　1%氯醛糖+10%氨基甲酸乙酯（即100ml生理盐水中加1%氯醛糖，10g氨基甲酸乙酯）混合麻醉剂或20%氨基甲酸乙酯，生理盐水，液状石蜡，棉球，纱布，30%过氧化氢溶液。

3. 对象　豚鼠。

【实验方法】

1. 仪器的连接和调试

（1）按图2-13所示连接仪器。

（2）仪器条件

①示波器：Y轴灵敏度，上线50mV/cm，下线与耳机正端相连，观察刺激波。扫描、外触发与刺激同步。X轴扫描速度10~50ms/cm。

②前置放大器：增益1000，高频滤波100Hz或1kHz，时间常数0.1s。

③刺激器：输出与耳机相连，波宽0.3~0.8ms，刺激频率1Hz，延迟适当，输出强度调至耳机中能发出最大响声为佳，触发输出连于示波器的外触发输入。

2. 麻醉　用已配好的混合麻醉剂（或氨基甲酸乙酯）以6ml/kg腹腔注射，待豚鼠被麻醉后将其放于实验桌上准备手术。

3. 手术　用手术剪剪去颅骨表面头顶部毛，在眼前缘水平，向后沿头顶正中切开皮肤3~4cm，分清颞区上1mm左右（矢状缝旁开约1cm，与冠状缝后约5mm会合处），将引导电极插入头骨，在其他任意区域也插入一引导电极，以备对照实验。吸干头骨表面的渗出液，滴上液状石蜡，并在引导电极和切开皮肤间垫一棉球，以防两者相碰而产生干扰。将接地电极与头皮切口相连，无关电极钉于颅骨正中冠状缝前1~2cm处。

4. 刺激形式　用电刺激器产生刺激脉冲使得耳机发声，声音刺激内耳产生耳蜗微音器电位（CM）和听神经动作电位，最终引起颞叶诱发电位。

5. 观察项目

（1）诱发电位的观察　调节好所有仪器，按刺激器"启动"钮，此时扬声器发出有节律的响声（或直接用电脉冲刺激听神经），在示波器上即可观察到刺激伪极后约8ms有一先正后负的诱发电位，但更多的情况只能出现正波，负波不明显。一般每三次声刺激或电刺激有一明确的诱发电位，则可认为插入部位正确。若诱发电位不明确，可改变引导电极位置，寻找较恒定的诱发电位部位。

（2）找到较恒定的诱发电位后，记录波形，并读出潜伏期与主反应正相的时程及幅值。

（3）停止刺激输出后观察有无电位变化。

（4）将引导线与另一对照电极相连，用同样方法记录该区电位变化。

【实验指导】

1. 预习要求

（1）复习自发脑电和诱发电位产生原理。

（2）复习听觉产生原理及听觉传导通路。

2. 操作要点

（1）熟练地调试仪器，注意必须将干扰信号清除掉。

（2）正确定位记录电极，寻找听神经管和分离听神经时要注意避免损伤听神经。

（3）本实验也可以连接计算机进行实验，连机方法同"神经干动作电位观察"实验，只是为了获得足够大的放大倍数，使生物电信号输出达到 A/D 卡的要求，可以将前置放大器 A、B 放大串联起来使用，这样最大放大倍数可达 10^6 倍。

3. 注意事项

（1）动物麻醉不宜过浅，否则由于自发脑电太大，影响诱发电位观察结果。

（2）消除干扰是本实验的关键，为了做到这一点，所有仪器必须接地良好，动物接地良好且屏蔽，扬声器也必须进行屏蔽并接地。

4. 报告要求

（1）记录刺激强度、波宽，并描绘诱发电位主反应图形，测量其潜伏期及正负波幅值。

（2）简述在颞区、枕区所记录到的电位为什么不同，以及本实验感觉传导途径。你是否认为在整个感觉传导途径上的电活动都一样？

（3）简述皮层自发电位和诱发电位的产生原理。

5. 思考题

（1）试分析诱发电位的潜伏期主要由哪几部分组成？

（2）试设计一个测定视觉诱发电位的实验方法。

（傅继华）

11　Evoked potentials of cerebral cortex

PURPOSE

To know the location of sensory function and electrical activity manifestation on the cerebrum cortex. Learn the recording method of evoked cortical potential.

PRINCIPLE

Evoked potential, is the electrical potential fluctuation recorded in the central nervous system as a response to the stimulation of receptors, peripheral nerves, sensory path, nuclei or other central structure. For example, peripheral stimulation can be recorded from the sensorimotor areas of the cortex, as is called primary evoked cortical potentials. Such potentials can be used to explore the location of sensory in the cortex. The test will prove that when stimulating acoustic nerves or stimulating ears by sounds electricity can bring out evoked potentials on the temporal lobe.

Since the cerebral cortex would give spontaneous electrical activity at any time, evoked potentials often stand out from the background of spontaneous activity, the lower amplitude of the spontaneous activity is, the higher the evoked potentials are. For this reason, we should choose deeper narcotic animals to depress the spontaneous electrical activity and to help the evoked potentials outstanding.

MATERIALS

1. Equipments   double – lines oscilloscope, pre – located direct current amplifier, inducing e-lectrode (stainless steal needles or mini – needles), stimuli electrode (d < 0. 3mm, cover with insu-lator, expose the tip), indifferent electrode (pin, andect.), injector (10ml), needle (6 size), scis-sors, tweezer, scalpel, triangle ruler, dropper, glass stick.

2. Solutions   1% Alphachloralose + 10% Ethyl carbamate (100ml normal saline with 1g al-phachloralose, 10g ethyl carbonate change into mixed anesthetic), normal saline, paraffin oil, cotton, gauzes, 30% hydrogen peroxide solution.

3. Object   cavy.

METHODS

1. Joint and Adjustment of the instruments

(1) connect the instrument as the Fig. 2 – 13.

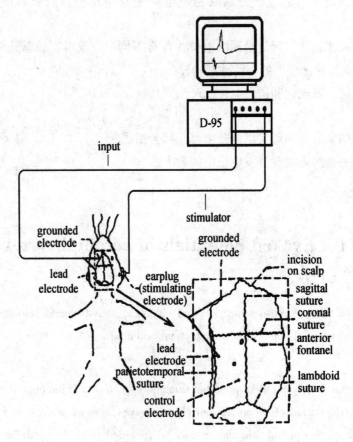

Fig. 2 – 13   Linking equipments

coordinates (– 10mm, – 5mm), take sagittal suture as Y axis, coronal suture as X axis, anterior fontanel as zero.

(2) Condition of the instruments

a. Oscilloscope: Y axis sensibility: up 50mV/cm, down connect with ear

        Electrode positive

        Observe stimulate wave

        Synchronize scan, speak, stimulation

        X axis scan rate 10 ~ 50ms/cm

88

b. Pre – located amplifier：enlargement 10000，high – frequency filter 100Hz or 1000Hz，Time constant 0. 1s.

c. Stimulation：connect ear – electrode with output wave width 0. 3 ~ 0. 8ms stimulate frequency 1Hz paper delay proper intensity.

2. Anesthesia　Intraperitoneal inject the narcotic 6ml/kg，make preparation for operation narcosis.

3. Operation　Clear the hair on the head，cut open the skin along the very middle at the level of the eyes. Locating temporal area 1mm or so，insert one induced – electrode into any place in order to check the result. Wipe off the water and give paraffin oil. In case of intervention caused by the touch of induced – electrode and skins，we should introduce cotton to separate them，connect the skins with the earth – electrode. Set the indifferent electrode in the front of the central coronal suture at 1 ~ 2cm.

4. Stimulation　Electrical stimulator gives impulses which make the ear – equipment give out sound. The sound influence on the inner ear and causes CM and acoustic action potential，finally evokes temporal potential.

5. Observation items

(1) Evoked potential　Adjust all the equipment，press START of the stimulator. The speaker give outrhythmic sound (or direct electrical impulse to the acoustic nerves). At the same time，the oscilloscope show evoked potential 8ms later. If improper evoked potential，you should change the place of induced electrode to another stable place.

(2) Record the wave shape after having had evoked placed well and write down the duration and intensity of the latent of major reaction positive.

(3) Observe the change of the electrical potential when you stop the output pf the stimulation.

(4) Connect the induced line with another reference electrode record the change of the electrical potential on the area.

GUIDANCE

1. Preview

(1) Review the spontaneous potential in the brain and mechanism of the evoked potential.

(2) Review the mechanism of sense of hearing occur and the path of the sense conduct.

2. Manipulation

(1) Adjust the equipment and clear interfering signal.

(2) Locate the record electrode accurately，be careful not to hurt the acoustic nerves when you search for nerve tube and separate the nerves.

(3) The test can be done by connecting to the computer directly. Turn pre – located amplifier A and B into series connection in order to fitting the A/D card.

3. Notices

(1) Keep the animals in the deep narcosis，otherwise，the huge brain electric activity will affect on the result of the evoked potential.

(2) Since the interference clearing is the key in the test，all the equipment must be earth and

the animals in well shield as well as the speaker.

4. Reports

（1）Write down stimulate intensity wave width, draw the evoked potential main action chart measure the latent duration and positive or negative wave strength.

（2）Tell the difference of the electrical potential recorded in temporal and occiput and the conduct path of the sense in the test. Do you think the electric activity is the same in the whole path?

（3）Tell the mechanism of the cortex spontaneous electrical potential and evoked potentials.

5. Questions

（1）Analyse the evoked electric potential latent duration's composition.

（2）Try to design a experiment to test visual evoked potential.

（Fu Jihua）

实验十二　小白鼠小脑损伤引起的共济失调

【实验目的】

本实验观察小白鼠一侧小脑损伤后出现的症状，以推断小脑与肌肉运动及肌紧张的关系。

【实验原理】

躯体的肌紧张与运动的协调受小脑控制，小脑损伤可引起共济失调。其表现为动物不能完成精巧动作，肌肉在完成动作时抖动而把握不住动作的方向，行走摇晃呈蹒跚状。

【实验材料】

1. 器材　蛙板，棉绳若干，小动物手术器械。

2. 对象　小白鼠。

【实验方法】

1. 取小白鼠一只腹位固定在蛙板上，将四肢用绳缚住（抓紧可先用镊子夹紧鼠尾，用手抓住耳朵与颈部皮肤，防止其咬人）。

2. 沿头部正中线剪开头皮，把附于枕骨上的肌肉往下剥离，即可经透明的颅骨看到小脑（图 2 - 14）。

3. 用探针插入（按图 2 - 14 上标志）伤其一侧小脑，注意切勿损伤中脑，然后将探针驱除，用棉球止血。

4. 放开缚绳，让小白鼠行走，观察其行为表现，有无旋转或翻滚动作。

【实验指导】

1. 预习要求

（1）复习小脑对运动调节的机制。

（2）复习锥体系调节肌肉运动的机制。

2. 操作要点 切开动物头皮后，可用左手食指和拇指将头顶部皮肤向两侧拉下，以便暴露颅顶，颅骨表面肌肉可用镊子刮离。

3. 注意事项

（1）抓握小鼠头部时要小心，防止被咬且抓握的力量要适度，以免动物窒息而死或将眼球挤出。分离肌肉也不能用力过大，以防过多的肌肉被损伤。

（2）损伤小脑时切勿损伤中脑，探针插入不宜过深，并正确损伤一侧小脑。

4. 报告要点 记述小脑损伤后的症状。

5. 思考题

（1）小脑分哪些区域，各有何功能？

（2）试述一侧小脑损伤后出现各种症状的机制。

（傅继华）

12　Ataxia induced by cerebellar injury in mouse

PURPOSE

The experiment focus on the symptom caused by one side of the cerebellar injury, in order to induce the relationship between the cerebellum and muscular tense.

PRINCIPLE

The cerebellum controls muscle tense and movement coordination. The cerebellum injury will lead to ataxia, as fail to achieve complex functions, lose the control of proper direction because of sick trembling muscles, walk staggeringly.

MATERIALS

1. Equipments Operating table, cotton thread (several), surgical equipments.

2. Object mouse.

METHODS

1. Fix the mouse on the operating table on abdomen, then binds the limbs with threads (We can to knead its tail as well as seize its ears and skins of the neck avoiding being bitten).

2. Cut open the skins of the head along the middle parts and clear the muscles attach to occipital at the same time. We can find the cerebellum through thetransparent cranial bone.

3. Stab in either side of the cerebellum and destroy it with probe, be careful not to do any harm to mesencephalon, then stop bleeding.

GUIDANCE

1. Preview

（1）The mechanism of morement regulation controlled by the cerebellum.

（2）The mechanism of muscular morement regulation controlled by pyramidal system.

2. Manipulation Pull the head skins down to both sides of the top with left thumb and index finger after cuts open the head skins in order to expose the cranial bones. Clear the muscles exist on the surface with tweezers.

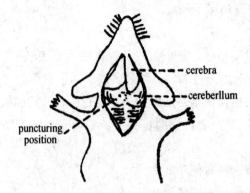

Fig. 2 – 14　Puncture to harm mouse's cerebellum

3. Notices

(1) Be careful of holding the head of the mouse and avoid bitten. Proper strength must be kept in mind for support normal breath and prevent from pressing the eyeball, and the same strength in separating the muscles for less injure.

(2) The probes should not stab extremely deep and only destroy one side of cerebellum, do not touch the mesencephalon.

4. Report　Write down the symptom after the cerebellum has been injured.

5. Questions

(1) How many area are there in the cerebellum, what are they and their functions?

(2) Please tell the mechanism of various symptoms brought by one side injured cerebellum.

(Fu Jihua)

第三章 血 液

Blood

实验十三 红细胞与白细胞计数

【实验目的】

用稀释法计数单位容积血液（立方毫米）内的红细胞数和白细胞数，学习红细胞和白细胞计数的方法和原理。

【实验原理】

由于血液中红细胞和白细胞数很多，无法直接计数，故需用适当溶液将血液稀释后，滴入血细胞计数板的计数室内，在显微镜下计数一定容积血液稀释液中的红细胞、白细胞个数，再将所得结果换算为 $1mm^3$ 血液中的红细胞、白细胞个数。

【实验材料】

1. 器材 血细胞计数板，显微镜，采血计，小试管，1ml 和 5ml 吸管，沙利吸血管，75% 酒精棉球。

2. 溶液 95% 酒精，乙醚，10% 氨水，蒸馏水，红细胞稀释液（NaCl 0.5g，Na_2SO_4 2.5g，$HgCl_2$ 0.25g 加蒸馏水至 100ml），白细胞稀释液（冰醋酸 1.5ml，10% 甲紫加蒸馏水至 100ml）。

3. 对象 人。

【实验方法】

1. 熟悉白细胞计数板结构 计数板（图 3-1）是由盖玻片和载物玻片构成。载物玻片中央有四条直槽，内侧两条直槽中间有一条横槽，把中间隔成两个长方形的平台，此平台与盖玻片之间的距离（即高度）为 0.1mm。在低倍镜下，平台中心部分各以 3mm 长、3mm 宽精确划分为 9 个大方格，称为计数室（图 3-2）。每个大方格长宽各 1mm，面积为 $1mm^2$，体积为 $0.1mm^3$。四角的大方格又分为 16 个中方格，适用于白细胞计数。计数白细胞时，数四角的 4 个大方格内白细胞数目，故被计数的稀释血液的容积为 $0.4mm^3$。中央的大方格则由双线划分为 25 个中方格，每个中方格面积为 $0.04mm^2$，体积为 $0.004mm^3$；每个中方格又各分成 16 个小方格，适用于红细胞计数。计数红细胞时，数中央大方格内四角及中央共 5 个中方格内红细胞数目，故被计数的稀释血液的容积为 $0.02mm^3$。

2. 稀释及采血

（1）稀释 用 1ml 吸管吸取 0.38ml 白细胞稀释液注入准备好的干燥小试管内备用，另

93

用 5ml 吸管吸取 3.98ml 红细胞稀释液注入准备好的干燥小试管内备用。

（2）采血 用 75% 酒精棉球消毒采血部位（耳垂或无名指指端）的皮肤，待酒精挥发后再采血。固定采血部位近侧，持已消毒采血针迅速刺入皮肤，深度为 2~3mm，见血液自动流出，擦去第一滴血，待流出第二滴血时，用沙利吸血管（图 3-3）吸血至刻度 20mm³ 处，将血液吹入盛有白细胞稀释液的试管内，吸上清液冲洗管壁上的残留血液。立即将吸管洗净，干燥备用。再用同样方法吸取血液至刻度 20mm³ 处，并将血液吹入盛有红细胞稀释液的试管内。轻轻摇动试管，混匀稀释血液。

3. 充液计数 将盖玻片平放在计数板上，用小吸管吸取摇匀的稀释血液，将一小滴滴在盖玻片边缘的载物玻片上，使稀释血液借毛细管现象而自动流入计数室内。如滴入过多，溢出并流入两侧深槽内，则使盖玻片浮起，体积改变，影响计数结果；如滴入过少，经多次充液易造成气泡。因此，滴入过多或过少，都必须洗净擦干，重新充液。红细胞和白细胞计数使用同一计数室，充液后，静置三分钟，在低倍镜下找到大方格，然后在高倍镜下（在低倍镜下计数亦可）计数。数白细胞时，数四角 4 个大方格的白细胞总数；计数红细胞时，数中央大方格的四角和中央共 5 个中方格的红细胞总数。计数时应循一定的路径，对横跨刻度上的白细胞依照"数上不数下，数左不数右"的原则进行计数（图 3-4）。计数白细胞时，如发现各大方格的白细胞数目相差 8 个以上；计数红细胞时，如各中方格的红细胞数目相差 20 个以上，表示血细胞分布不均匀，都必须把稀释液摇匀后，重新充液计数。

4. 计算

（1）白细胞数 将 4 个大方格内数的白细胞总数乘以 50，即得每 mm³ 血内的白细胞总数。因为：①稀释液 0.38ml 加入血 20mm³（1ml = 1cm³ = 1000mm³，故 20mm³ = 0.02ml），使血液稀释了 20 倍，换算成未稀释血液时应乘以 20；②计数四角上 4 个大方格内的白细胞总数，其容积为 0.4mm³，换算成每 mm³ 时应乘以 2.5。所以，把 4 个大方格内数得的白细胞总数乘以 50，即为每 mm³ 内的白细胞总数。

（2）红细胞数 将中央大方格中的 5 个中方格内数得的红细胞总数乘以 10000，即得每 mm³ 血内的红细胞总数。因为：①稀释液 3.98ml 加入血 20mm³（即 0.02ml），使血液稀释 200 倍，换算成未稀释血要乘以 200；②在计数室内只计数 0.02mm³（每个中方格容积为 0.004mm³），换算成每 mm³ 时应乘以 50，所以把 5 个中方格内数得的红细胞总数乘以 10000，即得每 mm³ 血液内的红细胞总数。

【实验指导】

1. 预习要求

（1）复习红细胞、白细胞正常值及生理功能。

（2）复习红细胞、白细胞的生成与破坏。

2. 操作要点

（1）准确吸取血液量 用中指和拇指捏住沙利氏吸管的橡皮囊，食指堵住囊上小孔，刻度朝向操作者，将吸血管倾斜，管口浸入血滴中，缓缓放松橡皮囊，将血吸到 20mm³ 处，然后先松食指，再松拇指和中指，这样血液就不会进入橡皮囊。用干棉球擦净管外的血液，如吸入血液超过刻度，可用左手指轻触管口数次，沾去多余的血液，动作要快，以防凝血。

（2）吸管洗涤法 弃去吸管内的血液稀释液，用蒸馏水洗三次，95% 酒精洗两次，以洗去管内水分，再用乙醚洗两次。如吸管内有血凝块，可置于 1% 氨水中浸泡，待血块溶解脱落后，再用流动水清洗，并按上述步骤清洗。

（3）计数板洗涤法　用自来水洗一次，蒸馏水洗两次，然后用擦镜纸擦干备用。不要用酒精、乙醚洗，以防损坏刻度。

3. 注意事项

（1）试管、沙利吸血管、计数板必须是干燥的，尤其在第二次使用前要洗净、干燥，否则影响结果的准确性。

（2）采血时不能刺得太浅，以能自然出血或轻轻挤压即可出血为度。若用力挤压，则会混有组织液或造成局部淤血而影响结果的准确性。

（3）注意中方格内红细胞的分布是否均匀，如差别过大，应重新充液后再计数。

4. 报告要点　写出每立方毫米血液中红细胞和白细胞数目，结合理论，讨论红细胞、白细胞的正常值及生理功能。

5. 思考题

（1）在红细胞、白细胞计数操作过程中，哪些因素可能会影响计数的准确性？怎样防止？

（2）计数时为什么要按一定顺序？为什么要"数上不数下，数左不数右"？

（3）红细胞和白细胞稀释液内各种成分的作用如何？

（吴玉林）

13　Counting of erythrocytes and leucocytes

PURPOSE

To study the methods and principles of erythrocytes and leucocytes counting, the dilution method is applied to counting the erythrocytes and leucocytes in a unit volume (cube millimeter) of blood in this experiment.

PRINCIPLE

There is no way to count the erythrocytes and leucocytes directly because there are so many erythrocytes and leucocytes in the blood. For this reason, the blood should be diluted by adequate liquid and dropped into the numerical chamber of Haemacytometer. The erythrocytes and leucocytes in the blood dilution of definite volume can be counted through a microscope. Then the results can be converted to the number of erythrocytes and leucocytes in the $1mm^3$ blood.

MATERIALS

1. Equipments　Haemacytometer, Microscope, Test Tube, Blood Taking Needle, Straws (1ml and 5ml), Sahli's Pipette

2. Solutions　75% Alcohol, 95% Alcohol, 10% Ammonia Water, Distilled Water, Erythrocyte Diluent (NaCl 0.5g, Na_2SO_4 2.5g, $HgCl_2$ 0.25g diluted by distilled water to 100ml), Leucocyte Diluent (acetic acid 1.5ml, 10% methylrosaniline chloride diluted by distilled water to 100ml).

3. Object　Human.

METHODS

1. Being familiar with the structure of haemacytometer　Haemacytometer is made up of cover glass and slide. There are four straight grooves in the center of the slide. There is a horizontal groove between the two medial grooves, which separates the center into two vectangular platforms and the distance between the platforms and the cover glass is 0.1mm high. The center of each platform is divided into 9 large checks, which are 3mm long and 3mm wide and are called the numerical chamber. Each large check is 1mm wide and long, of which the area is $1mm^2$ and the volume is $0.1mm^3$. Each large check on the quadrangular parts is divided into 16 middle checks, which can be used for leucocyte counting. When counting the leucocytes, the number of the leucocytes on the 4 quadrangular large checks is counted, so the calculated volume of the blood dilution is $0.4mm^3$. The central large check is divided into 25 middle checks by double lines. The area of each middle check is $0.04mm^2$ and its volume is $0.004mm^3$. Each middle check is divided into 16 little checks, which can be used for erythrocyte counting. When counting the erythrocytes, the number of the erythrocytes on the 5 quadrangular and central middle checks of the central large check is counted, so the calculated volume of the blood dilution is $0.02mm^3$.

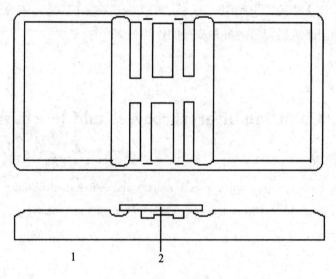

Fig. 3 – 1   Haemacytometer

1. slide   2. cover glass

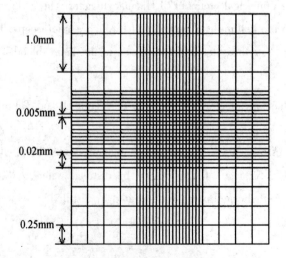

Fig. 3 – 2   Numerical chamber

2. Diluting and blood taking

（1）Diluting   For future use，0.38ml leucocyte diluent is sucked into a dry test tube by 1ml straw，and 3.98ml erythrocyte diluent is sucked into a dry test tube by 5ml straw.

（2）Blood taking   Disinfect the ear lobe or top of the forth finger with medical cotton and take blood after alcohol volatilizing. Sting a disinfected blood – taking needle into the skin quickly for a-bout 2 ~ 3mm deep. Wipe off the first drop of blood when it bleed out automatically. Use a Sahli's pi-pette to suck the second drop of blood to 20 mm^3. Blow the blood into the test tube with leucocyte diluent. Wash and dry the pipette immediately. Add 20 mm^3 blood into the test tube with erythrocyte diluent in the same way. Shake the tubes gently to mix up the blood diluent.

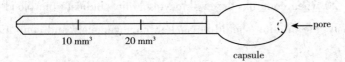

Fig. 3 – 3   Sahli's pipette

3. Filling up the dilution and counting   The cover glass is laid on the haemacytometer flat-ly. The blood dilution is shaken homogenously and is sucked by little straws. A drop is dribbled on the edge of between the slide and the cover glass，so the blood dilution can flow into the numerical chambers automatically relying on capillary phenomenon；if dribbling too much，the dilution flows outward and flows into the two – side deep grooves. The cover glass is floated，and the volume is changed. That will influence the counting results. If dribbling too less，air bubbles are ready to be produced because the dilution is filled up many times. Under both of the two circumstances，the haemacytometer have to be cleaned and dried and the dilution be re – filled up. A numerical cham-ber can be used respectively when counting the erythrocytes and leucocytes. After filling up the dilu-

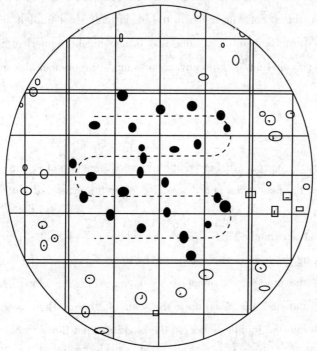

Fig. 3 – 4   Path of cells counting

tion, the haemacytometer is placed static for 3 minutes. The large checks are found through low power objective, and then the counting is done through high power objective (through low power objective as well). When counting the leucocytes, the total number of leucocytes on the four large checks of quadrangular parts should be counted; when counting the erythrocytes, the total numbers of erythrocytes on the quadrangular parts and the center of the central large check and on the five central middle checks should be counted. Counting should be done following some path. For instance, the blood cells across the scale are counted according to the principle that "counting the upward and left cells but not the downward and right ones". If the number of leucocytes in the largecheck differs by over 8 when counting the leucocytes; if the number of erythrocytes in the middle check differs from each other by over 20 when counting the erythrocytes, which indicate the blood cells are not dispersed homogenously, the dilution should be shaken homogenously and counting should be done again.

4. Calculating

(1) The number of leucocytes The total number of leucocytes on the four large checks of quadrangular parts is multiplied by 50 and the result is the total number of leucocytes per mm^3. The reasons are as follows: ①The 0.38ml dilution is added to $20mm^3$ blood ($20mm^3 = 0.02ml$), so the blood is diluted to 20 times. For conversion to the blood that is not diluted, the number should be multiplied by 20; ②When counting the total number of leucocytes on the four large checks of quadrangular parts, the volume is $0.4mm^3$. For conversion to mm^3, the number should be multiplied by 2.5 times.

(2) The number of erythrocytes The total number of erythrocytes on the five central middle checks is multiplied by 10,000 and the result is the total number of erythrocytes per mm^3. The reasons are as follows: ①The 3.98ml dilution is added to $20mm^3$ blood ($20mm^3 = 0.02ml$), so the blood is diluted to 200 times. For conversion to the blood that is not diluted, the number should be multiplied by 200; ②The total counting volume is $0.02mm^3$ in the numerical chamber (the volume of each middle check is $0.004mm^3$). For conversion to mm^3, the number should be multiplied by 50 times.

GUIDANCE

1. Preview

(1) Please review the normal number and physiological function of erythrocytes and leucocytes.

(2) Please review the generation and destruction of erythrocytes and leucocytes.

2. Manipulation

(1) Sucking blood accurately Firstly, pinch the rubber sac of Sahli's pipette by middle finger and thumb, and block up the pore in the rubber sac by index finger with the scales facing toward the operator. Secondly, tilt the pipette, and immerse its opening into the blood. Thirdly, please release the rubber sac slowly, and suck the blood up to the scale of $20mm^3$. Then loose the index finger before loosing the thumb and the middle finger, so the blood can not flow into the rubber sac. Finally, clean the remaining blood on the external surface of the pipette. If the blood volume sucked exceeds the scale of $20mm^3$, please touch the opening of the pipette lightly several times by fingers of left

hand in order to wipe out the superfluous blood. Perform quickly to prevent clotting.

（2）Washing the straw Please depose of the blood dilution in the straw, wash the straw with distilled water for 3 times and then with 95% alcohol for 2 times in order to wash out the water in the straw. At last, wash the straw with ethyl ether for 2 times. If there is blood clot in the straw, the straw should be soaked in the 1% ammonia water until the blood clotting is dissolved. Then it can be washed with current water and be washed according to the above steps.

（3）Washing the haemacytometer Please wash the haemacytometer with tap water for once and then with distilled water for twice before wiping dry with lens paper for future use. Do not wash with alcohol and ethyl ether in order to prevent from damaging the scales.

3. Notices

（1）Haemacytometers, test tubes and Sahli's pipettes should be kept dry, especially be washed and dried before second use, or the accuracy of the results would be affected.

（2）When taking the blood the needle should be sting deep enough for bleeding automatically or bleeding by gentle extrusion. The wound cannot be extruded roughly or it would result in local congestion or tissue fluid mixture. Thus the experimental results would not be accurate.

（3）Erythrocytes should be well – distributed in the chamber or the diluent should be filled and counted again.

4. Report Please give out the numbers of erythrocytes and leucocytes in the $1mm^3$ blood, and discuss the physiological functions of erythrocytes and leucocytes according to the curriculum.

5. Questions

（1）Which factors will affect the accuracy duying counting the erythrocytes and leucocytes? How to avoid them?

（2）Why should certain sequences be followed duying counting the erythrocytes and leucocytes? Why the cells should be "counted upward and left but not downward and right"?

（3）What is the function of every component in the cell diluents?

（WuYulin）

实验十四　血液涂片和染色

【实验目的】

熟悉血液涂片的制作和染色技术，并了解红细胞和白细胞的形态结构。

【实验原理】

红细胞内有血红蛋白，为有色无核的血细胞，而白细胞为无色有核的血细胞。因此，要观察血细胞的形态和结构，需用涂片复合染色的方法，并根据细胞的染色特征、有无颗粒、胞核形态及胞浆多少等特点，观察血细胞的形态和结构。血片复合染色剂由罗曼诺夫斯基（Romanovsky）创制，运用伊红和亚甲蓝两种溶液混合而成。现用的瑞（Wright）氏、姬姆萨（Giemas）等染色剂均由罗氏染色剂改良而成。瑞氏、姬姆萨染色剂基本染料是伊红和亚甲蓝，为了增强其水溶性，所用者为其中性盐。其染色原理如下：复合染料是由碱性亚甲蓝与酸性伊红钠盐混合而成的染色粉，当溶于甲醇后即发生解离，分成酸性染料和碱性染料两种。染色时，红细胞被染成粉红色或橙红色，粒细胞中的嗜酸物质即与酸性染料伊红结合而染成红色（嗜酸颗粒）；粒细胞中的嗜碱物质即与碱性染料美蓝结合而染成蓝色（嗜碱颗粒）；而粒细胞中嗜中性物质则同时结合酸、碱两种染料，染成红蓝混合的紫红色（嗜中性颗粒）。

【实验材料】

1. **器材** 消毒针，载玻片，酒精棉球，棉球。
2. **溶液** 75%酒精，甲醇，瑞氏染液，姬姆萨染液，蒸馏水。
3. **对象** 人或小鼠。

【实验方法】

1. 血液涂片

（1）主试者用手指按摩被试者的耳垂或无名指指尖，以加速局部血流，用75%酒精棉球消毒该处，待酒精挥发后用消毒针刺破皮肤，深约3mm。血液自动流出后，用消毒干棉球抹去第一滴血，然后用光洁玻片的一端，在穿刺处接触米粒样大小血液一滴（勿触及皮肤）。用小鼠实验时，剪去尾尖，待血液自动流出，取血液一小滴。

（2）另取边缘光滑平整之玻片为推片（最好磨去两角）放在血滴前方，然后稍向后拉，并向左右移动，使血滴由于推片移动作用形成一线，粘着推片边缘，再以20°～45°角度，由一端向另一端平稳地向前推动，直至血液推尽为止。角度大小可以控制血片之厚薄，推动时用力要均匀（图3-5）。血液涂片制成后，立即在空气中挥动，使之迅速干燥。

2. 血片染色法

（1）瑞氏染色法

①先将血片厚端用铅笔编号，并将血片置于染色架上。

②滴加瑞氏染液3～5滴盖满整张血膜。

③约1分钟（勿待甲醇成分完全蒸发）。另加2～3倍新鲜蒸馏水，小心摆动玻片，使染料充分混合。

④待2～5分钟后用水冲洗。

⑤将血片直立空气中干燥，或用吸水纸小心吸干。

（2）姬姆萨染色

①先将血片厚端用铅笔注明编号。

②用甲醇固定2分钟。

③将血片移置于染色架上，用新鲜配制的染色液盖满整张血膜，染色15～30分钟。

④用水冲洗，待干燥后镜检。

3. 血片镜检 先用显微镜的低倍镜观察血片，然后用油镜按一定的顺序观察红细胞、白细胞（中性粒细胞、嗜碱性粒细胞、淋巴细胞、嗜酸性粒细胞）的形态结构。

【实验指导】

1. 预习要求

（1）复习红细胞的形态结构。

（2）复习各类白细胞的形态结构。

2. 操作要点

（1）推血片要用力均匀、平稳，血滴不要太大，以免血涂片太厚。

（2）染色时间要准确控制，水冲洗时，应冲血膜玻片的背面，以免水的冲击破坏血膜。

（3）染液的配制

①瑞氏染液的配制

瑞氏染粉　　　　　　0.1g

甲醇（一级试剂 AR）　60ml

配制时，准确称取瑞氏染粉0.1g，放入清洁的研钵中研成细粉状，加少量甲醇继续研磨，使之充分溶解，然后倾注入有塞的棕色玻璃瓶中，再用其余甲醇把研钵中染料洗干净，一并贮入瓶内。

②姬姆萨染液的配制

姬姆萨染粉　　　　　0.5g

中性甘油（CP）　　　33ml

甲醇（AR）　　　　　33ml

配制时，先将姬姆萨染粉放入清洁研钵中，加甘油后研磨片刻，移置于 55～60℃ 水浴箱内 2 小时，经常用玻璃棒搅拌，使染粉溶解，再加入甲醇混合即为贮备液，临用时以 pH 6.8 的缓冲液或新鲜蒸馏水 10 份加贮备液 1 份配制即成。

③缓冲液的配制 1% KH_2PO_4、1% Na_2HPO_4 各30ml 加水至 1000ml。

3. 注意事项　先用低倍镜观察血片，然后用油镜观察。用油镜观察时，不用显微镜粗调调节焦距，而应该用微调调至细胞形态结构清晰为止，以避免损坏镜头。

4. 报告要点　画出红细胞、白细胞的图形，并说明它们在结构上的差异。

5. 思考题　用75%酒精消毒皮肤后，为什么要等酒精挥发后再用消毒针刺破皮肤取血？

（吴玉林）

14　Blood smearing and staining

PURPOSE

The purpose of this experiment is not only to be familiar with the manufacture process of blood smearing and the technology of staining, but also to understand the shapes and structures of erythrocytes and leucocytes.

PRINCIPLE

Erythrocytes are colored anuclear hemocytes in which there is haemoglobin, but leucocytes are achromic nuclear hemocytes. In order to observe the shapes and structures of hemocytes, the method of blood smearing plus staining should be adopted according to their staining specificities, and their characteristics of granules, nuclear shapes, and cytoplasm, etc. The compound stain for smearing is made by Mr. Romanovsky with mingling eosin and methylene blue together. Available stains at present are the Wright's stain and Giemsa stain, which both are the improved ones from Romanovsky's stain. The basic dyes of the Wright's stain and Giemsa stain are eosin and methylene blue, which neutral salts are used for increasing their characteristics of water solubility. The staining principle is as follows: the compound stain is dye powder by mixing acid eosin and basic methylene blue together. Once dissolved in the methanol, the stain is decomposed into two dyes, the acid one and the basic one. The erythrocytes are stained into red or orange. The acidophilic substances in the granulocytes conjugate with acid eosin, and then are stained into red (acidophilic granules); the basophilic substances in the granulocytes conjugate with basic methylene blue, and then are stained into blue (basophilic granules); but the neutral substances in the granulocytes conjugate both the acid and the basic dye, and are stained into purplish red (neutral granules).

MATERIALS

1. Equipments   Sterile Needle, Slide, Medical Cotton ball.

2. Solutions   75% Alcohol, Methanol, Wright's Stain, Giemsa Stain, Distilled Water.

3. Objects   Mice or human.

METHODS

1. Blood smearing

(1) The ear lobe or the fingertip of the volunteer is massaged by the trial person in order to speed up the local blood flow. These sites are disinfected with medical cotton dipped in 75% Alcohol, and the skin is not punctured about 3mm deep with sterile needle until the alcohol is volatilized. After the blood flows out automatically, the first drop of blood is wiped off with medical cotton. A ricey drop of blood is got with the end of a clean and dry slide at the puncture site, but the skin should not be touched. If a mouse is used as the experimental object, its tail tip is cut. Until the blood flows out automatically, a drop of blood is not taken.

(2) Another smooth and flat slide, the so-called push slide is placed in front of the blood drop, which two angles are better to be removed by grinding. It is drawn backward slightly, and is pushed forward left and right. Because of the movement of pushing slide, the blood drop is formed into a line. The smears are pushed ahead from one end to another end until the blood runs dry.

2. Smears staining

(1) Wright's Staining

① Number the smears with a pencil at their thick end and then put them on the staining bracket.

② Take 3 ~ 5 drops of Wright's Stain to cover the whole blood membrane.

③ After about 1 minute when methanol hasn't volatilized completely, add twice or three times of distilled water onto it, and then

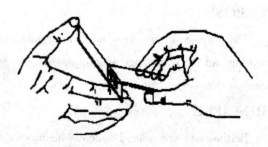

Fig. 3 – 5   Posture of pushing a smear

shake the smear gently to mix up the stain adequatly.

④Wash it with water after 2 ~ 5 minutes.

⑤Dry the smears by erecting them in the air or with a piece of filter paper.

（2）Giemsa Staining

①Number the smears with a pencil at their thick ends.

②Fix them with methanol.

③Put the smears on the staining bracket and cover the whole blood membrane with newly prepared stain for 15 ~ 30 minutes.

④Wash the smears with water and examine them by microscope after they are dry.

3. Microscopic examination for smears　First observe the smears under low power objective, and then observe the shapes and structures of erythrocytes and leukocytes (acidophilic granulocytes, basophilic granulocytes, neutral granulocytes, lymphocytes) under oil lens.

GUIDANCE

1. Preview

（1）Please review the knowledge on the shape and structure of erythrocyte.

（2）Please review the knowledge on the shape and structure of all kinds of leukocytes.

2. Manipulation

（1）Push the smears evenly and smoothly. Avoid a too big blood drop, or the smears might be too thick.

（2）Control the staining time accurately. When washing the smears, let the water falls onto back of the slides, or the blood membrane might be destroyed.

（3）Compound of the stains

a）Wright's Stain

Wright's stain powder　　　0. 1g

Methanol（A. R）　　　　60ml

Take Wright's stain powder 0. 1g and grind it into tiny powder. Add a little methanol in it and grind it to solve completely. Then put the solution into a capped brown glass bottle. Wash the grind instruments with the rest methanol and add it into the bottle.

b）Giemsa Stain

Giemsa stain powder　　　0. 5g

Neutral glycerine（C. P）　33ml

Methanol（A. R）　　　　33ml

Grind the Giemsa stain powder with glycerine for a while and then warm it up to 55 ~ 60℃ for 2 hours. Stir it often until it is solved. Finally add methanol into prepare the store solution. Mix 1 time of store solution with 10 times of buffer（pH6. 8）or distilled water for use.

c）Preparation of buffer

Dilute 1% KH_2PO_4 and 1 % Na_2HPO_4 of 30ml respectively to 1000ml with water.

3. Notice　First observe the smears with low power objective and then change to oil lens. Do not use the rough regulate switch when observing under oil lens. Do use the accurate regulate switch to focus until the cellular shape and structure are clear, or the lens might be destroyed.

4. Report Draw the figures of erythrocyte and leukocyte and explain their differences in structure.

5. Questions Why can the skin be sting to take blood only after alcohol volatilization when disinfected with alcohol?

(Wu Yulin)

实验十五 血红蛋白含量的测定

【实验目的】

用目前临床上常用的目视比色法，测定单位容积血液内血红蛋白的含量，了解用比色法测定的原理，并初步掌握操作技术。

【实验原理】

测定血红蛋白含量的方法很多，实验室常用比色法。其原理是在一定量的血液中，红细胞遇盐酸溶解释放出血红蛋白，血红蛋白经盐酸的作用，其中的亚铁血红素变成高铁血红素，呈现较稳定的棕黄色。其颜色深度与血红蛋白含量成正比。用水稀释后与标准色板进行比较，即可得出每 100ml 血液中血红蛋白的含量。

【实验材料】

1. 器材 沙利氏血红蛋白计，采血针，玻璃棒，滴管，滤纸片，酒精棉球。

2. 溶液 75% 酒精，95% 酒精，乙醚，0.1M 盐酸，蒸馏水。

3. 对象 人。

【实验方法】

1. 熟悉血红蛋白计 血红蛋白计主要有 $20mm^3$ 吸血管、比色计、比色管等部件（图 3–6）。比色计的左侧是标准玻璃片，右侧供插比色管用。比色管两侧有刻度，一行是血红蛋白的绝对值，以 g% 表示（即每 100ml 血液中含有血红蛋白克数），从 2 至 22 止。另一行是血红蛋白的相对值，以百分比表示（即相当于正常人血红蛋白平均值的百分数），从 10 至 150 止。临床常用血红蛋白的绝对值。

2. 采血及比色

（1）用滴管加 0.1mol/L HCl 到比色管刻度 2 处。

（2）采血 用前一实验同样方法采取耳垂或无名指指尖的血液，用血红蛋白吸血管吸血至刻度 $20mm^3$ 处（0.02ml）。

（3）制备比色液 用滤纸片拭净吸管外面的血液，将吸管很快插入血红蛋白比色管的盐酸内，将血液轻轻注入比色管中盐酸的底部，用上清液反复吸入、挤出，以洗净吸血管中的血液。摇匀或用小玻璃棒混合均匀后，放置 10 分钟，使盐酸与血红蛋白充分作用。

（4）比色读数 把比色管放入比色计座中，用滴管向比色管内边搅边加蒸馏水，对着光线比色，直到比色管内液体颜色与标准色板相同为止。读取比色管内液体凹面最低处所示的克数，即是 100ml 血液中血红蛋白的克数。

【实验指导】

1. 预习要求

（1）复习血红蛋白的基本组成及生理功能。

（2）复习正常人血红蛋白的正常值。

2. 操作要点

（1）准确吸取血液量。

（2）在加入蒸馏水稀释时，应逐滴加入，多做几次比色，以免稀释过量。每次比色时，应将搅拌用的玻璃棒取出，以免影响比色。

3. 注意事项

（1）注入血液至比色管及洗净吸管时，不宜用力过猛。

（2）由于操作过程过长而造成吸管内血液凝固、堵塞管孔时，则要按下列顺序冲洗吸管，即用蒸馏水→95%酒精→乙醚洗净吸管，干燥后备用。

（3）酸化时间 5~10 分钟。

（4）比色应在自然光下进行。

4. 报告要点

写出实验得出的血红蛋白值，讨论血红蛋白的生理功能及测定血红蛋白的实际意义。

5. 思考题

（1）血液中血红蛋白含量多少是否能反映机体的健康状况？为什么？

（2）哪些操作因素会影响血红蛋白的测定？怎样防止？

（吴玉林）

15　Assay of the hemoglobin content

PURPOSE

In order to determine the content of hemoglobin in the blood of unit volume, understand the principle of color contrast, and grasp the operating techniques initially, the method of color contrast by eyes is applied in this experiment, which is popular in clinical practice at present.

PRINCIPLE

There are many methods in assaying the hemoglobin content and the method of color contrast is usually applied in experiments. In certain volume of blood, erythrocytes are dissolved by hydrochloric acid to release hemoglobin. And then the hemoglobin will appears brown statically when its ferrous protoheme turns into ferric protoporphyrin after acted by hydrochloric acid. The color depth is relative to the hemoglobin content. The value of hemoglobin content in per 100ml blood can be achieved after diluting the colored hemoglobin solution and comparing it with the standard color contrasting plate.

MATERIALS

1. Equipments Sahli's Hemometer, Blood Taking Needle, Glass Stick, Dropper, Filter Paper Medical Cotton.

2. Solution 75% Alcohol, 95% Alcohol, Ethyl Ether, 0.1M Hydrochloric Acid, Distilled Water.

3. Objects Human.

METHODS

1. Familiar with the hemometer The hemometer is mainly composed of a $20mm^3$ straw, a color contrast meter and a color contrast tube, etc. In the left side of the color contrast meter there is a standard slide while in the right side of it the color contrast tube is inserted. There are scales along both sides of the color contrast tube. One is the absolute value of hemoglobin from 2 to 22 expressed as g% (namely the grams of hemoglobin in 100ml blood). The other is the relative value of hemoglobin from 10 to 150 expressed as percentage (namely the ratio in proportion to the average value of healthy people). The absolute value is generally applied in clinic.

2. Blood taking and color contrasting

(1) Add hydrochloric acid (0.1 mol/L) to scale 2 in the color contrast tube with a dropper.

(2) Blood taking: Take blood from ear lobe or fingertip with the same method in the last experiment, and then suck the blood to scale $20mm^3$ (0.02ml) in the hemoglobin straw.

(3) Preparing the color contrast solution: Clean the outer side with a piece of filter paper and quickly insert the straw into the hydrochloric acid in color contrast tube. Drop the blood in the bottom of the hydrochloric acid gently and then suck in and squeeze out the hydrochloric acid repeatedly to wash all the blood in the straw into the tube. Mix it up and set it static for 10 minutes until the blood has reacted sufficiently with the hydrochloric acid.

(4) Reading number of the color contrast: Insert the color contrast tube into the meter, and then stir it and add distilled water into it with a dropper. Contrast the color against the light until the color in tube becomes the same with that of standard color plate. Read the value instructing to the lowest point of solution surface in the color contrast tube and that is the grams of hemoglobin in 100 ml blood.

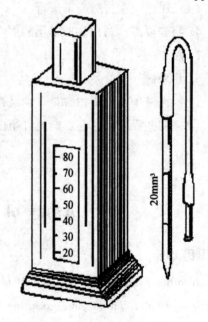

Fig. 3 – 6   **The hemometer**

GUIDANCE

1. Preview

(1) Review the knowledge on the standard components and physiological functions of hemoglobin.

（2）Learn the normal value of hemoglobin in healthy volunteers.

2. Manipulation

（1）Take the blood accurately.

（2）Add the distilled water drop by drop and contrast the colors for several times when diluting to avoid excessive water. Take out the stirring glass stick to avoid affecting the results when contrasting colors.

3. Notices

（1）Do not operate roughly when dropping blood into contrast tube or when washing the straws.

（2）When there is blood coagulation in the straws, they should be irrigated as the following order: distilled water→95% alcohol→diethyl ether. Dry the straws for use after cleaning them.

（3）Acidifying time is 5 ~ 10 minutes.

（4）Color contrast should be carried out under natural light.

4. Report Record the hemoglobin value in experiments and discuss the physiological functions of hemoglobin and the significant of assaying it.

5. Questions

（1）Can the hemoglobin content in blood affect the body conditions? Why?

（2）Which factors can affect the assay of hemoglobin content? How to avoid them?

（Wu Yulin）

实验十六　红细胞渗透脆性

扫码"学一学"

【实验目的】

通过红细胞渗透脆性实验，观察红细胞在不同渗透压的盐水中发生的变化，进而了解细胞外液渗透压的相对恒定对维持细胞正常形态与生理功能的重要性。

【实验原理】

生理状况下，哺乳类动物红细胞的渗透压与血浆的渗透压相等，约相当于 0.9% NaCl 溶液的渗透压。因此，将红细胞悬浮于等渗的 NaCl 溶液中，其形态和体积可保持不变。若将红细胞悬浮于低渗的 NaCl 溶液中，则水分过多进入红细胞，使之膨胀甚至破裂，血红蛋白释出，称为红细胞溶解。红细胞对低渗溶液具有不同的抵抗能力，即红细胞具有不同的脆性。故临床上常用不同浓度的低渗 NaCl 溶液来测定红细胞的渗透脆性。对低渗 NaCl 溶液抵抗力小，表示红细胞的渗透脆性大；对低渗 NaCl 溶液抵抗力大，表示红细胞的渗透脆性小。开始出现溶血时的 NaCl 溶液浓度，为红细胞的最大渗透抵抗力。正常人红细胞的最小渗透抵抗力为 0.42% ~ 0.46% NaCl 溶液，最大渗透抵抗力为 0.32% ~ 0.34% NaCl 溶液。刚成熟的红细胞渗透脆性较小，而衰老的红细胞渗透脆性较大。遗传性球形红细胞增多症及镰形红细胞增多症患者，红细胞渗透脆性增加。

【实验材料】

1. 器材 试管架，小试管，2ml 注射器，滴管，5ml 吸管。

2. 溶液 3.8%枸橼酸钠，1%和2% NaCl 溶液，蒸馏水。

3. 对象 兔。

【实验方法】

1. 制备不同浓度的 NaCl 溶液 取试管 11 支，做好编号，顺次排列在试管架上，按下表配制各种浓度的 NaCl 溶液，混匀。

试管编号	1	2	3	4	5	6	7	8	9	10	11
1% NaCl	—	1.2	1.4	1.6	1.8	2.0	2.2	2.6	3.6	4.0	—
2% NaCl	—	—	—	—	—	—	4.0	—	—	—	—
蒸馏水（ml）	4.0	2.8	2.6	2.4	2.2	2.0	1.8	1.4	0.4	—	—
管内 NaCl 浓度（%）	—	0.3	0.35	0.40	0.45	0.50	0.55	0.60	0.9	1.0	2.0

2. 兔血的制备 取兔血 2ml，加入盛有 3.8%枸橼酸钠 0.2ml 的试管中，混匀备用。

3. 红细胞悬液的制备 用滴管向每支试管中滴加兔血 1～2 滴，摇匀，静置半小时后观察各管的颜色，澄明度有何差别。

4. 观察结果 按下列标准判断有无溶血、不完全溶血或完全溶血。

（1）上层清液无色，管底为浑浊红色，表示没有溶血。

（2）上层清液呈淡红色，管底为浑浊红色，表示只有部分红细胞破裂溶解，为不完全溶血。这代表红细胞的最小渗透抵抗力。

（3）管内液体完全变成透明的红色，管底无细胞沉积，为完全溶血。这代表红细胞的最大渗透抵抗力。

【实验指导】

1. 预习要求

（1）复习红细胞的生理特征。

（2）复习血浆的理化特征。

2. 操作要点

（1）取兔血的方法 将兔装入兔箱内，将耳尖部位的毛剪掉，用手术刀将耳缘静脉划一横切口，血液自行流出，直接滴入试管中收集备用。或者用木棒将兔击昏后，颈部切开，颈总动脉放血。

（2）取血时一定要避免溶血。

3. 注意事项

（1）血液滴入试管后，立即混匀，避免血液凝固。滴加血液时，要靠近液面，使血滴轻轻滴入溶液中，以免溶血。

（2）试管一定要编号，避免混淆。

4. 报告要点 记录开始不完全溶血和完全溶血的 NaCl 溶液浓度，结合试验结果讨论红细胞的生理特性及血浆渗透压保持相对恒定的重要意义。

5. 思考题

（1）为什么在科研实验或临床上需用各种浓度的 NaCl 溶液？

（2）输液时为何要采用等张溶液？

（吴玉林）

16 Osmotic fragility of erythrocytes

PURPOSE

To observe the erythrocyte changes in different osmotic solutions and learn the significance of relative constant osmotic pressure of extracellular fluid in keeping the normal shape and functions of cells through this experiment on erythrocyte osmotic fragility.

PRINCIPLE

The osmotic pressure in the erythrocyte of mammalia equals to that in plasmaunder normal physiological conditions. That is approximately the pressure of 0.9% NaCl solution. Therefore, the shapes and volumes of erythrocytes can remain the same when suspended in isotonic NaCl solution. However, if the erythrocytes are suspended in hypotonic solutions, the water will permeate into the cells to make them bulge and break as well as the hemoglobin be released. This procedure is called hematoclasis. Erythrocytes have resistance to hypotonic solutions, which is called osmotic fragility. Hypotonic NaCl solutions of different concentrations are generally used to test the erythrocyte fragility in clinic. The smaller the erythrocytes resistances to hypotonic solutions are, the bigger their osmotic fragility will be. On the contrary, the bigger the erythrocytes resistances to hypotonic solutions are, the smaller their osmotic fragility will be. The concentration of NaCl solution when hemolysis first appears is the minimum osmotic resistance of erythrocyte. The concentration of NaCl solution when complete hemolysis appears is the maximum osmotic resistance of erythrocyte. Normal erythrocytes have a minimum osmotic resistance of 0.42% ~ 0.46% NaCl solution and a maximum osmotic resistance of 0.32% ~ 0.34% NaCl solution. The osmotic fragility of just mature erythrocytes is relatively small while that of senile erythrocytes is much bigger. The osmotic fragility of erythrocytes will increases in the patients with genetic spherocytic erythromatosis or drepanocytic polycythemia.

MATERIALS

1. Equipments tubes bracket, test tubes, syringe (2ml), dropper, straws (5ml).

2. Solutions sodium citrate solution (3.8%), NaCl solution (1% and 2%), distilled water.

3. Object Rabbit.

METHODS

1. Prepare NaCl solutions of different concentrations Take 11 test tubes and assemble them on the bracket after numbering them. Prepare NaCl solutions of different concentrations as the following table. Mix up the solutions.

No.	1	2	3	4	5	6	7	8	9	10	11
1% NaCl	—	1.2	1.4	1.6	1.8	2.0	2.2	2.6	3.6	4.0	—
2% NaCl	—	—	—	—	—	—	4.0				
Distilled water(ml)	4.0	2.8	2.6	2.4	2.2	2.0	1.8	1.4	0.4		
NaCl concentration in the tube(%)	—	0.3	0.35	0.40	0.45	0.50	0.55	0.60	0.9	1.0	2.0

2. Prepare rabbit blood　Take 2ml rabbit blood and mix it up with 2ml sodium citrate solution (3.8%) in a test tube.

3. Prepare erythrocyte suspension　Add 1~2 drops of blood into every test tube and shake the tubes respectively. Set the tubes static for half an hour, and then observe the color and transparency of every tube.

4. Observe standard　Judge whether there is a hemolysis according to the following:

(1)If the upper clear liquid is achromatic color and the bottom in the tube is turbid with red color, there is not a hemolysis.

(2)If the upper clear liquid is pale red and the bottom in the tube is turbid with red color, there is an incomplete hemolysis with part of erythrocyte dissolved. This represents the minimum osmotic resistance of erythrocyte.

(3)If the liquid in the tube is completely clear and red, and there are not any cells on the bottom, it is called complete hemolysis. This represents the maximum osmotic resistance of erythrocyte.

GUIDANCE

1. Preview

(1)Review the physiological characters of erythrocyte.

(2)Review the physical and chemical characters of plasma.

2. Manipulation

(1) Method of taking the rabbit blood: Put the animal into the rabbit fixture. Shear its hair on the ear top, and then make an incision across the vein in the edge of the ear. Collect the blood. Otherwise, beat the animal to faint and cut open its neck to take blood from the common carotid artery.

(2) Do avoid hemolysis when taking blood.

3. Notices

(1)Mix up the blood after dropping it into the test tubes to avoid coagulation. Approach to the liquid surface as near as possible when dropping the blood and let it drop into the solution gently to avoid hemolysis.

(2)Do number the tubes so as not to be confused.

4. Report
Record the concentrations of NaCl solutions when incomplete or complete hemolysis happens. Discuss the physiological characters of erythrocyte and the significance to keep the plasma osmotic to be relatively constant according to the experimental results.

5. Questions

(1)Why are the NaCl solutions of different concentrations needed in research experiments or in clinical?

（2）Why is the isotonic solution needed in clinical transfusion?

（Wu Yulin）

实验十七　血液凝固

【实验目的】

通过测定实验条件下的血液凝固时间，了解血液凝固的基本过程以及加速和延缓血液凝固的一些因素。

【实验原理】

血液凝固过程是血浆中许多凝血因子共同参与的化学连锁反应，其结果是使血液由流体状态变成胶胨状态。血液凝固系统可分为内源性凝血系统和外源性凝血系统。内源性凝血系统是指参与凝血的因子全部存在于血浆中，而外源性凝血系统是指在组织因子参与下的凝血过程。有组织因子参与的凝血时间较内源性激活途径引起的凝血时间为短。本实验采用兔颈总动脉插管放血取血，血液几乎未与组织因子接触。因此，凝血过程主要是由内源性凝血系统所发动。肺组织浸液含有丰富的组织因子，在血液中加入肺组织液，以观察外源性凝血系统的作用。

血液凝固受许多因素的影响。凝血因子可直接影响血液凝固过程。例如设法除去血液中的钙离子（Ⅳ因子），便可制止血液凝固。此外，血液凝固过程还受温度、接触面的光滑程度等因素的影响。

【实验材料】

1. 器材　兔血，兔手术台，哺乳动物手术器械，动脉夹，细塑料管，20ml 注射器，试管，小烧杯，竹签，冰块，棉花，肺组织浸液。

2. 溶液　20% 氨基甲酸乙酯，2% 草酸钾，8U/ml 肝素，液状石蜡，生理盐水，5% $CaCl_2$。

注：1. 肺组织浸液的制备：取兔肺剪碎，浸泡于 3~4 倍量的生理盐水中，放冰箱中过夜，过滤收集的滤液即肺组织浸液，存冰箱中备用。

2. 肝素的配制：取 12500U/2ml 肝素 1 支，加蒸馏水至 1563ml，即成 8U/ml 浓度的肝素。

3. 对象　兔。

【实验方法】

1. 麻醉、固定与手术　经兔耳缘静脉注射 20% 氨基甲酸乙酯（按 1g/kg 计算），麻醉后仰卧固定于兔手术台上，分离一侧颈总动脉，离心端用线结扎阻断血流，近心端夹上动脉夹，在靠近结扎线处剪一小口，插入细塑料管，结扎插管固定之。需要放血时，开启动脉夹即可。

2. 按下列要求准备试管 每管内加入血液约2ml；5、6、7、8、9号试管加入血液后，用拇指盖住试管口，将试管颠倒两次。

试管1 内放少量棉花。

试管2 用液状石蜡润滑整个内表面。

试管3 不做任何处理。

试管4 置于有冰块的小烧杯中。

试管5 内加生理盐水5ml。

试管6 内加肝素8U。

试管7 内加草酸钾1～2mg。

试管8 内加肺组织液0.1ml。

试管9 内加5% $CaCl_2$溶液1～2滴。

将多余的血盛于小烧杯中，并不断用竹签搅动直至纤维蛋白形成。

3. 记录凝血时间 每个试管加兔血约2ml后，立即开始计时，每隔15秒，将试管倾斜一次，观察血液是否凝固，至血液成为凝胶状不再流动为止，记下所需时间即凝血时间。小烧杯内加入血液后立即用竹签不断搅动，去除纤维蛋白。

【实验指导】

1. 预习要求

（1）复习血液凝固过程。

（2）复习加速和延缓血液凝固的影响因素。

2. 操作要点

（1）试管准备好后，应连续向每个试管内加血，且最先由插管内流出的血液应弃去。

（2）5、6、7、8、9号试管加入血液后，应混匀，以观察药物对血液凝固的影响。

3. 注意事项

（1）试管要编号，避免混淆，计时应及时准确。

（2）各试管口径及采血量要一致。

4. 报告要点 记录实验结果并按下表填写，分析解释实验结果。

编号	实 验 条 件		结果及凝血时间	解释
1	粗糙面的影响	预先在试管内放入少许棉花		
2		预先用液状石蜡润滑整个试管的内表面		
3	温度的影响	试管置于室温中		
4		试管置于有冰块的小烧杯内		
5	药物的影响	试管内预先加入生理盐水5ml		
6		试管内预先加入肝素8U		
7		试管内预先加草酸钾1～2mg		
8		试管内预先加肺组织浸液0.1ml		
9		试管内预先加 $CaCl_2$ 1～2滴		
烧杯	放血于小烧杯时用竹签不断搅动，约2分钟后取出竹签，用水洗净竹签上的血滴，观察纤维蛋白。烧杯内为去纤维蛋白血			

5. 思考题

（1） 血液从伤口流出，为什么会凝固？

（2） 测定凝血时间有何实际意义？

（吴玉林）

17　Blood coagulation

PURPOSE

In this experiment, the blood coagulation time is measured under different conditions to understand the basic procedure and effect factors in it.

PRINCIPLE

The blood coagulation procedure is chemical chain reactions involved many plasma coagulation factors, turning the blood from liquid into gel. It can be divided into endogenetic system and ectogenetic system. In the endogenetic system all the involved coagulation factors are in the plasma while in the ectogenetic system there are also tissue factors. The blood coagulation time involved in tissue factors are much shorter than that effected only by endogenetic system. In this experiment blood is taken out through a tube inserted into the common carotid artery and avoided from reaching the tissue, thus the coagulation is started mainly by the endogenetic system. The infiltration of lung tissue is abundant in tissue factors. It can be added into blood to observe the effects of ectogenetic system.

MATERIALS

1. Equipments　rabbit blood, rabbit operation table, operation instruments for mammalia, artery clip, fine plastic tube, syringe (20ml), test tubes, small breaker, bamboo chopsticks, ice cubes, medical cotton, infiltration of lung tissue (shatter the rabbit lung and soak it with 3 ~ 4 times of saline, then put it in fridge for half a day. Filter it and use the infiltration. Store it in fridge.)

2. Solutions　20% ethyl carbamate, potassium oxalate (2%), heparin (8U/ml, dilute a amp of 12500U/2ml heparin into 1563ml with distilled water), paraffin, saline, $CaCl_2$(5%).

3. Objects　Rabbits.

METHODS

1. Anesthesia and fixation　Weight the rabbit and inject 20% ethyl carbamate (1g/kg) into vein on the edge of an ear. After the disappearance of corneal reflex, fix the rabbit on operating table, and turn on the light at the table bottom to keep temperature. Separate the common carotid artery. At the end of the artery far from heart (as near as possible to the head), the common carotid artery is ligated with a silk thread. At the end of the artery near the heart (as near as possible to the heart), block the artery with an arterial clip. Then scissor an inclined cut towards the heart on the artery near the knot (the end far from the heart). Insert the arterial cannula into the artery from the cut, fix the top of the cannula with the silk thread, and the surplus thread is ligated on the side of cannula to avoid the slippage. Loose the artery clip whenever the blood is needed.

2. Prepare test tubes as the following Test tube No. 1:put a little cotton in it;

Test tube No. 2:lubricate its inside completely with paraffin;

Test tube No. 3:no any handling;

Test tube No. 4:be put in a small beaker in which is filled with ice cubes;

Test tube No. 5:put 5ml saline in it;

Test tube No. 6:put 1ml heparin (8U/ml) in it;

Test tube No. 7:put 1 ~ 2mg potassium oxalate (2%) in it;

Test tube No. 8:put 0. 1ml tissue infiltration in it;

Test tube No. 9:put 1 ~ 2 drops of $CaCl_2$ solution in it;

Every tube is added in about 2ml blood, and the tubes No. 5,6,7,8,9 should be reversed several times after blood added in. The rest blood is put in a small beaker to form fibrous protein by churning it with a bamboo chopstick, and then the fibrous protein is discarded.

3. Record of blood coagulation time Record the time as soon as blood is added into every tube. Slope the tubes every 15 seconds to make sure whether the blood is coagulated. Record the time when the blood turns into gel. The duration from blood being added into the tubes to it becoming gel is recorded as coagulation time.

GUIDANCE

1. Preview

(1) Review the knowledge on blood coagulation process.

(2) Review the knowledge on the factors in accelerating or postponing bloodcoagulation.

2. Manipulation

(1) Blood should be added into the tubes continuously and the blood, which initially flows out of the inserting fine tube, should be discarded.

(2) The blood added into test tubes No. 5,6,7,8,9 should be mixed up to observe the effects of certain drugs on blood coagulation.

3. Notices

(1) Test tubes should be numbered clearly; recording should be accurate and in time.

(2) Diameters of the tubes and volumes of the blood samplings should be almost identical.

4. Report Record the experimental results in the following table and explain them.

No.	Experimental conditions		Results & coagulation time	Explanation
1	Effects of rough surface	A lttle cotton in it		
2		Lubricate inside with paraffin		
3	Effects of temperature	Under the room temperature		
4		Among ice cubes in a beaker		
5	Effects of drugs	5ml saline be added firstly		
6		8U heparin be added firstly		

content

No.	Experimental conditions		Results & coagulation time	Explanation
7	Effects of drugs	1～2ml potassium oxalate be added firstly		
8		0.1ml tissue infiltration be added firstly		
9		1～2 drops of CaCl₂ solution be added firstly		
Small beaker (about 10ml blood)	Blood in the beaker is churned with a bamboo chopstick continuously. Take out the chopstick 2 min later and wash the blood off to observethe formed fibrous protein on it. What left is difibrinated blood.			

5. Questions

（1）Why blood will coagulate when leaking out of wound?

（2）What is the practical significance of determining coagulation time?

（Wu Yulin）

实验十八　血型鉴定

扫码"学一学"

【实验目的】

通过观察红细胞凝集反应，了解 ABO 血型鉴定的原理及测定血型的方法和意义。

【实验原理】

血型是根据红细胞膜表面存在的特异性抗原（镶嵌于红细胞膜上的糖蛋白和糖脂）来确定，这种血型抗原或凝集原由遗传基因决定。抗体或凝集素存在于血清中，它能与相应的凝集原或抗原发生凝集反应，最后使红细胞溶解。由于这种现象，临床上在输血前必须进行血型鉴定，以确保安全输血。

【实验材料】

1. 器材　显微镜，小滴管，牙签，载玻片，刺血针，棉球，酒精棉球。

2. 溶液　A 型、B 型标准血清，生理盐水。

3. 对象　人。

【实验方法】

1. 用蜡笔将一干净玻片在中间划为两半，左上角注"A"，表示 A 型血清；右上角注"B"，表示 B 型血清。

2. 用小滴管吸 A 型标准血清（含抗 B）一滴加入左侧中央。用另一小滴管吸 B 型标准血清（含抗 A）一滴加入右侧中央。

3. 消毒耳垂或无名指皮肤，用消毒刺血针深刺约 2mm，出血后分别用牙签刮取一小滴血，立即加入玻片两侧的血清中，并用牙签搅拌，使每侧血清和血液混合。每侧用一支牙签，切勿混用。

4. 室温下静置 10 分钟后，用肉眼观察有无凝集现象。例如只是 A 侧发生凝集，则血型为 B 型；若只是 B 侧凝集，则血型为 A 型，若两侧均凝集，则血型为 AB 型。若两侧均未发生凝集，则血型为 O 型（图 3-7）。这种凝集反应的强度因人而异，所以有时需借助显微镜才能确定是否出现凝集。

【实验指导】

1. 预习要求

（1）复习 ABO 血型系统。

（2）复习血型系统与临床输血的关系。

2. 操作要点及注意事项

（1）滴加在两侧的血清不要混匀，左侧 A 型血清，右侧 B 型血清，严防两种血清相互接触。

（2）每侧用一根牙签加入血液一滴，不能用同一根牙签。

3. 报告要点 将观察到的现象进行简单描述，并结合课本内容讨论血型鉴定的原理及临床意义。

4. 思考题

（1）根据自己的血型，说明你能接受输血的血型和给何种血型的人输血，为什么？

（2）如何区别血液凝集、血液凝固与红细胞叠连，其机制是否一样？

（吴玉林）

18　Identification of blood group

PURPOSE

The principle, method and significance of ABO blood group identification are learned by the observation of erythrocyte agglutination.

PRINCIPLE

Blood group is determined by specific antigen, which is made up of glycoprotein and glycolipids locating in the erythrocyte membrane. Gene decides the blood group antigen or agglutinogen. Antibody or agglutinin, which is in serum, can cause agglutination with antigen or agglutinogen and result in erythrocyte haemolysis. Thus in clinical blood group should be identified before blood transfusion.

MATERIALS

1. Equipments microscope, blood taking needle, straws, small bamboo needle, slide, medical cotton.

2. Solutions 75% alcohol, saline, standard serum A & B.

3. Object Human.

METHODS

1. Divided a clean slide along the midline with a pen; mark the left as "A" and the right as

"B" to indicate serum A & B respectively.

2. Put a drop of standard serum A (containing antibody B) with a straw in the middle of the left side of the slide; and put a drop of standard serum B (containing antibody A) with another straw in the middle of the right side of the slide.

3. Disinfect the skin of ear lobe or the forth finger tip, and then make it bleedingby sting into the skin for about 2mm with a disinfected needle. Scrape a drop of blood with a bamboo needle and add it into the serum A or B respectively. Mix up the blood and serum with the bamboo needle. Do use different bamboo needles for different serums.

4. Put the slide in static under room temperature for 10 minutes and observe whether there is a agglutination with naked eyes. If the agglutination only happens on "A" side, the blood group is "B". If the agglutination happens only on "B" side, then the blood belongs to group "A". If the agglutination happens on both "A" and "B", the blood group is "AB". And when the blood is group "O", none agglutination can be observed. The extend of agglutination is different in

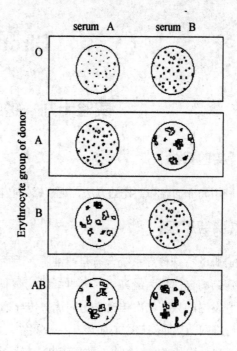

Fig. 3 – 7　Test agglutination reaction of ABO group

different people, so microscope should be used to determine it whenever needed.

GUIDANCE

1. Preview

(1) Review the knowledge on ABO blood group.

(2) Review the knowledge on the relations of blood group and clinical bloodtransfusion.

2. Manipulation

(1) Do not mix the serum: put the serum A on the left and the serum B on the right. Do prevent them from contacting with each other.

(2) Use different bamboo needles to add blood into the serum. Avoid the cross contamination.

3. Report　Describe the observed phenomena simply and discuss the principle and clinical significance of blood group identification according to text.

4. Questions

(1) According to your own blood group, try to explain which group of blood you can receive or people with which blood group can receive your donation? Why?

(2) How to distinguish the blood agglutination, blood coagulation and erythrocyte aggregation? What are their mechanisms?

(Wu Yulin)

第四章 循环系统

Circulation

实验十九 蟾蜍心起搏点分析

【实验目的】

利用局部加温和结扎的方法，观察蟾蜍心正常起搏点，并比较心脏不同部位自律性的高低。

【实验原理】

心脏的特殊传导系统含有自律细胞，因而具有自动节律性，但各部分的自律性高低不同，以窦房结的自律性为最高，浦肯野纤维为最低。正常情况下，窦房结是哺乳动物的心脏起搏点，它发出的兴奋依次传给心房内优势传导通路、房室交界、房室束（希氏束）及其分支、浦肯野纤维网，从而使整个心脏发生一次兴奋。两栖类动物的心起搏点是静脉窦，如将心室与心房、心房与静脉窦之间的兴奋传导阻断，静脉窦以外的其他自律性细胞的自律性就会显示出来。

【实验材料】

1. **器材** 蛙类手术器械，蛙板，温度计，小试管，滴管，丝线。
2. **溶液** 任氏液。
3. **对象** 蟾蜍或蛙。

【实验方法】

1. 取蟾蜍一只，毁脑和脊髓后，背位固定于蛙板上，用剪刀剪开胸腔，暴露心脏，参照图 4 - 1，识别静脉窦、心房和心室。

2. 观察项目

（1）局部加温，用盛有 40℃ 左右热水的小试管依次接触心室、心房和静脉窦，观察心率有何变化？

（2）用丝线沿房室沟做第二斯氏结扎后，分别观察心房、心室的跳动频率有何变化。

（3）用玻璃分针将心脏翻向头端，在静脉窦和心房交界处可见一白色半月形沟（窦房沟），沿此沟用丝线做第一斯氏结扎后，分别观察静脉窦和心房的跳动频率有何变化。

（4）放置 30 分钟后再观察心房和心室是否能恢复跳动？两者的频率有何差别？

【实验指导】

1. **预习要求**
（1）心脏特殊传导系统的组成。

（2）窦房结对潜在起搏点的控制方式。

2. 操作要点

（1）当温热小试管接触心室、心房时，整个心脏的跳动频率不受影响。只有当接触静脉窦时，才使心跳频率加快，说明静脉窦的自律性控制了整个心脏的兴奋性，因此可证明静脉窦是蟾蜍心脏的正常起搏点。

（2）做第一、第二斯氏结扎后，心房、心室可停搏长达半小时才表现出其自身的自律性。其原因可能是心房、心室的特殊传导组织虽然也有自身的自律性，但在正常情况下受到心脏正常起搏点的抑制作用而未能表现出来，在做第一、第二斯氏结扎后，由静脉窦发出的兴奋虽不能下传到心房、心室，但潜在起搏点的自律性一时尚不能从抑制中解脱出来，故心房、心室会出现较长时间停搏的现象。

3. 注意事项

（1）局部加温时，试管放置的位置要准确，接触面不宜过大，接触时间不宜过长。否则会由于热的传导和辐射作用，造成对心房和心室的加温，也会出现心跳加快的假象。

（2）结扎部位要准确。

（3）实验过程中，要经常用任氏液湿润标本，以保持组织的兴奋性。

4. 报告要点　根据心脏不同部位自律性的高低，分析蟾蜍心脏起搏点的部位。

5. 思考题

（1）为什么正常起搏点能主导心脏的节律性活动？

（2）试讨论窦房结的起搏离子流基础。

（颜天华　刘冰冰）

19　Analysis of heart pacemaker in toad

PURPOSE

To observe the normal heart pacemaker in toad and to compare the auto – rhythmicity in different part of the heart by means of part heating and deligation.

PRINCIPLE

The special conducting system of heart contains auto – rhythmic cells, so it has auto – rhythmicity. However, the different parts of the heart has its own auto – rhythmicity, the highest the sinoatrial node, the lowest the Purkinje fiber. In normal condition, the sinoatrial node is the mammal's heart pacemaker. The excitation emitted by it transmits to preferential pathway in atrium, atrioventricular junction, atrioventricular bundle (Hisbundle) and its branches, Purkinje fiber one by one, making the whole heart excite once. The amphibian animal's heart pacemaker is sinus venous. If the excitation conduction is prohibited between ventricle and atrium, atrium and sinus venous, the auto – rhythmicity of the auto – rhythmic cells except sinus venous will be shown.

MATERIALS

1. Equipments　operational plate for toad, frog board, thermometer, little test tube, dropper, suture.

2. Solutions   Ringer's solution.

3. Object   toad or frog.

METHOD

1. Take a toad and destroy its brain and spinal cord and put it on frog board. Open the thorax and make heart exposed (Fig. 4 – 1), to recognize the sinus venous, autrium, and ventricle.

2. Observation Items

(1) Touch the ventricle, autrium and sinus venous with the little test tube containing about 40℃ warm water. Observe the difference of the heart rate.

(2) Make the first deligation by using suture across the atrioventricular groove, and then observe the difference of autrium, ventricles subsultus frequency respectively.

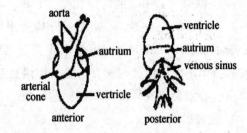

Fig. 4 – 1   The construction of toad heart

(3) Turn up heart by glass needle, to find out the crescent – shaped groove (sinoatrial) in the relay between sinus venous and autrium, and make the second deligation across the groove by suture, then observe the difference of sinus venous and autrium subsultus frequency respectively.

(4) Observe autrium and ventricle, to see if the heartbeat can be recovered after 30 minutes. Note the difference of the heartbeat frequency between the former and the latter.

GUIDANCE

1. Preview

(1) The consistence of the special heart conducting system.

(2) The methods of sinoatrial node controlling the potential pacemaker.

2. Manipulation

(1) When the warm little test tube touch autrium and ventricle, the subsultus frequency of the whole heart does not change. But as the sinus venous is warmed up, the heart rate will get faster, it proves that the auto – rhythmicity of the sinus venous controls the excitability of the whole heart. So it is established that sinus venous is the normal heart pacemaker in toad.

(2) The autrium's and ventricle's auto – rhythmicity cannot be seen until half an hour of cardiac arrest after the first、second deligation. The reason may be that the special conducting tissue of the autrium and ventricle has its own auto – rhythmicity, but it can not be exposed by the normal heart pacemaker's inhibition under normal conditions. After the the first, second deligation, the excitation emitted by sinus venous can not be transmitted to autrium and ventricle. However, the auto – rhythmicity of the potential pacemaker is inhibited, so the cardiac arrest will last for long time.

3. Notice

(1) When heating, the placement of test tube should be accurate, the contact surface should not be large, and the contact time should not be longer. Otherwise, under the condition of heat conduction and irradiation, which might warm up the autrium and ventricle, the false image of the heart faster beat would appear.

（2）Make an accurate deligation.

（3）During the experiment, wet the sample by Ringer's solution from time to time, to keep the excitability of tissue.

4. Report　According to the auto－rhythmicity of different part of heart, make an analysis of the heart pacemaker in toad.

5. Questions

（1）Why does the normal pacemaker can master the heart rhythmicity?

（2）Discuss the basis of sinoatrial node's pacemaker current.

（Yan Tianhua, Liu Bingbing）

实验二十　蟾蜍心室期前收缩和代偿间歇

扫码"学一学"

【实验目的】

通过期前收缩和代偿间歇的观察，验证心肌有效不应期长的特征，从而加深了解心肌兴奋性的周期性变化规律和特点。

【实验原理】

心肌每发生一次兴奋后，其兴奋性会发生一系列周期性变化，与其他可兴奋组织相比，其特点是有效不应期特别长，几乎相当于整个收缩期和舒张早期。在此期中，任何强大的刺激均不能引起心肌兴奋而收缩。但在舒张中晚期内，给予心室一次阈上刺激，便可在正常节律性兴奋到达心室之前，引起一次扩布性兴奋和收缩，称为期前收缩。期前收缩也具有不应期，因此，当静脉窦传来的正常节律性兴奋落在期前收缩的有效不应期内时，则不能引起心室的兴奋和收缩，心室停留于舒张状态，直至下一次正常节律性兴奋到达时，才恢复正常的节律性收缩，此较长的舒张期称为代偿间歇。

【实验材料】

1. 器材　BL－420F生物信号采集与分析系统，刺激电极，张力换能器，铁支架，双凹夹，蛙板，蛙类手术器械，蛙心夹，棉线，小烧杯，滴管，探针。

2. 溶液　任氏液。

3. 对象　蟾蜍或蛙。

【实验方法】

1. 用探针毁蟾蜍的脑和脊髓后，将其仰卧固定于蛙板上。从剑突下将胸部皮肤向上剪开，然后剪掉胸骨，打开心包，暴露心脏。

2. 将与张力换能器相连的蛙心夹在心舒期夹住心尖约1mm。刺激电极固定于铁支架上，使心室处于电极的两极之间。按图4－2连接并调整好记录装置。

3. 接通BL－420F生物信号采集与分析系统，进入期前收缩记录界面。调整好走纸速度，进行观察记录。

4. 观察项目

（1）先记录一段正常心动曲线，辨认代表收缩期和舒张期的曲线部分。

（2）在心室收缩期给予单个刺激，观察有什么变化？

（3）在心舒期的早、中、晚期，分别给予单个刺激，观察有无期前收缩和代偿间歇出现？结果见图 4-3。

【实验指导】

1. 预习要求

（1）预习心肌的生理特征。

（2）预习 BL-420F 生物信号采集与分析系统的操作方法。

2. 操作要点　刺激电极应与心室密切接触，可按心脏心室部分置于电极两极之间或者将两极均置于心室一侧壁。

3. 注意事项

（1）毁脑、脊髓必须彻底。

（2）操作过程中必须经常滴加任氏液，以防心脏组织干燥。

（3）引起期前收缩后，须间隔一段时间后再给予第二次刺激。

4. 报告要点　将实验记录曲线注字剪贴，每个同学均应有一份记录曲线，并解释产生期前收缩和代偿间歇的原因。

5. 思考题

（1）叙述心肌的生理特性与兴奋性周期性变化的关系，并和神经、骨骼肌进行比较。

（2）以上述结果推测心室有效不应期的长度，并说明有何生理意义。

（3）期前收缩后，是否一定出现代偿间歇？

（颜天华　刘冰冰）

20　Premature contraction and compensatory pause of toad ventricle

PURPOSE

To confirm characteristics of cardiac muscle's effective refractory period through observing premature contraction and compensatory pause, and try to get a further knowledge of the periodicity regulation of cardiac muscle's excitability.

PRINCIPLE

Once cardiac muscle excites, its excitability will change periodically. And its effective refractory period is comparatively much longer, almost equals to the whole systole and pre-diastole. During this period, any stronger stimulus can not cause the cardiac muscle excite and contract, but during the last period of diastole, given a ventricle over threshold stimulus, it can cause excitation and contract once before the normal rhythmicity excitation arrives at ventricle. It is called premature contraction. Premature contraction has also refractory period. So if the normal rhythmicity excitation transmitted by sinus venous is in the effective refractory period of premature contraction, it can not lead to ventricle's excitation and contraction, and ventricle is in diastole. It is not until the next normal rhythmicity excitation arrives that the ventricle recovers to normal rhythmicity contract. This long period diastole is called compensatory pause.

MATERIALS

1. Equipments BL – 420F biological signal acquisition and analysis system, stimulate electrode, tension transducer, iron bracket, double cave clamp, operational plate for toad, frog board, toad heart clip, beaker, dropper, suture, probe.

2. Solutions Ringer's solution.

3. Object toad or frog.

METHOD

1. Destroy the toad's brain and spinal cord by probe, and put the toad on frog board. Open the thoracic cavity, and cut pericardium to make heart exposed.

2. Clip apex of the heart for 1mm in the diastole with a toad heart clip connected with tension transducer. Fix the stimulate electrode at iron bracket with ventricle between the two poles of electrode, and then connect the heart to recording equipment (Fig. 4 – 2).

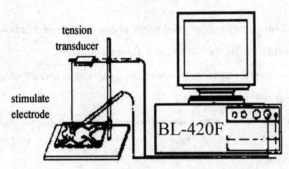

Fig. 4 – 2   The connection of recording equipment

3. Open BL – 420F biological signal acquisition and analysis system, so that the record of premature contraction will be exposed. Adjust the speed of paper, so as to make an observation and recording.

4. Observation Items

(1) Record a period of normal cardiac curves, to recognize the curve of systole and diastole.

(2) Make single stimulate in ventricle systole to observe the contraction of the ventricle.

(3) During the first, middle, last period of diastole, make single stimulation respectively to see if the premature contraction or compensatory pause comes. (the results are shown in Fig. 4 – 3).

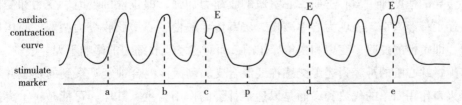

Fig. 4 – 3   The cardiac contraction curve of premature contraction and compensatory pause on toad

E. premature contraction P. compensatory pause a, b. stimulation in absolute refractory period

C, d, e. stimulation in relative refractory period

GUIDANCE

1. Preview

（1）Preview the physiological characteristics of cardiac muscle.

（2）Preview the operation methods of BL－420F biological signal acquisition and analysis system.

2. Manipulation　Stimulate electrode should be contact to ventricle，and ventricle should be put between two pole of electrode，or dispose the two pole at the same lateral wall of the ventricle

3. Notice

（1）Thoroughly destroy the brain and spinal cord.

（2）Add Ringer's solution time and again during the operation to prevent heart tissue from dehydration.

（3）Once premature contraction happens，be sure to make the second stimulation later in a period of time.

4. Report　Mark，Clip and paste the experiment record curve. Each student should have one copy of it and with its help try to account for the premature contraction and compensatory pause.

5. Questions

（1）State the relationship between physiological characteristic of cardiac muscle and excitation periodicity，and compare them with the nerve，and skeletal muscles.

（2）According to the above results，speculate the length of ventricle effective refractory period，and state the physiological meaning.

（3）Is the compensatory pause a necessary process after premature contraction？

（Yan Tianhua，Liu Bingbing）

扫码"学一学"

实验二十一　蟾蜍心脏的神经支配

【实验目的】

观察电刺激迷走交感混合神经对心脏活动的影响，以了解心脏的神经支配。

【实验原理】

心脏受交感神经和迷走神经双重支配。心交感神经兴奋，表现为心率加快，兴奋经房室交界传导的速度加快，心房肌、心室肌的收缩力加强，即正性的变时、变力和变传导作用。心迷走神经兴奋，表现为心率减慢，房室传导减慢，心房肌收缩力减弱，心房肌不应期缩短，即负性的变时、变力和变传导作用，而对心室肌收缩力的影响不大。

支配蟾蜍心脏的神经为迷走交感神经混合支。刺激该混合神经观察到的现象并不是两种神经兴奋作用简单的代数和，而是以迷走神经的作用为主。其原因可能是：①突触前调制作用。在肾上腺素能神经纤维末梢表面存在着胆碱能 M 受体，和这些末梢直接接触的胆碱能纤维所释放的乙酰胆碱与上述 M 受体结合，可使肾上腺素能纤维末梢释放的递质减少，乙酰胆碱对肾上腺素能纤维末梢的这种作用，称为突触前调制作用。②迷走神经潜伏期短。

③混合支中迷走神经占主导地位。因此，刺激迷走交感混合神经，主要表现为心率减慢甚至停搏。在刺激后期或加大刺激强度，可表现为交感神经兴奋的作用。

【实验材料】

1. 器材　BL-420F 生物信号采集与分析系统，张力换能器，刺激电极（钩状保护电极），铁支架，双凹夹，蛙板，蛙类手术器械，蛙心夹，丝线，小烧杯，滴管，探针。

2. 溶液　任氏液。

3. 对象　蟾蜍或蛙。

【实验方法】

1. 用探针毁蟾蜍的脑脊髓后，仰卧位固定于蛙板上。在一侧下颌角与前肢之间剪开皮肤，分离下面的结缔组织，暴露肩胛骨提肌，将其剪断，在其下面可见到一血管神经束，其中有颈总动脉、颈静脉、迷走交感混合神经，用玻璃分针仔细分离迷走交感混合神经，穿线备用（图4-4）。

2. 打开胸腔，暴露心脏，在心舒期用蛙心夹夹住心尖约 1mm，并使蛙心夹的连线与张力换能器相连。

3. 将保护电极置于迷走神经干下，并通过刺激输出线与微机相连，调整好 BL-420F 生物信号采集与分析系统。

4. 观察项目　描记一段正常的心动曲线，然后以适宜的方波刺激迷走交感混合神经，观察心跳的变化。

5. 实验结果

（1）心率减慢甚至停搏。

（2）心率减慢，心收缩力加强。

（3）起初心脏停搏，而后出现心跳，心收缩力逐渐加强。

总之，刺激迷走交感混合神经，对心脏的影响是复杂的、多重性的，应具体问题具体分析。一般来说，早期以迷走神经的作用为主，后期又逐渐转变为交感神经的作用。

【实验指导】

1. 预习要求

（1）复习心脏的神经支配。

（2）复习心血管活动的调节机制。

2. 操作要点

（1）要准确寻找迷走交感混合神经，该神经位于肩胛舌骨肌内侧缘且与之伴行，横跨于肩胛骨提肌上方，它与前肢臂神经丛不同，臂神经丛位置较低，且粗大色白，有光泽，通往两侧前肢。

（2）蛙心夹安放于心尖部位，尽量少损伤心脏组织。

3. 注意事项

（1）采用保护电极，以避免电流刺激周围组织而影响记录。

（2）经常用任氏液湿润神经，以防组织干燥而失去功能。

（3）刺激电极间的组织液须用棉球吸干，以防短路或电流扩散。

扫码"看一看"

（4）一次刺激的时间不能过长，两次刺激之间必须间隔 3～5 分钟，以防损伤神经。

4. 报告要点　用配有文字说明的记录曲线表达实验结果，根据实验结果讨论心脏活动的调节。

5. 思考题

（1）心脏的神经支配及其作用机制。

（2）刺激迷走交感混合神经时，为什么以迷走神经兴奋为主?

（颜天华、刘冰冰）

21　The innervation of toad heart

PURPOSE

To observe the effects of vagosympathetic stimulation on heart action, so as to have a good knowledge of the innervation of the toad heart.

PRINCIPLE

Heart action can be regulated by two sets of nerves, the vagus nerve and the sympathetic nerve. Sympathetic stimulation can cause the effects of increased heart rate, increased conduction of impulses through atrioventricular node, increased strength of atrial and ventricular contraction. The effects are also called positive chronotropic action, positive inotropic action, positive dromotropic action. Vagal stimulation can cause the effects of decreased heart rate, decreased conduction of impulses through the atrioventricular node, decreased strength of atrial contraction, decreased refractory stage of atrial muscle. The effects are also called negative chronotropic action, negative inotropic action, negative dromotropic action, being poor on vigor of ventricular contraction.

Heart function of the toad is controlled by vagosympathetic mixed nerve. The effects of vagosympathetic mixed nerve are mainly the effects of the vagus nerve, not simply the sum of the vagus nerve and sympathetic nerve. The phenomena maybe be caused by three reasons：①presynaptic modulation. M cholinergic receptor exists in adrenergic nerve terminal, which contacts some cholinergic nerves releasing acetylcholine and the acetylcholine interacts with the M receptor, causing the number of neurotransmitter from the adrenergic nerve terminal to decrease. This is called presynaptic modulation. ②The latent period of impulse in vagus nerve is shorter than that in sympathetic nerve. ③ Vagus nerve is a primary part in mixed nerve. Therefore, the effects of vagosympathetic mixed nerve are mainly decreased heart rate or ceased heart beat. In the later stage or when augmenting intensity of stimulation, the effects of vagosympathetic mixed nerve can be the effects of sympathetic stimulation.

MATERIALS

1. Equipments　BL – 420F biological signal acquisition and analysis system, stimulate electrode (hemate shield electrode), tension transducer, iron bracket, double cave clamp, operational plate for toad, frog board, toad heart clip, beaker, dropper, suture, probe.

2. Solutions　Ringer's solution.

3. Object　toad or frog.

METHOD

1. Follow the complete destruction of the brain and the spinal cord by inserting dissecting needle (probe), and fix the toad lying on the back to toad board. Cut the skin between angle of mandible and forelimb in one side of body, and separate the connective tissue exposing levator scapulae and cutting off the muscle, to find out the vascular bundle and the nerve tract including the carotid artery, jugular vein and vagosympathetic mixed nerve, all of which run together. (Fig. 4 – 4) Separate the vagosympathetic mixed nerve carefully with a glass probe and the thread should be ready to retrieve the nerve for stimulation.

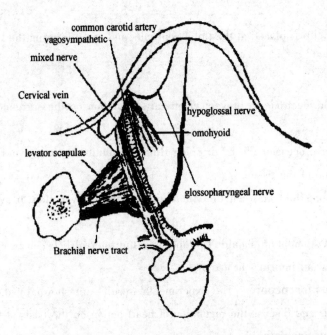

Fig. 4 – 4　The anatomic position of vagosympathetic mixed nerve in toad

2. Open the thoracic cavity to expose the heart, and clip the tip of the ventricle about 1mm by toad heart clip, then connect the clip with tension transducer by a thread.

3. Place shield electrode under the stem of vagosympathetic nerve, and connect shield electrode to the output terminals of the stimulator, then connect the stimulator to the computer. Open BL – 420F biological signal acquisition and analysis system and let it work well.

4. Observation items　Record a normal contraction curve, and stimulate the vagosympathetic nervewith adequate square waves to observe the changes in heart beat.

5. Experimental Results

(1) Heart rate become slow or heart arrest is even observed.

(2) Strength of cardiac contraction is increased.

(3) In the beginning heart block is observed, then heart beat appears gradually and Strength of cardiac contration is gradually increased, too.

In summary, the effects of vagosympathetic stimulation on the heart are complex and multiplex, which should be treated practically. Generally, the effects of vagus nerve are obvious in early stage and the effects of sympathetic nerve become prominent in later stage.

GUIDANCE

1. Requirements for preparation

(1) Review the innervation of the heart.

(2) Review the mechanism of regulation on cardiovascular action.

2. Requirements for manipulation

(1) Search the vagosympathetic nerve correctly. The nerve is at the interior edge of omohyoid following the muscle, stretching across levator scapulae. The nerve is different from forearm nerve plexus. Position of forearm nerve plexus is low, which is big, white, bright and reaches to two fore-limbs.

(2) Toad heart clip is placed at the tip of ventricle, and avoid injuring the heart as far as possible.

3. Notice

(1) Apply shield electrode to prevent electrical stimulation on the surrounding tissue to cause incorrect recording.

(2) Wet the nerve occasionally by dripping Ringer's solution on it to avoid loss of the function because of desiccation of the tissue.

(3) Dry the tissue fluid between the stimulating electrode by cotton to avoid short circuit or current diffusion.

(4) The time of stimulation shouldn't be too long, the interval between two stimulating is 3 ~ 5 minutes in order to avoid injuring the nerve.

4. Requirements for peport

The experimental results are shown by the curve noted with some necessary words and discuss the regulation of heart action on the basis of the results.

5. Consideration problems

(1) What is the innervation of the heart and its mechanism?

(2) Why are the effects of vagus nerve primary in mixed nerve when the vagosympathetic nerve is stimulated?

(Yan Tianhua, Liu Bingbing)

实验二十二　心电与收缩活动的时相关系

【实验目的】

了解心电和收缩的时相关系，兴奋与收缩是通过什么联系，了解横管系统在兴奋－收缩耦联中的作用。

【实验原理】

心脏的起搏点为窦房结（两栖类为静脉窦），兴奋沿特殊传导途径传导到整个心脏，分别引起心房肌和心室肌兴奋，心肌细胞的兴奋可通过兴奋－收缩耦联引起细胞内肌丝滑行产生收缩。兴奋 – 收缩耦联需要 Ca^{2+} 参与，所需的 Ca^{2+} 主要由细胞外供给，因此细胞外 Ca^{2+} 浓度对心肌的兴奋 – 收缩耦联影响很大。

细胞外 Ca^{2+} 主要通过横管系统进入细胞内，甘油任氏液能可逆性地破坏心肌的横管系统，阻止细胞外 Ca^{2+} 进入细胞内，从而阻断兴奋 – 收缩耦联，使心肌的兴奋活动不能引起其收缩活动。

【实验材料】

1. 仪器　BL – 420F 生物信号采集与分析系统（或二道生理记录仪），蛙手术器械，蛙心夹，蛙心插管，双凹夹，长滴管，木质试管夹，蛙板，铁架台，万能滑轮，叉形记录电极。

2. 药品　任氏液，25% 高渗甘油任氏液。

3. 对象　蟾蜍。

【实验方法】

1. 仪器连接和调试

（1）如图 4 – 5 所示连接好仪器。

（2）仪器条件　心电记录测量范围 0.5mV/cm，时间常数 2s，滤波 100Hz；心肌收缩测量范围 10mV/cm，滤波 100Hz，DC。使心电图和收缩曲线的基线稳定，灵敏度适中，先以慢纸速描记，当各波皆能充分显示后才以 25mm/s 的纸速记录。

2. 手术

（1）取蟾蜍一只，破坏脑和脊髓，剪开心包暴露心脏。

（2）在主动脉下穿双线，用玻璃针穿过主动脉干，将心尖翻向头端，然后将预先穿入的一条线沿静脉窦与后腔静脉交界处结扎（注意勿结扎半月沟和静脉窦），心脏恢复原位，立即做蛙心插管，方法同《化学物质对蟾蜍离体心脏活动的影响》实验，使心脏保留在原来位置，蛙心插管与蛙体表成 15°角（也可将心脏离体后进行实验）。

（3）用连线蛙心夹在舒张期夹住心尖，将线连至换能器，换能器输入线连至记录仪二道。

（4）用注射针头插入蟾蜍右前肢与左下肢，分别连接导线正负极，然后引入记录仪一道，把地线夹在插入右下肢的针头上（Ⅱ导联）。

3. 观察项目

（1）正常心电图和心肌收缩活动观察　正常任氏液灌注，先用纸速 10mm/s 记录，然后调用 25mm/s，观察心电发生在前，收缩发生在后。

（2）25% 甘油任氏液灌注结果观察　用 25% 甘油任氏液灌流，纸速 10mm/s，此时心电存在，收缩曲线不出现。

（3）正常任氏液灌注结果观察　用正常任氏液灌注，观察心电及重新出现的收缩曲线。

【实验指导】

1. 预习要求

（1）复习心肌兴奋和传导的原理。

（2）复习骨骼肌的超微结构。

（3）复习骨骼肌兴奋－收缩耦联的原理和肌丝滑行学说。

（4）复习心电图的产生原理。

2. 操作要点

（1）熟练地调试仪器，正确安装仪器，排除干扰。本实验干扰来源主要有两方面：①由于接地不良可产生干扰；②可因实验动物过于潮湿而产生干扰。

（2）精心制作标本　正确进行蛙心插管。实验过程中可能产生插管口堵塞，灌流不畅，其原因可能有二：①结扎静脉时未扎紧，致有血液流入心室，凝固而堵塞插管口；②插管口位置不合适，致使插管口紧贴心室内壁而堵塞。因此实验时，应洗尽心室内血液，正确进行蛙心插管并尽量使心室纵轴方向与插管方向一致。

3. 注意事项

（1）排除干扰，蛙板及动物必须保持干燥。

（2）甘油任氏液灌注时出现变化立即换洗，否则心脏将不能恢复活动。

4. 报告要点

（1）正确记录实验结果并观察 ECG 和心肌收缩前后顺序，分析其产生原理。

（2）讨论心电和收缩活动的时相关系及兴奋－收缩耦联中横管系统的作用。

（3）简述心肌兴奋至收缩的整个过程。

5. 思考题

（1）怎样用实验来证明心肌兴奋－收缩耦联的 Ca^{2+} 主要来源于细胞外？

（2）你有办法让心肌一直处于收缩状态而无舒张吗？

（傅继华）

22　The relationship compare with myocardial contraction in time

PURPOSE

To know the cardiac – electric and contraction phase, excitation – contraction coupling, transverse tubular system.

PRINCIPLE

Heart pacemaker is sinoatrial node, (or venous sinus in amphibian). The excitation spreads to the whole heart by particular conduct path, and affect on myocardium of atria and ventricles, which can reach at contraction from intracellular sliding filament. Ion Ca^{2+} plays an important role in the process of the excitation – contraction coupling, and ion Ca^{2+} required come from extracellular mainly, as a result, the density of extracellular ion Ca^{2+} have great effect on myocardial excitation – contraction coupling.

Extracellular ion Ca^{2+} flows into cell through the transverse tubular system while Ringer's glycerite solution can destroy myocardial T system reversibly and prevent extracellular ion Ca^{2+} flowing into cell, which can stop excitation – contraction coupling and let myocardial electric activity fail to introduce contraction.

MATERIALS

1. Equipments BL – 420F biological signal acquisition and analysis system (or two – channel physiological recorder) , surgical equipment, toad heart clip, toad heart cannula, double cave clamp, long dropper, wooden tube holder, operating table, iron bracket, universal pulley, Y – eletrode

2. Solutions Ringer' s solution, 25% hypertonic glycerite Ringer' s solution.

3. Object toad.

METHODS

1. Joint and regulation of the equipments

(1) Connect the equipments as the fig. 4 – 5.

(2) Condition: myocardial electricity record range: 0. 5mV/cm, time constant: 2s, frequency: 100Hz, DC. You can' t record until the graph and wave base – line keep steady, the sensibility is acceptable, and all kinds of waves show clearly. First choose slow speed, then 25mm/s.

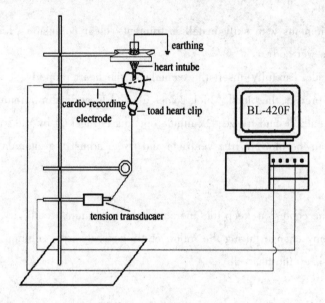

Fig. 4 – 5   The apparatus installment of the isolated toad heart

2. Operation

(1) Get a toad, destroy its brain and spinal cord. Open the thoracic cavity and expose the heart.

(2) Introduce double threads below the aorta, and turn over the bottom upwards with glass stick. A strong ligature is passed around the boundary between venous sinus and postcaval vein to be tied (Be careful not to tie venous sinus vein and semilunar gulf. The toad heart cannula and the toad table are at an angle of 15°. (Or isolated heart.)

(3) The clamp which link to thread clip the bottom of heart when it in diastole, then connect the thread with force – displacement transducer, transduce link to physical grapher.

(4) Needles inserted into the right fore – leg and left hind – leg name positive and negative respectively. Then connect to the one channel recorder, insert the earth into the right hind leg.

3. Observation items

(1) Normal ECG and myocardial contraction: normal Ringer's solution, first paper speed

10mm/s, then turn to 25mm/s. You can first find out the ECG to come into being before the contraction.

(2) Ringer's glycerite solution 25% : paper speed 10mm/s, ECG is still there, while contraction waves disappear.

(3) Normal Ringer's solution : Repeat the normal Ringer's solution and observe whether ECG and contraction waves come back.

GUIDANCE

1. Preview

(1) Mechanism of myocardial excitation and contraction.

(2) micro – structure of Skeletal muscle.

(3) Skeletal muscle excitation – contraction coupling and Sliding – Filament theory.

(4) Mechanism of the ECG.

2. Manipulation

(1) Adjust equipments with skill : install instruments, clear confusion which originates from : ① wrong earth; ② too wet body.

(2) Work on model carefully : insert the cannula in the heart properly; sometimes the cannula may be blocked and prevent the blood. which comes from : ① loose ligature around the vein that causes blood flow into ventricle and freeze; ② cannula opening is blocked by the wall of ventricle. In a word, you should clean the blood in the ventricle and try to adjust the cannula direction along the ventricle ordinate axis.

3. Notices

(1) Eliminate the confusion, keep the operating table and animal body dry.

(2) If there is any change during the inflow of Ringer's glycerite solution, you should replace the fluid in time for keep the heart alive.

4. Reports

(1) Write down the results, the actual order of the ECG and myocardial contraction. Tell the mechanism.

(2) Discuss phase relationship to the ECG and myocardial contraction, function of transverse tubular system in the excitation – contraction coupling.

(3) Tell the whole process from the excitation to contraction in the heart.

5. Questions

(1) How to prove Ca^{2+} which promote excitation – contraction coupling in heart originate from extracellular mainly.

(2) Would you raise some methods to force the heart in systole without diastole?

(Fu Jihua)

实验二十三　化学物质对蟾蜍离体心脏活动的影响

扫码"学一学"

【实验目的】

本实验沿用 Straub 氏法灌流离体蛙心，观察钠、钾、钙三种离子，肾上腺素、乙酰胆碱等因素对心脏活动的影响。

【实验原理】

作为两栖类动物蟾蜍或蛙心起搏点的静脉窦，能自动产生节律性兴奋。将失去神经支配的离体蛙心保持在适宜的理化环境中，在一定时间内仍能保持节律性兴奋，产生节律性收缩。因此，心脏正常的节律性活动依赖于内环境理化因素的相对稳定。改变灌流液的成分，可以引起心脏活动的改变。

【实验材料】

1. 器材　BL – 420F 生物信号采集与分析系统，张力换能器，蛙心夹，滑轮，木质试管夹，铁支架，双凹夹，蛙心插管，蛙类手术器械，滴管，搪瓷杯，缝线

2. 溶液　任氏液、0.65% NaCl、1% $CaCl_2$、1% KCl、1：10000 肾上腺素溶液和 1：10000 乙酰胆碱溶液

3. 对象　蟾蜍或蛙。

【实验方法】

1. 离体蛙心制备

（1）取蟾蜍一只，破坏脑和脊髓后，将其仰卧固定在蛙板上，从剑突下将腹部皮肤向上剪开，然后剪掉胸骨，打开心包，暴露心脏。

（2）在两根主动脉下方引 2 根线。一条在左主动脉上端结扎作插管时牵引用；另一根则在动脉圆锥上方，系一松结用于结扎固定蛙心插管。

（3）左手持左主动脉上方的结扎线，用眼科剪在松结上方左主动脉根部剪一倒"V"形小口（不能剪断动脉），右手将盛有少许任氏液的大小适宜的蛙心插管由此剪口处插入动脉圆锥。当插管头到达动脉圆锥时，再将插管稍稍后退，并转向心室中央方向（左后方）。左手用镊子轻提房室沟周围的组织，右手小指或无名指轻推心室，在心室收缩期将插管插入心室。切忌用力过大和插管过深。如果蛙心插管已经进入心室，则插管内的任氏液液面可随心室的舒缩而上下波动。用滴管吸去插管内的血液，换任氏液冲洗 1 ~ 2 次。把预先准备好的松结扎紧，并固定在蛙心插管的侧钩上，以免蛙心插管滑出心室。剪断两根主动脉。

（4）轻轻提起蛙心插管以抬高心脏，用一线在静脉窦与腔静脉交界处作一结扎，结扎线应尽量下压，以免伤及静脉窦。在结扎线外侧剪断腔静脉，游离蛙心。

（5）用滴管吸取新鲜任氏液换洗蛙心插管内液体数次，直至蛙心插管内灌流液无血色为止。此时离体蛙心已制备成功，可供实验。

2. 仪器装置　按图 4 – 6 示方法连接 BL – 420F 生物信号采集与分析系统。先用木质试

扫码"看一看"

管夹夹住蛙心插管，再将木质试管夹通过双凹夹固定在铁支架上。用一端带有长线的蛙心夹在心室舒张期夹住心尖，并将蛙心夹的线头连至张力换能器的应变梁上（也可通过滑轮）。通过调节滑轮的位置以使此线具有适当的紧张度。

3. 观察项目

（1）描记正常的蛙心搏动曲线。注意观察心跳频率及心室的收缩和舒张程度。

（2）把蛙心插管内的任氏液全部更换为 0.65% NaCl 溶液，观察心跳变化。

（3）把 0.65% NaCl 吸出，用新鲜任氏液反复换洗数次，待曲线恢复正常时，再在任氏液内滴加 3% $CaCl_2$ 1～2 滴，观察心跳变化。

（4）将含有 $CaCl_2$ 的任氏液吸出，用新鲜的任氏液反复换洗，待曲线恢复正常后，在任氏液中加 1% KCl 1～2 滴，观察心跳变化。

（5）将含有 KCl 的任氏液吸出，用新鲜的任氏液反复换洗，待曲线恢复正常后，再在任氏液中加 1∶10000 的肾上腺素溶液 1～2 滴，观察心跳变化。

（6）将含有肾上腺素的任氏液吸出，用新鲜的任氏液反复换洗，待曲线恢复正常后，再在任氏液中加 1∶10000 的乙酰胆碱溶液 1～2 滴，观察心跳变化。

【实验指导】

1. 预习要求

（1）复习有关心脏活动的神经、体液调节理论。

（2）复习心肌的四大生理特性及其影响因素。

2. 操作要点　本实验的难点是将蛙心插管插入心脏的心室内。插管时要认真、细心，要在心室的收缩期将插管插入。因为此时主动脉瓣处于开启状态。另外，在静脉窦与前后腔静脉之间结扎时，切勿扎及静脉窦（起搏点所在）。可一人结扎，另一人用镊子将线结下压，然后再结扎。

3. 注意事项

（1）游离蛙心时，勿伤及静脉窦，要连静脉窦一起取下。

（2）吸新鲜任氏液的滴管要与吸插管内液体的滴管要分开，以免影响观察实验现象和分析结果。

（3）蛙心插管内液面应保持恒定（约2cm），以免影响结果。

（4）进行各观察项目时，作用明显后应立即用新鲜任氏液换洗，以免心肌受损使心跳难以恢复。待心跳恢复正常频率和幅度后方能进行下一步实验。

（5）滴加药品时，要及时标记，以方便观察分析。

（6）化学药物作用不明显时，可再适当加量。

4. 报告要点

（1）附记录曲线，并对实验现象进行描述。

（2）根据结果分析 Na^+、Ca^{2+}、K^+、肾上腺素、乙酰胆碱对心跳各有什么影响？机制如何？

5. 思考题

（1）简述心肌细胞动作电位产生机制。

（2）有哪些因素影响心肌兴奋性、自律性、传导性及收缩性？

（丁启龙）

23 Effects of chemical substances on the activity of the isolated toad heart

PURPOSE

Using Straub's infusing method, observe the effects of three ions (sodium, potassium and calcium) and two chemical substances (acetylcholine and adrenaline) on the activity of the heart in vitro.

PRINCIPLE

The vein sinus, which is the pacemaker of the heart in the amphibious animal, such as toad or frog, can automatically produce the rhythmic stimuli. The isolated heart in a simulated physiological environment, despite out of the nerve control, can also keep the rhythmic stimuli and produce rhythmic constriction in a time. Therefore, the normal rhythmic activity of the isolated heart depends on the stability of the inside environment. Alteration of the component in the infuse liquid can change the activity of the isolated heart.

MATERIALS

1. Equipments   BL – 420F biological signal acquisition and analysis system, tension transducer, operational instruments of frog, toad heart clip, pulley, tube clip, iron stand, double cave clamp, toad heart cannula, operational plate for toad, dropper, beaker, suture.

2. Solutions Ringer's   solution, 0. 65% NaCl, 1% $CaCl_2$, 1% KCl, 1 : 10000 adrenalin and 1 : 10000 acetylcholine.

3. Object   toad or frog.

METHODS

1. Preparation of the isolated heart

(1) Take a toad, after damaging its brain and spinal cord, lay it on back and fix it on the toad plate. Cut the skin of the upper abdomen near the xiphoid, then shear the breastbone, open the pericardium, and expose the heart.

(2) Put two lines under the two aortas. One, made a knot at the superior extremity of the left aorta, is used to tow when intubation; the other is above arterial cone, joined a slipknot to ligate and fix the cannula of the heart.

(3) The left hand holds the ligature above the left aorta, shears a reversed "V" shaped incision with ophthalmological scissors at root of the left aorta and above the slipknot (doesn't cut off the aorta); the right hand inserts a proper cannula of toad heart that contains a little Ringer's solution into the artery cone from the cut position. When the top of the cannula reaches the arterial cone, withdraw the cannula a little, and turn it to the direction of the ventricle central (left rear). The left hand holds up the tissue around atrioventricular groove with a forceps, the little finger or the ring finger of right hand pushes the ventricle gently. Insert the cannula into the ventricle at the systole. Avoid overexerting or intubing deeply. If the cannula has already entered the ventricle, the sur-

face of Ringer's solution in the cannula would fluctuate up and down following the diastole and contraction of the ventricle. Take out the blood in the cannula with a dropper, and wash it 1 ~ 2 times with fresh Ringer's solution. Ligate the prepared slipknot tightly, and fix it on the side hook of the cannula to prevent the cannula to slip out of the ventricle. Cut off two aortas.

（4）Hold up the cannula gently to raise heart, make a ligation at the boundary of the venous sinus and the vena cava. In order to avoid harming the venous sinus, the ligation should be made as low as possible. Cut off the vena cava at the nether side of the ligation; dissociate the heart from the toad.

（5）Take the fresh Ringer's solution with a dropper to exchange the liquid in the cannula several al times, until the infused liquid isn't red. At this time an isolated toad heart has already been made successfully and can be supplied for experiment.

2. Apparatus installment   Link the BL − 420F biological signal acquisition and analysis system according to fig. 4 − 6. At first clamp the cannula with a wooden tube clip, and then the wooden tube clip is fixed on the iron bracket by a double cave clamp. Clamp the tip of the heart at ventricle diastole with a toad heart clip that is linked with a long line in the other end, and then link the line to the adaptive bridge in the tension transducer (also can be linked to a transducer through a pulley). Regulate the position of the pulley or the double cave clamp in order that the tensility of line is appropriate.

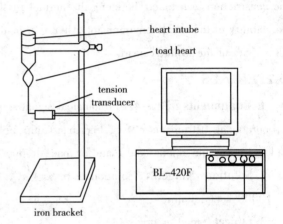

Fig. 4 − 6   **The apparatus installment of the isolated toad heart**

3. Observation items

（1）Record the normal curve of the diastole and constriction of the isolated heart. Pay attention to observing the frequency and the amplitude of the heartbeat.

（2）After the Ringer's solution in cannula is all replaced by 0.65% NaCl solution, observe the change of the heartbeat.

（3）Take out the 0.65% NaCl solution, wash it several times repeatedly with fresh Ringer's solution. When the heartbeat recovers to normal, add 1% $CaCl_2$ 1 ~ 2 drops to the Ringer's solution in the cannula, and then observe the change of the heartbeat.

（4）Take out the Ringer's solution including $CaCl_2$, wash it several times repeatedly with fresh Ringer's solution. After the curve recovers to normal, add 1% KCl 1 ~ 2 drops in the Ringer's solution in the cannula, observe the change of the heartbeat.

（5）Take the Ringer's solution including KCl, wash it several times repeatedly with fresh Ringer's solution. After the curve recovers to normal, then add 1 : 10000 adrenalin 1 ~ 2 drops in the Ringer's solution in the cannula, observe the change of the heartbeat.

（6）Take the Ringer's solution including adrenalin, wash it several times repeatedly with fresh Ringer's solution. After the curve recovers to normal, add 1 : 10000 acetylcholine 1 ~ 2 drops in the

Ringer's solution in the cannula, observe the change of the heartbeat.

GUIDANCE

1. Preview

(1) Review the theory of nerve and humoral regulation on the heart activity.

(2) Review the four physiological characteristics of the cardiac muscle and their influencing factors.

2. Manipulation
The difficult point in the experiment is how to insert the cannula into the ventricle. Be serious and careful when intubating. Insert the cannula at ventricular systole, because the aortic valve is in open condition at this time. Moreover, when ligating between the venous sinus and the vena cava, don't ligate the venous sinus (pacemaker position). When one is ligating, the other presses down the line knot with a forceps, then ligate it tightly.

3. Notices

(1) When isolating the heart, don't harm the venous sinus, take out the toad heart with the venous sinus together.

(2) The dropper to take the fresh Ringer's solution and the dropper to take the liquid in cannula should be separated lest affecting observation of the experiment phenomenon and analysis of results.

(3) Keep the stable height (2cm) of the liquid in cannula lest affecting results.

(4) When observing each item, wash the cannula with fresh Ringer's solution after the effect becomes obvious lest harming the cardiac muscle and recovering the heartbeat hardly. Don't turn to the next item until the heartbeat recovers to normal.

(5) As dropping a drug, mark it in time in order to observe and analyze expediently.

(6) When the action of a drug is not obvious, add a little again.

4. Reports

(1) Attach the recorded curve on the experimental report and describe the experiment phenomenon.

(2) Analyze the effects of Na^+, Ca^{2+}, K^+, adrenine and ACh on the heartbeat according to the results. What is the mechanism?

5. Questions

(1) What is the mechanism that the myocardial cells produce the action potential?

(2) Which factors affect the excitability, autorhythmicity, conductivity and contractility in the myocardial cells respectively?

(Ding Qilong)

实验二十四　豚鼠心室肌细胞动作电位测定

【实验目的】

通过学习单个心肌细胞动作电位的记录方法，从而加深对心肌细胞电生理特征的理解。

【实验原理】

心肌细胞与其他可兴奋细胞一样，在静息状态下其细胞的膜内外存在电位差，内负外正，呈极化状态。当心肌细胞受到外来刺激或在体心脏的心肌受到传导而来的兴奋时，也可产生动作电位，但动作电位的形状和特征与其他可兴奋细胞的电活动有明显区别，其时程可长达几百毫秒。通常将心肌细胞的动作电位分 0～4 五个时相：0 时相包括除极化和超射，其最大上升速率 V_{max} 可达 800～1000V/s；早期复极化的 1 时相快速而短暂，占时约 10ms；2 时相又称平台期，其电位持续于 0mV 左右，历时 100～150ms，是整个动作电位持续时间长的主要原因；3 时相是一快速复极化过程，膜内电位逐步向静息电位的水平恢复，历时可达 100～150ms；4 时相是极化状态的恢复，膜电位稳定于静息电位水平。

本实验应用细胞内微电极技术，结合微机自动分析，观察豚鼠心肌细胞动作电位的形态特征。

【实验材料】

1. 器材 微电极放大器 1，微电极操纵器 1，双通道电子刺激器及隔离器 1，微分器 1，前置放大器 1，双线长余辉示波器 1，微型计算机 1，钢瓶（内含 95% O_2 + 5% CO_2），屏蔽及防震实验台，有机玻璃肌槽，超极恒温水浴 1，电子蠕动泵 1，玻璃微电极（电阻 10～30MΩ，其内充灌 3M 的 KCl 溶液），铂金丝双电极，Ag－AgCl 乏极化电极，硅橡胶块，长约 0.5cm 的不锈钢小针若干，哺乳动物手术器械一套。

2. 药品 台氏液成分（mmol/L）：NaCl 136.7，KCl 5.4，$CaCl_2$ 1.8，$MgCl_2$ 1.05，$NaHCO_3$ 11.9，NaH_2PO_4 1.1，Glucose 5.5。

3. 动物 豚鼠 1，体重 300～400g。

【实验方法】

1. 仪器连接和调试

（1）按图 4－7 示意连接仪器。

（2）由 Ag－AgCl 电极引导出电位，经微电极放大器放大后分三路：一路送至示波器上线进行肉眼观察或拍照记录；一路经前置放大器 A 通道后再经转换开关 R（拨至 A）送达微机；最后一路送入微分器，对动作电位的 V_{max} 进行微分。经过微分后的电信号又分成两路，一路送至示波器下线观察，另一路经前置放大器 B 通道后再经转换开关 R（拨至 B）送入微机，微机由刺激器触发采样并分析动作电位的各项参数，将结果打印输出。

（3）调试各仪器参数

①刺激器，频率 60 次/分，波宽 1ms，输出强度 10V 档级，同步输出触发示波器扫描。

②微电极放大器，高频滤波 10kHz，增益 10 倍。

③前置放大器，增益 100 倍，高频滤波 100kHz。

④微分器，∧校正 200V/s，高频滤波 100kHz，时间常数 20μs。

⑤示波器，DC 输入，y 轴增益 20mV/cm，x 轴扫描为 10s/cm 档级进行微调。

⑥微机系统，放大倍数 50，0 相采样同期 t 为 20μs，整个动作电位采样同期 T 为 2ms，校正值（d）为 200V/s（本实验室采用 Doctor－1 软件系统）。

2. 标本制作　用木锤击昏豚鼠后迅速取出心脏，用台氏液冲洗后，投入充有 $95\% O_2 +$ $5\% CO_2$ 饱和的台氏液培养皿中（温度为 15℃ 左右），剪开右心室取下乳头肌标本，将标本以水平方向用不锈钢细针固定于肌槽的硅橡胶上，以 $95\% O_2 + 5\% CO_2$ 饱和的台氏液循环灌流，温度为 $37 \pm 0.5℃$，流速为 4ml/min，pH7.2～7.4。

3. 刺激标本　在解剖显微镜下，调节刺激电极操纵器，将一对刺激电极移至乳头肌根部上方，轻压标本，调节刺激强度起搏心肌，以 150% 阈值的刺激强度持续刺激 1 小时后开始记录动作电位。

4. 安装微电极　将充满 3MKCl 的玻璃微电极用蒸馏水冲洗外壁后，取滤纸将外壁吸干，其末端吸去 3～4mm KCl 溶液，插入一根 Ag－AgCl 引导电极，最后将微电极固定在微电极操纵器上，调节转角锁紧旋钮，使微电极与台氏液液面垂直，再调节水平面的 x 轴和 y 轴的拖板，使微电极对准乳头肌，旋转 y 轴粗调，将微电极下降并使尖端与台氏液接触，参考电极直接放入槽内台氏液中，与微电极放大器探头上的接地端相连。

5. 调节微电极放大器　微电极与台氏液接通后，调节微电极放大器"零平衡"旋钮，使微电极放大器与示波器 y 轴均显示零电位，此时表示极化补偿完毕。

按下"阻抗"钮，此时示波器上显示一串方波，测量方波高度，从而计算电极电阻（MΩ/mV），选择电阻为 10～30MΩ 的电极进行穿刺。

将参考电极与微电极放大器探头上的校正端相连，按下"校正"钮，此时示波器上呈现一串方波，调节"容量补偿"钮，使方波的上升沿与方波的顶边成直角，此时表示高频补偿完成。

6. 校正信号采集　如采用微分器分析 0 相上升速率，则需给微机提供一个 0 相最大速率的校正值。将微分器输入选择开关拨至"校正"，"Λ校正"选择 200V/s，此时微分器输出一个三角波信号，该信号经微电极再引入微分器，经微分后，在微机上可采到一矩形波，该矩形波的高度即表示速率为 200V/s。校正完毕，输入选择拨至"Λ"。

7. 测定心肌细胞动作电位　向下转动微操纵器，微电极尖端一插入心肌细胞内，即可见到示波器上线向下跳动约 90mV（微电极放大器显示 -90mV 左右），此即静息电位，当给予适宜电刺激时，即可见动作电位图形（图 4-8）。

8. 观察项目

（1）在示波器上测量静息电位幅度（mV）、动作电位幅度（mV），0 相最大速率（V/s）、动作电位时程（ms），并与微机分析结果比较。

（2）测定有效不应期　在基础频率为 1Hz 的基础上，每 8 次刺激插入一次期前刺激，期前刺激波的波宽和强度均为基础节律刺激的 2 倍，改变期前刺激和基本节律刺激之间的时间间隔，以期前刺激能引起动作电位产生的最短时间间隔为有效不应期，比较有效不应期与 90% 动作电位时程之间的关系。

（3）改变刺激频率，分别以 0.5、1、2、3Hz 刺激标本，上述各参数动作电位的时程有何规律性变化。

【实验指导】

1. 预习要求

（1）心脏细胞跨膜电位的形成机制。

（2）有关仪器的原理和使用说明。

2. 操作要点

（1）用于拉制玻璃微电极的玻璃毛坯，预先要在王水中浸泡 8 小时左右，然后用清水冲洗，冲洗干净后再用蒸馏水煮三遍，烘干。

（2）在制备 Ag – AgCl 乏极化电极时，银丝表面应光滑，并用酒精脱脂。镀 AgCl 时，电流控制在 0.4mA 左右，以保证所涂 AgCl 牢固，不易脱落。

（3）要严格控制台氏液 pH，每次实验前均应调定 pH 在 7.2 ~ 7.4 范围内。

3. 注意事项

（1）实验室要有良好的屏蔽措施，远离磁场。

（2）应有专门的接地线，保证一点接地。

（3）标本制备要迅速、轻柔。标本固定以自然长度为准，避免过度牵拉。

（4）避免微电极内高浓度的 KCl 滴入肌槽内。

4. 报告要点

（1）分析动作电位图形。

（2）讨论心肌细胞动作电位的电生理基础。

5. 思考题

（1）试讨论温度或药物对心肌细胞动作电位的影响。

（2）刺激频率改变对动作电位的时程有何影响？有什么生理意义？

注：由于各实验室条件不同，所以应根据实际情况严格按照仪器使用说明书进行操作。

（颜天华　刘冰冰）

24　Action potential of ventricular cell in guinea pig

PURPOSE

To learn the methods of recording action potential of single ventricular cell, so as to have a good knowledge of the electrophysiological characteristics of cardiac muscle cell.

PRINCIPLE

It exists potential difference between inner membrane and outer membrane in resting condition of cardiac muscle cell like other excitable cells. The potential of outer membrane is positive and the potential of inner membrane is negative. Whencardiac muscle cell is stimulated or the excitement is conducted to cardiac muscle cell in vivo, action potential appears in cardiac muscle cell. The characteristics of action potential in cardiac muscle cell are different with other excitable cells. The period of action potential is more than ten centiseconds. The action potential in cardiac muscle cell is divided into 0 ~ 4 phase; 0 phase includes the depolarization and overshoot potential, the maximal rising velocity (V_{max}) can reach to 800 ~ 1000V/s; 1 phase includes the early repolarization which is short and rapid, the period is 10ms; 2 phase is also called platform period, the potential is about 0mV and is unchanged, the period is 100 ~ 150ms; 3 phase includes the repolarization which is rapid, the potential of inner membrane come back to resting potential, the period is 100 ~ 150ms; 4 phase is polarized state again, the membrane potential is stable at resting potential.

The microelectrode technique and the automatic analytical microcomputer are used to observe the shape characteristics of action potential in cardiac muscle cell in the experiment.

MATERIALS

1. Equipments microelectrode amplifier, microelectrode manipulator, doublechannel stimulator and isolato, differentiator, preamplification, double beam memory synchroscop, microcomputer, steel bottle ($95\% O_2 + 5\% CO_2$), board for shield and shock proof, lucite muscular socket, water bath, electronic shake pump, glass microelectrode (it is filled with 3M KCl solutions, electric resistance $10 \sim 30M\Omega$), platinum bipolar electrode, Ag – AgCl non – polarizable electrode, silastic mass, Stainless steel pins (0.5cm), an operational tool for mammal.

2. Solutions Turk's solution component: NaCl 136.7, KCl 5.4, $CaCl_2$ 1.8, $MgCl_2$ 1.05, $NaHCO_3$ 11.9, NaH_2PO_4 1.1, Glucose 5.5.

3. Experimental object Guinea pig (body weight $300 \sim 400g$).

METHOD

1. preparation of the recorder

(1) Refer to Fig. 4 – 7 and connect the devices.

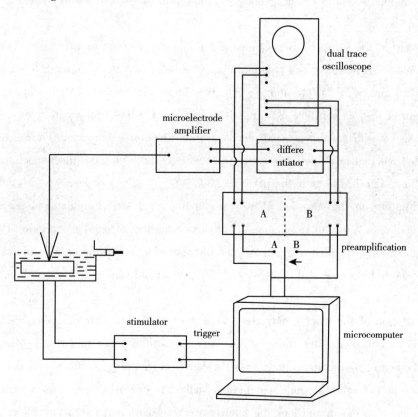

Fig. 4 – 7　abridged general view of device installation

(2) Connect the Ag – AgCl electrode to the microelectrode amplifier. Connect the microelectrode amplifier with three devices: superior part of the oscillograph for observing or taking photographs. A – channel of the preamplification, and the switcher is moved to A so as to the electric signal is sent to the microcomputer. the differentiator, and V_{max} of action potential is differentiated, then the electric signal is sent to two devices: inferior part of the oscillograph for observing. B – channel of the preamplification, and the switcher is moved to B so as to the electric signal is sent to the micro-

computer, the computer carries out sampling action by the trigger of stimulator and analyzes parameters of action potential, then prints the results.

（3）Adjustment of device parameters

①stimulator: The frequency is 60 times one minute, the width of waves is 1ms, the intensity of output is 10V step and the output triggers the scanning of the oscilloscope.

②microelectrode amplifier: The high – frequency of waves which are filtered is 10kHz, the gain is 10 times.

③preamplification: The gain is 100 times, the high – frequency of waves which are filtered is 100kHz.

④differentiator: The " $\wedge$ correction" is 200V/s, the high – frequency of waves which are filtered is 100kHz, the time constant is 20μs.

⑤synchroscope: The input current is direct current, the gain of Y – axis is 20mV/cm, the gain of X – axis is about 10s/cm, please readjust.

⑥microcomputer: The amplifying power is 50, the time of sampling action in 0 phase is 20μs, the time of sampling action in action potential is 20ms. (Doctor – 1 soft – ware system is used in the laboratory)

2. Makeup of the sample　Beat guinea pig to fall into a swoon by a hammer. Take the heart out quickly and wash it with turk's solution. Place the heart into the culture dish which is full of turk's solution saturated by 95% O_2 and 5% CO_2 (the temperature is about 15℃). Open right ventricle with a pair of scissors and take away papillary muscles. Fix the papillary muscles on the silastic of muscular socket with a stainless small needle whose direction is horizontal. Perfuse the papillary muscles with circulated turk's solution saturated by 95% O_2 and 5% CO_2 (the temperature is 37 ± 0. 5℃ , the flow – rate is 4ml/min, the pH is 7. 2 ~ 7. 4)

3. Stimulation on the sample　Control stimulating electrode manipulator under an anatomic microscope and move a pair of stimulating electrodes on the root of papillary muscles. Press the papillary muscles gently. Regulate the intensity of stimulation to excite the cardiac muscle. Stimulate the cardiac muscle for a hour at the intensity of 150% threshold value, then record the action potential of cardiac muscle.

4. Installation of the microelectrode　Wash the exterior of glass microelectrode full of 3M KCl solutions with distilled water, then dry the exterior with filter paper and suck 3 ~ 4mm KCl solutions from the end of the microelectrode, insert a Ag – AgCl guiding electrode into the end, fix the microelectrode on the microelectrode manipulator, make the microelectrode form a right angle with the surface of turk's solution and lock the knob, move the board to make the microelectrode aim at the papillary muscles, rotate the y – axis knob to descend the microelectrode in order to contact the tip with turk's solution, put reference electrode into turk's solution and connect it with the earth clamp of detecting head in the microelectrode amplifier.

5. Adjustment of the microelectrode amplifier　Turn on microelectrode power and set the "zero – balance" button of the microelectrode amplifier to make the microelectrode amplifier and the y – axis of oscilloscope show "zero potential". It is the time that the polarization has been compensated.

Press the "impedance" button and a string of square waves are showed on the oscilloscope, record the height of square waves in order to calculate the electric resistance of the electrode (MΩ/mV), puncture the microelectrode into the papillary muscles when the electric resistance is $10 \sim 30$MΩ.

Connect the reference electrode with the correction tip of the detecting head in the microelectrode amplifier, press the "correction" button and a string of square waves are showed on the oscilloscope, set the "capacity compensation" button to make the rise line of square waves form a right angle with the top line of square waves. It is the time that the high frequency has been compensated.

6. Correction of the signal collection　It is necessary to input a correction value of 0 – phase maximum velocity when the differentiator is used to analyze 0 – phase maximum velocity. Turn the "input selection" switch to "correction" and turn the " $\wedge$ correction" switch to 200V/s to result that the differentiator output a triangular wave signal. Input the signal to the differentiator through the microelectrode. After the signal is differentiated, record a rectangular wave whose height indicates the velocity is 200V/s on the microcomputer. Turn the "input selection" switch to " $\wedge$ " when the correction of the signal collection is over.

7. Determination of action potential on cardiac muscle cell　Turn down the microelectrode manipulator. When the tip of the microelectrode is inserted into cardiac muscle cell, the height of the top line decreases (it is showed the potential is about 90mV on the microelectrode amplifier), the potential is resting potential. When electric stimulation is adequate, the figure of action potential is showed (Fig. 4 – 8).

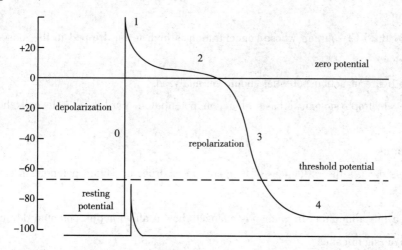

Fig. 4 – 8　resting potential and action potential of single cardiac muscle cell the down line shows 0 – phase maximal rising velocity

8. Observation items

(1)Measure the range of resting potential and action potential, 0 – phase maximum velocity, action potential duration on the oscilloscope. Compare them with the analytical results of microcomputer.

(2)Determinations of effective refractory period: When the basic frequency of stimulation is 1Hz, insert a extra stimulation whose wave width and intensity is two times of basic frequency stimulation each eight basic frequency stimulation to show up action potential, change the interval between

143

extra stimulation and basic frequencystimulation to result in the shortest interval which is effective refractory period. Compare effective refractory period with 90% action potential duration.

（3）When the frequency of stimulation is 0.5,1,2,3Hz,observe action potential duration to find some rules.

GUIDANCE

1. Preview

（1）Review the principle of transmembrane potential.

（2）Review the theory and introduction of the equipments.

2. Manipulation

（1）Soak the glass which is in primitive state in universal solvent for about 8 hours in advance, which is used to produce glass microelectrode,wash them with clean water and boil them three times with distilled water,toast them to dryness.

（2）Defat the silver wires whose surface is smooth with alcohol when the Ag – AgCl non – polarizable electrode is produced. Limit the current to about 0.4mA to firm the AgCl plating when the AgCl is plated.

（3）Set the pH value of turk's solution to the range of 7.2 ~ 7.4 before the experiment.

3. Notice

（1）The laboratory is shielded very well and is far away to magnetic field.

（2）The laboratory has earth wires which are used specially to connect the floor at a point.

（3）Produce the sample quickly and gently,fix the sample to the standard of natural length to avoid drag strongly.

（4）Avoid the KCl solution whose concentration is high to be dripped in the muscular socket.

4. Report

（1）The figure of action potential should be analyzed.

（2）The electrophysiological basis of action potential in cardiac muscle cell should be discussed.

5. Questions

（1）Please discuss the influences of temperature or drugs on action potential in cardiac muscle cell.

（2）When the stimulation frequency is changed,how it affect action potential duration? What is the physiological significance?

Note：Operate the experiment according to the specifications of the equipments at the basis of the condition of every laboratory because the condition of every laboratory is different.

（Yan Tianhua　Liu Bingbing）

实验二十五　人体心电图描记

【实验目的】

通过本实验了解人体正常心电图各波的波形及其生理意义，学习心电图机的使用方法

扫码"学一学"

和心电图波形的测量方法。

【实验原理】

心脏在收缩之前，首先发生电位变化。心电变化由心脏的起搏点——窦房结开始，经传导系统最后到达心室肌，并引起心肌的收缩。心脏犹如一个悬浮于容积导体中的发电机，其综合电位变化可通过体内组织和体液这一容积导体反映在体表。用体表电极所引导的这种电位变化，经心电图机的放大和记录，成为心电图。心电图可以反映心脏内综合性电位变化的发生、传导和消失过程，但与心脏的机械收缩活动无直接关系。正常人心电图包括P、QRS、T 三个波形。P 波表示心房去极化，QRS 波群表示心室去极化，T 波表示心室复极化。

【实验材料】

1. 器材　心电图机，诊断床，导电糊，酒精棉球。

2. 对象　人。

【实验方法】

1. 熟悉心电图机的基本结构与使用性能。心电图机的型号繁多，样式各异，但基本结构相似，有三个主要部件：①电流计，可以反映心脏不断变化的电流；②放大器，可以将心脏兴奋时的微弱电流加以放大，再引入电流计，以便记录或观察；③记录装置，一般采用热笔直接描记，将电流计中测出的电流在心电图纸上记录出来。

心电图机的主要控制旋钮及其作用如下：①导联选择开关，作为选择导联用，一般有Ⅰ、Ⅱ、Ⅲ、aVR、aVL、aVF、V1、V2、V3、V4、V5、V6 数挡。②记录开关：一般分为3 档，即"准备""观察"和"记录"。"准备"时，热笔电源切断，放大器输入封闭，热笔不偏转。在"观察"时，热笔接通电源，放大器开放，热笔偏转。在"记录"位时，开始走纸。使用前后及变换导联时，应置于"准备"位。③定标电压钮：按压此钮可得到方形标准电压。④衰减开关：分"2""1"和"1/2"三档。一般将"1"档按下。按下"1/2"档时，灵敏度减小一半。"1"档时，1mV 定标电压偏转 10mm。⑤走纸变速开关：一般有25mm/s 和 50mm/s 两档，多选用 25mm/s；大、小白鼠心率较快，宜选用 50mm/s。⑥基线调节钮：旋动此钮时，基线上下移动，一般将描笔置于中间位置。⑦热笔温度调节：可调节热笔的温度，顺时针转动使温度升高。此外，还有电源插孔和地线插孔。心电图机必须良好接地，以避免交流电干扰，保护受试者安全。

2. 按上述要求将心电图机面板上各控制钮置于适当位置，在妥善接地后心电图机接通电源，预热 5～20 分钟，同时令受试者安静平卧于诊断床，全身肌肉放松。

3. 安放电极，连接导联线。把准备安放电极的部位先用酒精棉球脱脂，再涂上导电糊，以减少皮肤电阻。电极应安放在肌肉较少的部位，一般应在两臂的腕关节上方（屈侧）约3cm 处，两腿的小腿下段内踝上方约 3cm 处。然后夹上电极夹。务必使电极夹与皮肤接触严密，以防干扰和基线漂移。之后，正确连接联线。一般有 5 种不同颜色的导联线插头与身体相应部位的电极相连，上肢：左黄、右红；下肢：左绿、右黑；胸白。胸部常用电极有 6 个，其位置如图 4 - 9 所示。

4. 调节基线，旋动基线调节钮，使基线位于中间。再输入标准电压，重复按动 1mV 定标电压按钮，调节灵敏度（或增益）旋钮，使标准方波上升10mm，开动记录开关，描记标准电压曲线。

5. 记录心电图，将"导联选择"分别拨到Ⅰ、Ⅱ、Ⅲ、aVR、aVL、aVF、V1~V6，逐一记录各导联上的心电图。

标准Ⅰ、Ⅱ、Ⅲ导联或称为双极肢导联。Einthoven规定Ⅰ导联为右臂–左臂、Ⅱ导联为右臂–左足、Ⅲ为左臂–左足之间所引导的记录。胸（V）导联的接法系由右臂、左臂、左足三连线各接一5KΩ的电阻，然后连接在一起作为参考电极（又称为Wilson中心电站），探测电极分别置于V1~V6诸位置。标准导联记录的是心动周期中，心电活动分别在各导联连线的投影；而V导联所引导的，则为所在处体表下心室表面的电位变化。如果以Wilson中心电站为参考电极；而探测电极在相应的肢体上，则称为单极肢体导联。因记录的电位很小，故将中心电站中所探测的联线取消，再将探测电极置于相应的肢体，可提高记录电压1.5倍，而图像不变。称此种导联为单极加压肢体导联。分别以aVR（右臂）、aVL（左臂）、aVF（左足）表示，以资区别。

标准导联所记录的心电图图形如图4–10。

6. 实验完毕，将心电图机面板上的各控制旋钮转回原处，切断电源。取下电极，擦净电极夹。

7. 心电图的测量与计算

（1）波幅测量　凡向上（正波）的波幅应从基线的上沿量到波的顶点，负波（基线以下的波）则应从基线的下沿量到波的最低点。若标准电压为1mV/10mm，则心电图上1mm代表0.1mV。

（2）心电图间期的测量　一般心电图记录时的走纸速度为25mm/s，每一小格代表0.04s。

P–P间期即两个P波之间的时间，代表一个心动周期的时间过程，可用来计算心率。也可用R–R间期来计算心率。由于R波峰较高尖，易于判定，故多用。

$$心率 = \frac{60}{P–P间期（s）或R–R间期（s）}$$

P–R间期（或P–Q间期）是从P波开始到R或Q波开始的间期，代表兴奋从心房传到心室的时间，正常为0.12~0.2s。

S–T间期　为QRS波终了到T波起点，代表心室完全去极化持续时间，此段通常位于零电位线，持续时间0.05~0.15s，视心率快慢而定。

Q–T间期　为Q波开始到T波结束，代表心室去极化到复极化的时间。

【实验指导】

1. 预习要求　预习心电图产生原理及各波形的生理意义，了解各波形的形状、大小及正常值范围。

2. 操作要点　用心电图机记录心电图，最主要的是消除干扰。一般要去除被记录者身上的金属物品，人体各部分肌肉放松，保持电极与人体、机器与大地接触良好。

3. 注意事项

（1）肌肉放松以消除肌电干扰。

（2）心电图机要良好接地。

4. 报告要点

（1）正确记录实验结果。

（2）按步骤 7 测量标准导联 Ⅱ 中各波的电压和各间期所占时间，写出其具体数值，并算出心率。

（3）根据心电观察结果，讨论心电波形产生原理，并说明各波形的生理意义。

5. 思考题

（1）P-R 间期与 Q-T 间期的正常值与心率有什么关系？

（2）试用心肌细胞电位来解释心电图各波及间期的形成。

（丁启龙）

25　Electrocardiogram in man

PURPOSE

The purpose of this experiment is to observe each wave of electrocardiogram（ECG）in man, to understand its physiological meaning, and to study the usage of the ECG machine and the measurement of waves.

PRINCIPLE

Before constringency, the electric activity in heart takes place first. The electric activity in the heart begins from sinus – atria node that is the pacemaker of the human heart, to the ventricle muscle along special conduction system and finally results in the constringency of the cardiac muscle. The heart resembles a generator suspending in a dimension conductor. Its integrated potential can be reflected on the surface of the body through the tissue and body fluid. This potential, introduced by the electrode on the surface of the body, is demonstrated as ECG through the enlarging and recording of ECG machine. The ECG can reflect the occurrence, conduction and disappearance of the integrated potential in the heart, but has no direct relation with the mechanistic constriction of the heart. The normal ECG in human includes three wave clusters, namely P, QRS and T wave. The P wave represents the depolarization of the atrium. The QRS wave cluster represents the depolarization of the ventricle. The T wave represents repolarization of the ventricle.

MATERIALS

1. Equipments　electrocardiogram machine, diagnosis bed, conducting electric paste, alcohol cotton ball.

2. Object　human.

METHODS

1. The basic construction and usage of ECG machine　Though there are numerous models and different styles for electrocardiogram machine, the basic construction of ECG machine resembles with three main parts：①amperemeter, reflecting the continuous current change in the heart；②amplifier, enlarging the weak current in the heart, and then inducting it into the amperemeter in order to record or observe；③the record device, recording the current in the amperemeter on the electrocardiogram paper by a electric heat pen.

The main manipulative knobs of the electrocardiogram machine and their functions are as follows: ①the lead choice switch, which can choose the leads such as Ⅰ, Ⅱ, Ⅲ, aVR, aVL, aVF, V1, V2, V3, V4, V5, V6 and so on. ②the record switch, is generally divided into 3 classes, namely "preparation", "observation" and "recording". When in "preparation", the power supply of the heat pen is cut off, the importation of the amplifier is closed, and the heat pen does not drifted. When in "observation", the power supply of the heat pen is turned on, the importation of the amplifier is opened, and the heat pen can be drifted. When in "recording", the recording paper is moving. The lead choice switch should be placed to the "preparation" before or after the usage and during the alteration of the lead. ③the standard voltage knob, pressed to get a square standard voltage. ④the attenuation switch, set into 3 classes, namely "2"、"1" and "1/2". Generally, the "1" class is chosen. When "1" class is pressed, the heat pen will drift 10 mm for 1 mV of standard voltage. When pressing the "1/2, the sensitivity will be attenuated to a half. ⑤the shifting switch of recording paper, with two classes of 25 mm/s and 50 mm/s. The 25 mm/s is been chosen in most instances. 50 mm/s is chosen properly in rat and mice because their heart rates are too high. ⑥the regulation knob of the base line, by moving which the base line is placed in the middle on the paper. ⑦the regulation knob of the heat pen temperature, which can adjust the temperature of the heat pen. When turning the knob clockwise, the temperature increases. Furthermore, there are still the power supply socket and the ground line socket in the machine. The electrocardiogram machine must be well connected to the ground in order to avoid the AC interference and to protect the examinate.

2. Placement of knobs　Place each knob on the front – panel in appropriate position according above requiremeuts. Turn on the machine afterconnecting to the ground, and warm up it for 5 ~ 20 minutes. The volunteer should lie on the diagnosis bed and relax whole muscles.

3. Emplace the electrodes and link the lead lines　Use some alcohol cotton balls to wipe the skin where the electrode will be placed in order to degrease. Then conduct electric paste should be coated to those positions in order to reduce the skin electric resistance. These electrodes should be placed where the muscle is less. Generally the positions are roughly 3 cm upper wrist joint in the front at two arms and roughly 3 cm upper ankle joint in the medial side at two legs. Then fix the electrode to the positions. It must be ensured that the contact between the electrode nip and the skin is tight against the interference and the excursion of base line. After electrode nips being emplaced, connect lead lines withthe nips. Generally, each lead line of 5 different colors should be plugged into the corresponding electrode nip: arms: left – yellow, right – red; Limbs: left – green, right – black; chest: white. The chest leads have 6 electrodes, their positions are showed in the Fig. 4 – 9.

V1: the intersection of the fourth rib space and the right edge of the breastbone. V2: the intersection of the fourth rib space and the left edge of the breastbone. V3: the middle point between V2 and V4. V4: the intersection of the middle line across the left collarbone and the fifth rib space. V5: the point on the left armpit front line and the same height as V4. V6: the point on the left armpit middle line and the same height as V4.

4. Regulate the base line　Move the regulating knob of the base line, and locate the base line in the middle.

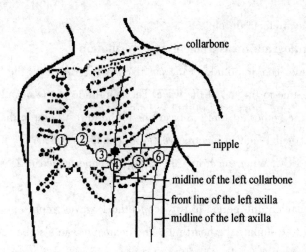

collarbone

nipple

midline of the left collarbone
front line of the left axilla
midline of the left axilla

Fig. 4 – 9 The emplacement position of chest electrodes

Input the standard voltage, repeatedly pressing the button of 1 mV standard voltage, and regulate the sensitivity knob (or the gain knob) to make the standard square wave rise 10 mm. Then start the recording switch and record the standard voltage curve.

5. Record the electrocardiogram Ⅰ, Ⅱ, Ⅲ, aVR, aVL, aVF, V1 ~ V6 are chosen by "lead choice" respectively, record the ECG of all the leads one by one.

Standard Ⅰ, Ⅱ, Ⅲ lead are also called the double pole limb lead. Einthoven prescribes: ECG of Ⅰ lead, Ⅱ lead and Ⅲ lead is the voltage change between the right arm – left arm, right arm – left foot or left arm – left foot respectively. The recording method of the chest (V) lead is to connect lines of right arm, left arm and left foot as a reference electrode (named Wilson center electric station) after linking each, line to a 5 kΩ resistance, and then place the probe electrodes on the V1 ~ V6 points respectively. The ECG recorded in standard leads is the projection of the heart electric activity on each lead line in cardiac cycle; While in V leads, the ECG is the voltage change of the ventricle surface under the surface of the body where the probe electrode is placed on. If the Wilson center electric station serves as a reference electrode and the probe electrode is placed on the corresponding limb, these leads are named single pole limb lead. Because the record voltage is very small, the line linked with the center electric station is cancelled and then the probe electrode is placed on the corresponding limb, thus the recorded voltage will be increased to 1. 5 times with the same image. These leads are named single pole adding voltage limb lead, expressed as aVR (right arm)、aVL (left arm) and aVF (left foot) respectively.

The ECG waves recorded in standard leads are showed in the Fig. 4 – 10.

6. Recover of knobs After the experiment being completed, turn each control knob on the front – panel to the original place, and cut off the power supply. Take

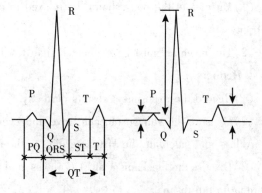

Fig. 4 – 10 The measurement method of the ECG waves

down electrodes and clean electrode nips.

7. The electrocardiogram measurement and calculation

(1) Wave amplitude. The amplitude of the positive wave (wave over the base line) is from the upper edge of the base line to the top of the wave. The amplitude of the negative wave (wave under the base line) is from the nether edge of the base line to the lowest point of the wave. If the standard voltage is 1mV/10mm, then 1 mm in electrocardiogram equals to 0.1mV.

(2) Interphase in ECG. When recording the ECG, the paper speed is 25 mm/s, and each small pane is 0.04s.

P – P interphase, namely the period of two sequential P waves, represents the time of a cardiac cycle, and can be used to calculate the heart rate. The heart rate can also be calculated with the R – R period. Because of R wave peak being high, tine and apt to judge, it is often used.

$$\text{Heart rate} = \frac{60}{\text{P – P interphase(s) or R – R interphase(s)}}$$

P – R interphase (or P – Q interphase), namely the period between the P wave starting point and the R or Q wave starting point, represents the stimuli spreading from the atrium to the ventricles. Its normal value is 0.12 ~ 0.2s.

S – T interphase, namely the period between the QRS wave terminal point and the T wave starting point, represents the entire depolarization duration of the ventricle. This interphase, usually locating in the zero potential line, is 0.05 ~ 0.15s and relates with the HR.

Q – T interphase, namely the period between the Q wave starting point and the T wave terminal point, represents the time from depolarization to repolarization of the ventricle.

GUIDANCE

1. Preview   Prepare the ECG mechanism and the physiological meaning of each wave in ECG. Understand the shape, size and normal value scope of each wave.

2. Manipulation   The main problem is how to eliminate the interference during recording the ECG. A general requirement is to take away any metal articles on the body, to keep each muscle of human body relaxing and to maintain good contacts between the electrodes and the body as well as the machine and the Earth.

3. Notices

(1) Muscles in the body should be relaxed in order to eliminate the interference of the muscle electricity.

(2) The machine must be connected rightly with the ground.

4. Reports

(1) Record the experiment results correctly.

(2) Measure the voltage of each wave and every interphase time in the standard Ⅱ lead, then write values and calculate the HR according to the methods in step 7.

(3) Discuss the mechanism of ECG waves, and explain the physiological meaning of every wave according to the results.

5. Questions

(1) What is the relation between the HR and the values of P – R interphase or Q – T inter-

phase?

（2）Try to explain the mechanism of the waves and interphases in ECG with the electrophysiology of cardiac muscle cells.

（Ding Qilong）

实验二十六　几种动物心电图描记

【实验目的】

学习几种动物心电图的描记方法，了解两栖类和哺乳类动物正常心电图的波形。

【实验原理】

在动物进化过程中，虽然心脏的结构和功能不断变化、逐渐完善，但心肌细胞的基本电活动却大同小异。整个心脏的综合电变化也可以通过心脏周围的导电组织传导到动物体表，通过心电图机记录出来。动物的心电图与人的心电图相似，基本包括P波、QRS波群和T波。但在某些动物心电图的QRS波群中，Q波较小或缺少；在变温动物中，心率受温度和其他因素的影响较大。

【实验材料】

1. 器材　心电图机（或示波器），动物手术台，蛙手术器械一套，蛙板，针形电极，探针，粗棉线。

2. 溶液　3%戊巴比妥钠。

3. 对象　蟾蜍，家兔，大白鼠。

【实验方法】

1. 动物的麻醉与固定　除大白鼠外，其余动物都可在不麻醉的情况下，进行心电活动的描记。根据不同动物的不同特点，采用不同的固定方法。

（1）蟾蜍　仰卧位固定于蛙板上，开始时出现挣扎，故在固定后需要安静20min左右方可进行描记。亦可先毁脑、脊髓，后再进行仰卧位固定。

（2）家兔　将清醒家兔取仰卧位固定于手术台上，常规固定其头部和四肢，但需拉紧缚带。开始固定时，动物挣扎较厉害，一般亦需安静20min左右，方可进行心电描记。

（3）大白鼠　用3%戊巴比妥钠按40mg/kg腹腔注射。麻醉后即可用粗棉线缚其四肢，仰卧位固定于手术台上。

2. 电极的安放与导线连接

（1）蟾蜍　以针形电极刺入蟾蜍四肢皮下，描记胸前导联时，可将电极刺入心尖部皮下。

（2）兔　前肢两针形电极分别插入相当于人肘关节上部的前臂皮下，后肢两针形电极分别插入相当于人膝关节上部的大腿皮下。胸导联V1～V6可参照人的相应部位安放。

（3）大白鼠　前后肢的四个针形电极同兔。大白鼠一般测以下四个导联：标准导联Ⅰ、

Ⅱ、Ⅲ和CF导联（即胸与大腿之间的电位差），胸部电极可置于心前区皮下。

如果使用心电图机描记，可参看人心电描记连接导线，也是5种不同颜色的导联线插头分别与动物体相应部位的针形电极连接：右上红、左上黄、左下绿、右下黑、胸前白。

如不使用心电图机，使用示波器也可观察心电图。示波器选用"AC"双端输入，灵敏度为1mV/cm，扫描速度可根据心率的快慢选定，导联选择标准肢体导联。将其导联的两条导联线连接示波器的输入端，即可在荧光屏上显示该导联的心电图波形。

3. 仪器调试　按照要求将心电图机面板上各控制钮置于适当位置，在妥善接地后通电。预热5分钟。调节基线于中间位置，确定走纸速度。输入标准电压，一般1mV/10mm，开动记录开关，记下标准电压曲线。

4. 记录心电图　旋动导联选择开关，依次记录Ⅰ、Ⅱ、aVR、aVL、aVF，如果描记胸导联，则可拨至V处进行描记。毁脑、脊髓蟾蜍在描记正常心电图波形后，可将心脏连同静脉窦一起剪下取出，观察是否仍能记录到心电图；再将心脏放回原位或倒置，观察心电图波形有无变化。

5. 记录完毕　取下针形电极，将心电图机面板上各控制钮复位后关机，并切断电源。

注　心电图的测量、计算与分析：

三种动物心电图如图4-11所示。大白鼠正常心电图与其他小哺乳类动物相似，有以下三个特点：①通常在导联Ⅰ和Ⅱ中P波是直立的，且易于读出，在导联Ⅲ中则可出现直立或倒立的波形；②没有明显的T波存在，当T波出现时，又缺乏等电位的ST段；③QRS波比较复杂，难以分析。出现上述特点的原因是小动物心率较快，P-P间期和QRS持续时间较短的缘故。

动物体重越轻，越小，心率有越快的倾向。冷血动物心率最慢，低温可降到10次/分，而在高温下不超过150次/分，ECG中，QRS为0.02~0.06s，与心率无关，但ST段随心率减慢而相应延长。

QRS波在任一种动物的ECG中均可见到，大动物T波非常低。在高温下，冷血动物的T波增高，处于冬眠时的低温条件下，T波消失。一般讲，氨基甲酸乙酯麻醉对动物的心率没有什么影响。仰卧位固定后，只要保持体温不变，在麻醉30~40min后开始的2~3h内，心率极其稳定，此后开始徐徐变动。戊巴比妥钠对心脏有一定抑制作用，特别是当静脉注射快时，可加快心率，使ST段移位，T波倒置。吸入性麻醉药如三氯甲烷对心脏毒性大，除非为引起心律失常，不可用于描记心电图实验动物的麻醉。乙醚能加快心率，三氯甲烷减慢心率。

【实验指导】

1. 预习要求　见人体心电图描记。

2. 操作要点　清醒动物记录ECG时，应待动物静止后进行，以防肌电干扰。动物ECG各波电压小，定标电压拟定1mV/20mm；心率快的，纸速应置于50mm/s。

3. 注意事项

（1）在清醒动物上进行心电描记，必须保证动物处于安静状态，否则动物挣扎，肌电干扰甚大。为此，在固定动物后需让其稳定一定时间，再进行描记。

（2）针形电极与导联连接必须紧密，如有松动，则出现干扰。

（3）记录过程中，每次变换导联时，必须先切断输入开关，待导联改变后再开启。每换一次导联，均须观察基线是否平稳及有无干扰。如基线不稳或有干扰存在，须调整或排除后再做记录。

4. 报告要点

（1）说明心电图各波的生理意义，按人的心电计算方法分析、计算动物的心电图，并与人的心电图做比较。

（2）若用蟾蜍做心电描记，请描述取出心脏、将心脏放回原处或倒置心脏时心电波形的变化。

5. 思考题

试分析不同动物心电图的特点。

（丁启龙）

26　Electrocardiogram in some animals

PURPOSE

The aims of the electrocardiogram（ECG）experiment in a few animals are to study the record method and to understand the normal ECG waveform in amphibious and mammal animal.

PRINCIPLE

Although the construction and function of heart are changing continuously and perfecting gradually in the evolving process, but the basic electric activity of myocardial cells is alike with minor differences.

The integrated electric activity in whole heart can be conducted to the surface of the animal by electric conductive tissue around the heart and be recorded by a electrocardiograph. The electrocardiogram of the animal resembles the ECG in the human, including P wave, QRS wave cluster and T wave. But in QRS cluster of ECG in a few animals, Q wave is small or lack. The heart rate of the poikilothermal animal is affected by temperature and other factors.

MATERIALS

1. Equipments　electrocardiogram machine（or oscillograph）, animal operation table, operational instruments of frog, frog plate, needle electrode, metal probe, cotton thread.

2. Solutions　3% sodium pentobarbital.

3. Objects　toad or frog, rabbit, rat.

METHODS

1. Anesthesia and fixation of animals　Except for rat, the ECG of other animals can be recorded in conscious state. Difference fixation methods are adopted according to different animals.

（1）Toad　Toad is put back on the frog plate and fixed. Because the toad appears flounder during the starting of the fixation, ECG cannot be recorded until 20 minutes after fixation. ECG can also be recorded after destroying brain and spinal marrow of the toad.

（2）Rabbit　A conscious rabbit is taken on its back to the surgical operation table and fixed. Its head and limbs are fixed as routine regulations, and the fixation cords should be tensed. Because the rabbit appears flounder during the starting of the fixation, ECG cannot be recorded until 20 minutes after fixation, too.

(3) Rat   Injecting 3% sodium pentobarbital (40 mg/kg) into the abdominal cavity. After placing its back on the table, binding its limbs with cotton thread.

2. Electrode emplacement and electrical wire connection

(1) Toad   The needle electrodes are inserted into the skin of the toad limbs. When recording ECG of chest lead, the electrode should be inserted into the skin of the chest near the heart.

(2) Rabbit   Two needle electrodes are inserted into the upper skin of forelegs, as corresponding that of human elbowjoint; two needle electrodes are inserted into the thigh skin, as corresponding that of human knee joint. The positions of needle electrodes of chest lead V1 ~ V6 can be determined referring to the ECG record in human.

(3) Rat   The positions of four needle electrodes in forelimbs and hind legs are the same as those in rabbit. Four leads are recorded in rat generally: standard lead Ⅰ、Ⅱ、Ⅲ and CF lead which represents the voltage between the chest and leg. The electrode in chest should be inserted into the skin near the heart.

If an ECG machine is chosen, you may connect the electric wire referring to methods in human ECG record. Those plugs of five lead lines with different colors are connected with needle electrodes inserted into the skin of animal respectively: right upper limb – red, left upper limb – yellow, left lower limb – green, right lower limbblack, chest – white.

If there is no ECG machine, the oscillograph can be used to observe the electrocardiogram. The "AC" double input in oscillograph may be chosen. The sensitivity is 1mV/cm; the scan speed is chosen according to heart rate; and the standard limb lead is chosen. The two lines of the lead are connected to the importer in oscillograph, and then the ECG wave is showed on the fluorescence screen immediately

3. Debugging of the electrocardiogram machine   Set each knob on the front – panel in the ECG machine in the appropriate position according to the operating request, and switch the machine on after appropriately connecting to the ground. Warm up 5 minutes. Regulate the base line in the middle position and determine the paper speed. Input the standard voltage with 1mV/10 mm. Start to record the standard voltage curve.

4. Recording ECG   Move the lead choice switch, record the ECG of the Ⅰ, Ⅱ, Ⅲ, aVR, aVL and aVF in turn. If recording ECG of the chest lead, move the lead choice switch to the V and then record. After recording the normal ECG in the toad ruined brain and spinal marrow, take out the heart with vein sinus, observe whether the ECG can be recorded. Then put the heart back in the primary position or set it upside down, observe the change of the waves.

5. After recording   Dismantle the needle electrode, restore each control knob on the front – panel of electrocardiogram machine to the primary position, and cut off the power supply.

Notes   ECG measurement, calculation and analysis:

Electrocardiogram in three kinds of animals is showed in Fig. 4 – 11.

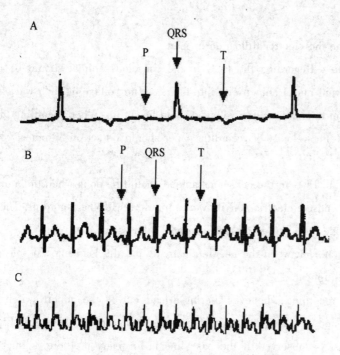

Fig. 4-11 ECG in 3 kinds of animal (Ⅱ lead)

A:toad. B:rabbit. C:rat. (1mV = 10mm)

The normal electrocardiogram in rat is similar to that in the other small mammals. It possesses the following three characteristics:①The P wave is upright in Ⅰ and Ⅱ lead usually, and can be read out easily. But in the lead Ⅲ, the P wave may be either erect or upside down. ②There is not an obvious T wave. And even when T wave emerges, there is no S – T segment of the equal potential. ③The QRS wave cluster is too complicated to analyze.

The emergence of the above characteristics attributes to the high heart rate and the short P – P interval and QRS duration in the ECG of these small animals.

There is a tendency that the smaller animal weight is, the higher its heart rate is. The heart rate of cold – blooded animal is the slowest, and it can decline to about 10 beats/min under low temperature, but do not exceed 150 beats/min under high temperature. In the ECG, QRS (0. 02 ~ 0. 06s) is irrelevant with the heart rate, but ST segment is correspondingly extended with heart rate slowing.

QRS wave can be seen in the ECG of any animals. T wave of the ECG in big animal is very low. However, in the cold – blooded animals, T wave rises under high temperature, but disappears under low temperature in dormancy.

Generally, the heart rate is not influenced by ethylurethane. When the animal is on its back and with constant body temperature, its HR is extraordinarily stable during the 2 ~ 3 hours from 30 ~ 40 min after anesthesia, and then begins to change. The pentobarbital sodium has an inhibition on the heart with heart rate quickening, which includes ST segment shifting and T wave upside down, especially when fast injected intravenously. Because of their serious toxicity, the inhalational anesthetic medicines, such as chloroform, can't be used for anesthesia in recording ECG experiment unless for causing arrhythmia. The HR can be accelerated by aether, but slowed down by chloroform.

GUIDANCE

1. Preview   See the electrocardiogram in man.

2. Manipulation   Recording the ECG in the conscious animal should be done in the calm state in order to prevent muscle electricity interference. The voltage of each wave in animal ECG is low, so 1mV/20mm of the demarcation voltage should be set up. When recording the ECG in the animal with a high HR, the velocity of recording paper should be set on 50mm/s.

3. Notices

(1) Recording the ECG in the conscious animal should be done when the animal is calm. If the animal struggles, the muscle electric activity would interfere with the recording. Therefore the recording should not be done until the animal is fixed and calms down.

(2) The conjunction between the needle electrode and the lead must be close, or AC interference with 50 Hz will appear.

(3) During the recording, whenever altering a lead, cut off the import switch first, then change the lead and finally open the switch again. After every change of the lead, stability of the base line and interference must be observed. If the base line is unsteady or there is interference, the ECG could be recorded only after adjustment or removal.

4. Reports

(1) Elucidate the physiological meaning of each wave of ECG. According to the calculation method in human ECG, analyze and compute the ECG, and then compare it with that in man.

(2) If the animal for recording ECG is toad, please describe varieties of waves in ECG during taking out the heart and putting the heart back in the original place or setting the heart upside down.

5. Question   Try to analyze the characteristics of ECG in different animals.

(Ding Qilong)

实验二十七　家兔动脉血压的神经体液调节

扫码"学一学"

【实验目的】

本实验是用直接测量和记录动脉血压的急性实验方法，观察神经和体液因素对动脉血压的调节作用。

【实验原理】

在生理情况下，人和其他哺乳动物的血压相对稳定，这种相对稳定是通过神经和体液因素的调节而实现的。神经调节中以颈动脉窦 – 主动脉弓压力感受性反射（减压反射）尤为重要。此反射既可在血压升高时降压，又可在血压降低时升压。此反射的传入神经为主动脉神经和窦神经。家兔的主动脉神经为独立的一条神经，称减压神经，易于分离和观察其作用。在人、犬等动物，主动脉神经和迷走神经混为一条，不能分离。调节心血管运动的体液因素最重要的是肾上腺素和去甲肾上腺素。本实验通过压力换能器把压力转化成电

156

信号，输入到计算机，利用 BL-420F 直接显示动脉血压及其波动。

【实验材料】

1. 器材　BL-420F 生物信号采集与分析系统、压力换能器、保护电极、兔手术台、哺乳动物手术器械、铁支架、双凹夹、试管夹、气管插管、塑料动脉插管、动脉夹、注射器（10ml、5ml、1ml）、丝线、棉花、纱布。

2. 溶液　20% 氨基甲酸乙酯，肝素（1000U），1∶10000 肾上腺素，1∶10000 乙酰胆碱，含 0.5% 肝素的生理盐水。

3. 对象　兔。

【实验方法】

1. 实验装置　如图 4-12 连接安装好实验装置，要求压力换能器的高度与心脏在同一水平为准。

2. 动物的麻醉与固定　家兔称重，从耳缘静脉缓慢注射 20% 氨基甲酸乙酯（1g/kg）进行麻醉，待动物角膜反射消失后，将其仰卧位固定于兔手术台上，打开手术台底面电灯保温。

扫码"看一看"

3. 手术　颈部剪毛，暴露手术野，在紧靠喉头下缘沿颈部正中线切开皮肤 5~7cm，用止血钳分离皮下组织，暴露胸骨舌骨肌，再用止血钳于正中线分开肌肉，即可暴露气管，进行气管插管。用止血钳拉开气管上方皮肤、肌肉，即可在气管两侧见到与气管平行的左、右颈总动脉。颈总动脉旁有一束神经与之伴行，这束神经中包含有迷走神经、交感神经及减压神经。小心分离颈动脉鞘，仔细识别三条神经，迷走神经最粗，交感神经较细，减压神经最细且常与交感神经紧贴在一起。一般先分离颈总动脉及迷走神经，然后分离减压神经与交感神经。每条神经分离出 2~3cm，在各条神经下穿一条不同颜色的丝线以便区分。颈动脉下亦穿一条丝线备用。本实验分离左侧颈总动脉以测量血压，分离右颈总动脉和右侧神经分别作阻断血流和刺激用。

4. 动脉插管　首先从耳缘静脉注入肝素（500U/kg 体重）以防凝血，然后在已连接塑料动脉插管的压力换能器内注满肝素生理盐水。

在分离出来的左侧颈总动脉远心端处（尽可能靠头端），用丝线将动脉结扎。在颈总动脉近心端（尽可能靠心端），用动脉夹将动脉夹住。于两者之间另穿一线，打一活结；在紧靠远心端结扎处，用锐利的眼科剪在动脉上沿向心方向做一斜形切口，约切开管径的一半，将准备好的动脉套管由切口插入动脉内，用备好的丝线将套管尖端固定于动脉管内，并将余线结扎于套管的侧管上，以免滑脱。保持套管与血管方向一致，以防扭转或套管尖端刺破动脉管壁见图 4-13。

5. 观察项目　在实验装置准备妥当，手术完毕以后，慢慢放松动脉夹，即可见有少量血液自颈总动脉冲向动脉插管。如不漏血，即可观察记录血压。

（1）描记一段正常曲线。识别一级波（心搏波）与二级波（呼吸波）。一级波是由心脏舒缩而引起的血压波动，二级波是由呼吸时肺的扩张和缩小引起的血压波动。见图 4-14。

（2）用动脉夹夹闭右侧颈总动脉 15 秒，观察血压变化。

（3）刺激减压神经，调节电刺激器的输出强度于 10V，用频率为 8~16Hz，波宽 2~5ms 的连续刺激，通过保护电极刺激一侧减压神经，观察血压有何变化。然后进行双结扎，在两结扎线之间切断神经，以上述同样强度的电流依次刺激减压神经的向中端和离中端，观察记录血压变化。

（4）结扎右侧迷走神经，于结扎线头端将神经剪断，用同样强度的电流刺激迷走神经离中端，观察血压变化。

（5）从耳缘静脉注入 1：10000 肾上腺素 0.3ml，观察血压变化。

（6）从耳缘静脉注入 1：10000 乙酰胆碱 0.3ml，观察血压变化。

【实验指导】

1. 预习要求　复习心血管活动的神经体液调节理论，特别是减压反射在维持动脉血压稳定过程中的重要作用。

2. 操作要点

（1）仔细分离血管、神经，防止扯断。

（2）动脉套管的尖端应圆钝。插管时可用手术刀柄垫于切口处血管的下方。打开动脉夹时不要急于移走，观察插管处有无漏血，如有血喷出，可用动脉夹重新夹住，重新插管，固定或进行其他处理后才能打开。

3. 注意事项

（1）手术过程中若有出血应及时止血。

（2）在实验过程中，需保持动脉套管与颈动脉平行，以免刺破动脉。

（3）注意保温。

（4）每一观察项目进行后必须等血压恢复正常，才能进行下一个项目的观察。

4. 报告要点　将实验描记的血压变化曲线剪贴在报告本上，简述实验结果，并分析其机制。

5. 思考题

（1）短时夹闭对侧颈总动脉对全身血压有何影响？为什么？假如夹闭部位在颈动脉窦以上，影响是否相同？

（2）刺激减压神经向中端与离中端对血压有什么影响？为什么？

（3）迷走神经为何要切断并刺激离中端，结果如何？为什么？

（丁启龙）

27　The neurohumoral regulation of the artery blood pressure in anesthetics rabbit

PURPOSE

The aims of this experiment are to measure and record the arterial blood pressure (BP) and to observe effects of the neural and humoral regulating factors on artery blood pressure.

PRINCIPLE

In physiological state, the blood pressures of human and other mammals are relatively stable, which are realized through neural and humoral regulation, especially the carotid sinus – aortic arch baroreceptor reflex. The reflex not only lowers blood pressure when BP rises, but also raises the blood pressure when BP lowers. The afferent nerve of this reflex is the aortic nerve and the sinus nerve. The aorta nerve in rabbit is an independent nerve named aortic depressor nerve and is apt to be separated and observed. In human and dog, the aortic nerve and the vagus can't be separated since they join to a strip. The blood pressure is turned into an electric signal by a pressure transducer in the experiment, and then the signal is imported into the computer. The changes of blood pressure are displayed and recorded by BL – 420F computer experimental teaching system.

MATERIALS

1. Equipments BL – 420F biological signal acquisition and analysis system, pressure transducer, protective electrode, operating instruments of mammalia, iron stand, artery clip, biconcave clamp, operating table of rabbit, artery cannula, tracheal cannula, syringe (1,5,10ml), coloured silk thread.

2. Solutions 20% ethyl carbamate, heparin solution (1000U/ml, in 0.9% sodium chloride), 1 : 10000 adrenalin, 1 : 10000 acetylcholine.

3. Object Rabbit.

METHODS

1. Emplacement of equipments Install experimental equipments as Fig. 4 – 12. The height of the pressure transducer should be set at the same level with the rabbit heart.

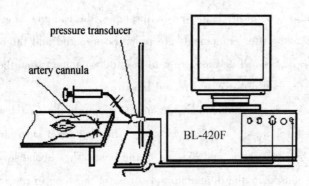

Fig. 4 – 12 the apparatus installment in measuring the blood pressure in rabbit

2. Anesthesia and fixation Weighs rabbit. 20% ethyl carbamate (1g/kg) is injected into vein in the edge of an ear. After the disappearance of the corneal reflex, fix the rabbit on operating table, and turn on the light at the table bottom to keep temperature.

3. Operation Shear the fur in cervical part in order to expose operative field. Cut a 5 – 7cm incision on the skin along the midline of cervical under the inferior border of larynx. Separate subcutaneous tissue with haemostatic forceps and expose the sternohyoid muscle. And separate the muscles in midline with haemostatic forceps, then expose trachea, intubate the tracheal cannula into the trachea. Pull apart the skin and muscles above the trachea with haemostatic forceps, then the left and right common carotid artery paralleling with the trachea can be seen on both sides of the trachea. A bundle of nerves goes along with the common carotid artery. The bundle of nerves includes a vagus, a sympathetic nerve and a depressor nerve. Separate the sheath of carotid artery, and distinguish three strips of nerve carefully. Among them, the vagus is the thickest, the sympathetic nerve is thin, and the depressor nerve is the thinnest and often adheres to the sympathetic nerve. Generally, first separate the common carotid artery and the vagus, and then separate the depressor nerve and the sympathetic nerve. Every nerve is separated out of 2 ~ 3cm. Put different colored silk threads under different nerves to distinguish them. Also put a silk thread under the carotid artery for further use. The left common carotid artery separated is used to measure blood pressure, and the right common carotid artery and right – side nerve are to be blocked up and to be stimulated respectively. Pay attention to hemostasia in the operation.

4. Artery intubation Inject (500U/kg) heparin solution into vein in the edge of an ear to prevent from cruor, then inject the solution full into the transducer that connects to a plastic artery cannula.

At the end of the artery far from heart (as near as possible to the head), the left common carotid artery is ligated with a silk thread. At the end of the artery near the heart (as near as possible to the heart), block the artery with an arterial clip. Then cross a thread between the knot and the clip under the artery, join a slipknot. At the end of the artery near the knot (the end far from the heart), scissor an inclined cut towards the heart on the artery with a sharp ophthalmological scissors, about half diameter of the artery. Insert the arterial cannula into the artery from the cut, fix the top of the cannula with the silk thread, and the surplus thread is ligated on the side of cannula to avoid the slippage. Keep the direction of the cannula along with that of blood vessel in order to avoid the cannula turning round or the wall of the artery being cut by the top of the cannula (Fig. 4 – 13).

5. Observation items After equipments are properly prepared and the operation is finished, loose the artery clip slowly, see a little blood rush to the artery cannula from the common carotid artery. If blood doesn't leak, then observe and record blood pressure.

(1) Record normal curves of the blood pressure. Distinguish the first level wave (heart beat wave) and the second level wave (respiratory wave). The first level waves are fluctuations of the blood pressure caused by constriction and diastole of the heart. The second level waves are fluctuations of blood pressure caused by the dilatation and shrink of the lung in respiratory (Fig. 4 – 14).

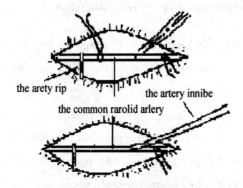

the arety rip

the artery innibe

the common rarolid arlery

Fig. 4 – 13 The sketch map of the artery intube

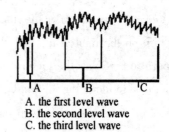

A. the first level wave
B. the second level wave
C. the third level wave

Fig. 4 – 14   The curve of the blood pressure
in the common carotid artery

(2) Nip closely the right common carotid artery for 15 seconds with the artery clip, then observe the change of blood pressure.

(3) Stimulate the right depressor nerve by a protective electrode, then observe the change of

blood pressure. The parameters of successive stimulation are as follows: the stimulation intensity is 10V, the frequency is $8 \sim 16$Hz, the wave breadth is $2 \sim 5$ms. And then make two knots on the middle of the nerve, cut off the nerve between the two knots. Stimulate the depressor nerve at the end near the centrum and the end away from centrum respectively, and then observe changes of the blood pressure.

(4) Ligate the right vagus, cut off the nerve at head end of the knot, stimulate the vagus at the end away from centrum, and observe change of the blood pressure.

(5) Inject 1 : 10000 adrenalin 0.3 ml into the vein in an edge of the ear, observe change of the blood pressure.

(6) Inject 1 : 10000 acetylcholine 0.3ml into the vein in an edge of the ear, observe change of the blood pressure.

GUIDANCE

1. Preview Review the theory of the neurohumoral regulation of the cardiovascular activity, especially the important effect of the depressor reflex in maintaining stable arterial blood pressure.

2. Manipulation

(1) Carefully separate blood vessels and nerves to prevent from injuring them.

(2) The top of the arterial cannula should be round and blunt. Underlay the blood vessel with the handle of a scalpel when cutting the artery and intubating. When opening the artery clip, don't move it away quickly. First observe whether there is a blood leaking in the cannula position. If the blood spurts out, clamp the vessel and intubate again. Open the clip only after fixation or other disposal is done.

3. Notices

(1) Stop bleeding immediately whenever it takes place in operation.

(2) Keep the arterial cannula and the common carotid artery in parallelism to avoid artery being cut in experiment.

(3) Pay attention to keeping temperature.

(4) Don't observe the next item until the blood pressure restores to normal level after each item is finished.

4. Report Print and scissor the change curves of the blood pressure, and then paste it on the report book. Try to state the result in brief and analyze its mechanism.

5. Questions

(1) What is the effect on blood pressure when clamping the common carotid artery on the opposite side for a short time? Why? If the clamping location is above the carotid sinus, are the effects the same?

(2) What is the effect on blood pressure when stimulating the decompression nerve near the centrum and away from the centrum respectively? Why?

(3) Why should the vagus be cut and stimulated at the end away from the centrum? What is the result? Why?

(Ding Qilong)

扫码"学一学"

实验二十八 人体动脉血压测定及其影响因素

【实验目的】

学习间接测定人体动脉血压方法，观察人体在运动后和体位变化时脉搏和血压的变化，以了解人体在运动和体位变化时，通过神经和体液调节，使循环功能发生一系列适应性变化。

【实验原理】

人体血压是用血压计与听诊器间接测定的，测量部位通常为上臂肱动脉。一般采用 Korotkoff 氏听诊法，即根据从外部压住动脉所必须的压力来确定该动脉的血压，测出收缩压和舒张压。通常血液在血管内流动时并没有声音。如果血流经过狭窄处形成涡流时，则可发生声音。当用橡皮气球将空气打入缚于上臂的袖带内，使其压力超过收缩压时，完全阻断了肱动脉内的血流，此时以听诊器探头按于被压的肱动脉远端，听不到任何声音，也触不到桡动脉的搏动，如徐徐放气减低袖带内压，当其压力低于肱动脉的收缩压而高于舒张压时，血流将陆续地流过受压的血管，形成涡流而发出声音，此时即可在被压的肱动脉远端听到声音，亦可触及桡动脉搏动。如果继续放气，以致外加压力等于舒张压时，则血管内血流便由断续变为连续，声音突然由强变弱或消失。因此，动脉内血流刚能发出声音时的最大外加压力相当于收缩压，而动脉内血流声音突然变弱时的外加压力则相当于舒张压。在运动和体位变化时，可通过神经和体液调节，使循环功能发生一系列适应性变化而改变收缩压和舒张压。

【实验材料】

1. 器材 听诊器，血压计。

2. 对象 人。

【实验方法】

1. 熟悉血压计的结构 血压计由检压计、袖带和气球三部分组成。检压计是一个标有 $0 \sim 260mm$ 刻度的玻璃管，上通大气，下端和水银槽相通。袖带是一个外包布套的长方形橡皮囊，借橡皮管分别与检压计的水银储槽及橡皮球相通。气球是一个带有螺丝帽的球状橡皮囊，供放气或充气用。

2. 测量前准备

（1）让受试者脱去一臂衣袖，静坐桌旁 5 分钟以上。

（2）松开血压计上橡皮球的螺丝帽，驱出袖带内残留的气体，然后将螺丝旋紧。

（3）让受试者前臂平放于桌上，手掌向上，使前臂与心脏位置等高。将袖带缠绕在该上臂，袖带下缘位于肘关节上方至少 2cm，松紧须适宜。

（4）将听诊器两耳器塞入操作者外耳道，务必使耳器的弯曲方向与外耳道一致。

（5）在肘窝内侧先用手触及被检者肱动脉搏动所在部位，然后将听诊器胸器放于该处。

3. 观察项目

（1）测量安静时动脉血压

①测收缩压：用橡皮球将空气打入橡皮袖带内，使血压表上水银柱逐渐上升到听诊器听不到脉搏声音为止（一般升至180mmHg左右），随即松开气球螺丝帽，徐徐放气，减少袖带内压力，在水银柱缓慢下降的同时仔细听诊；在开始听到"蹦蹦"样的第一声脉搏音时，这时血压表上所示水银柱刻度即代表收缩压。

②测舒张压：继续缓慢放气，这时声音有一系列变化，先由低而高，而后由高突然变低，最后完全消失。在声音突然由强变弱的这一瞬间，血压表上所示水银柱刻度即代表舒张压；有时亦可以声音突然消失时血压计所示水银柱刻度来代表之（二者相差5～10mmHg）。可同时记录这两个读数。

（2）观察运动对血压和脉搏的影响

①受试者左上臂缠上袖带，在安静环境中静坐，不讲话，也不要注意操作过程及水银柱的波动，每隔2分钟测量血压、脉搏各一次（测15s的脉搏数乘以4作为每分钟值），直至测量数据连续三次稳定（血压波动小于4mmHg、脉搏波动小于2次/分），取最后三次数据，分别算出脉搏、血压的平均值。

②做蹲下起立运动，以每2s 1次的速度进行20次，在运动后即刻、3min、5min时各测定脉搏与血压一次。

注：健康人在蹲下起立运动试验中，运动刚停止时，心跳数增加30次以上，收缩压增加20～40mmHg，舒张压增加不到10mmHg，在3min内恢复至安静状态。而心功能不全者运动刚结束时，心跳数增加30次以上，收缩压仅有轻度增加，舒张压则显著增高，心跳、血压恢复至安静状态都需要5min以上。

（3）观察体位变化对脉搏和血压的影响

①受试者卧床安静10～30min后，每隔1min测定其血压和脉搏数，直至稳定为止。

②受试者下床站立于地上。起立后1min内，每隔30s测定其血压和脉搏数，以后每隔1min测定其血压和脉搏数直到起立后10min为止。

注：起立试验阳性反应判断的标准及生理相临床意义：脉压减小16mmHg以下，收缩压降低12mmHg以上，脉搏数增加21次/分以上，符合以上一项者即为阳性反应。本实验阳性反应系交感神经紧张度欠佳所致。有时由于脑贫血，可出现头晕与昏厥。

【实验指导】

1. 预习要求 预习有关动脉血压形成及其调节、影响因素。

2. 操作要求

（1）袖带置于肘关节上方，下缘离肘关节一定距离。

（2）找准肘关节屈侧肱动脉搏动位置。

3. 注意事项

（1）室内必须安静以利听诊。

（2）测量前嘱受试者休息5～10min。

（3）袖带应包绕得松紧适宜。

（4）上臂位置应与心脏在同一水平，血压计袖带应缚在肘窝以上。

（5）听诊器胸器放在肱动脉搏动位置，不能压得太重，也不能压在袖带底下进行测量。必须注意胸器与皮肤接触不能过松，以免听不到声音。

（6）发现血压超出正常范围时，可让受试者休息10min后复测。

（7）1mmHg = 133.322Pa。

4. 报告要点

（1）记录受试者安静时的收缩压与舒张压。血压记录常以收缩压/舒张压 mmHg 表示。例如 120/75 ~ 70mmHg，120mmHg 代表收缩压值，75mmHg 代表声音由强变弱时舒张压值，70mmHg 代表声音消失时的舒张压。

（2）将运动和体位变化试验的血压和脉搏数据填入下表。

（3）根据上述试验结果，分析血压升降、脉搏变化及其恢复时间情况。

5. 思考题

（1）试评价你组同学测出的血压值是否正常。

（2）采用触诊法和听诊法测肱动脉收缩压有无差异？为什么？

（3）影响测量血压准确性的操作因素有哪些？

（4）讨论运动及改变体位后引起血压、脉搏变化的可能原因。

（5）心功能不全或交感神经紧张度欠佳者，运动及体位变化后引起的心血管反应与正常人有何区别？为什么？

（丁启龙）

28　Measurement and influence factors of the blood pressure in human

PURPOSE

Learn how to measure the arterial blood pressure in human indirectly. Observe changes of the pulse and the blood pressure in human and a series of adaptive alteration in circulatory system, and then understand the neurohumoral regulative mechanism in sport and change of body position.

PRINCIPLE

Human blood pressure is measured indirectly with a sphygmomanometer and a stethoscope. Usually the measurement position is at the humeral artery in arm. Korotkoff's auscultation is adopted generally that the arterial blood including the systolic pressure and diastolic pressure is decided according to the requisite pressure to suppress the artery from outside. Usually it is noiseless when the blood flows in blood vessels. But it sounds when the blood flows through a narrow place and a vortex current is formed. When air is filled into the rubbery cuff tied on upper arm, its pressure exceeds to the systolic pressure and blocks the blood flow in the humeral artery completely. At this moment, no sound could be heard from the stethoscope with its chest piece placed on the terminal of the humeral artery and the pulse of the radial artery also could not be touched. Discharge the gas slowly to reduce the pressure in cuff. When the pressure is lower than systolic pressure of the humeral artery and higher than diastolic pressure, the blood will flow interruptedly through the pressed blood vessels, form eddy current and produce sound. At this moment, sound could be heard from the stethoscope at the distal of the humeral artery and the pulse of the radial artery could be touched. Continuously discharge the gas till the outside pressure equals to the diastolic pressure, the blood flow in the humeral artery will become continuous, and the sound will weaken or disappear. So the maximal additional pressure equals to the systolic pressure when the blood in theartery just produces sound, and the additional pressure equals to the diastolic pressure when the sound produced by the blood flow in the artery suddenly becomes weak. In sport or change of the body position, there occurs a series of adaptive change in the circulatory function through the nervous and humoral regulation and further the diastolic pressure and systolic pressure are affected.

MATERIALS

1. Equipments　stethoscope, sphygmomanometer.

2. Object　Person.

METHODS

1. Understand the structure of sphygmomanometer　A sphygmomanometer is constituted of a manometer, a cuff and a balloon. The manometer is a glass tube that marked with a scale of 0 ~ 260mm. The upper end is opened to the atmosphere; the nether end is communicated with a mercury groove. The cuff, a rectangular rubber bag packed with cloth, is communicated with a rubber ball and the mercury groove of manometer by rubber tubes. The balloon is a globed rubber bag with a nut to deflation and inflation.

2. The preparation before measurement

(1) The volunteer takes off a sleeve, and calmly sits down beside the table for more than 5 minutes.

(2) Loose the nut of the rubber ball, and lustrate the remaining gas from the cuff, and then twist the nut tight.

(3) Lay the forearm on the table with palm upwards, keeping the height of forearm equals to the position of heart. Wind the cuff on the forearm with proper tightness. The nether border of the cuff should be 2cm above the elbow joint at least.

(4) Stuff both ear pieces of the stethoscope into the external auditory canals; keep the curvature of the ear pieces concordant with that of external auditory canals.

(5) Touch the pulse point of the humeral artery in the elbow fossa, then put the chest piece of the stethoscope there.

3. Observation items

(1) Measurement of the arterial blood pressure in calm status

①Measurement of the systolic pressure: Use the rubber ball to pump gas into the rubber cuff. The mercury column in the glass tube rises gradually. When no sound can be heard from the stethoscope, stop pumping gas (generally near to 180mmHg). Whereat loosen the nut in the balloon, and slowly deflate the gas in order to decrease the pressure in the cuff. While the column of mercury declines slowly, carefully listen to the sound. When hearing the pulse sound likes "peng, peng", please pay attention to the height of the mercury column. The scale beside the height expresses the systolic pressure.

②Measurement of the diastolic pressure: Continue deflating the gas slowly. At this time there occurs a series of variety in the sound: first from low to high, then from high to low suddenly, and at last disappears completely. When the sound changes from strong to weak suddenly, the scale of mercury column of sphygmomanometer represents the diastolic pressure. Sometimes the scale also represents diastolic pressure when the voice suddenly disappears (the difference between the two reading numbers is 5 ~ 10mmHg). Both of the reading numbers can be recorded.

(2)Observe the influence sport on the blood pressure and the pulse

①The volunteer, left forearm winded up by the cuff, sits quietly in a peaceful environment. Don't talk or pay attention to the operative process and the fluctuation of the mercury column. Measure the blood pressure and the pulse every 2 minutes (the number of pulse in 15 second multiplied by 4 is minute pulse), till the measured data are stable in successive three times (the fluctuation of the blood pressure is within 4mmHg, and that of the pulse is within 2 beats/min). Take the data of the last three times, calculate the means of blood pressure and pulse respectively.

②Squat down and stand up twenty times with the frequency of once every two seconds, measure the pulse and the blood pressure at 0min, 3min, 5min after the sport respectively.

Note In this sport test of squatting down and standing up, the heart beats of the health volunteer increases more than 30 times, the systolic pressure increases 20 ~ 40mmHg, the diastolic pressure increases less than 10 mmHg. And in 3 min after stopping sport, these indexes recover to normal values in peaceful status. But for the person with a heart failure, when the sport is just over, the heartbeat increases more than 30 times, the systolic pressure increases slightly, and the diastolic pressure increases remarkably. The heartbeat and blood pressure recover entirely to normal values over 5 minutes.

(3)Observe the effects of body position change on the pulse and the blood pressure

①After the volunteer lies in a bed for 10 ~ 30min, measure the blood pressure and pulse once every two minutes till stabilization.

②The volunteer gets off the bed and stands up on the ground. Measure the blood pressure and pulse once every thirty seconds in one minute, and once every two minutes till ten minutes later.

Note The judgmental standard of positive reaction and the meanings in clinic and physiology

In the test of standing up, the result is positive if it suits to any items following: the difference between systolic pressure and diastolic pressure reduces more than 16mmHg, the systolic pressure lowers over 12mmHg, the pulse increases over 21beats/min. The positive reaction of the test is caused by the shortage of the sympathetic tonicity. Sometimes the volunteer appears dizzy and faint because of the cerebral ischemia.

GUIDANCE

1. Preview　Study the relevant theory on the formation, regulation and influence of the arterial pressure.

2. Manipulation

(1)The cuff is winded over the elbow joint, and its nether border is away from the elbow joint.

(2)Seek the pulse point of the humeral artery in the elbow fossa correctly.

3. Notices

(1)Keep the room in silence in order to auscultation.

(2)Tell the volunteer to rest for 5 ~ 10 mins before the measurement.

(3) The tightness of the cuff winded should be proper.

(4) The position of the forearm and the heart is at the same level, and the cuff of the sphygmomanometer should be winded above the elbow fossa.

(5) The chest piece of stethoscope is put on the pulse position of the brachial artery, can't be pressed heavily, and also can't be pressed under the cuff. Pay attention that the chest piece may be touched to the skin too loosely to hear nothing.

(6) When the blood pressure exceeds the normal scope, let the volunteer have a rest for 10 minutes and measure again.

(7) 1mmHg = 133. 322Pa.

4. Reports

(1) Record the systolic pressure and diastolic pressure of the volunteer in quiet state. The record of the blood pressure is often expressed as systolic pressure/diastolic pressure mmHg. For example, 120/75 ~ 70 mmHg, the 120 mmHg represents the value of the systolic pressure, 75 mmHg represents the value of the diastolic pressure when the sound turns from strong to weak, 70 mmHg represents the diastolic pressure when the sound disappears.

(2) Fill the following table with the data of the blood pressure and the pulse in tests of sport and body position change.

(SBP: systolic pressure; DBP: diastolic pressure)

(3) According to above results, analyze the variety of the blood pressure, the pulse variety and their recovery time.

5. Questions

(1) Try to evaluate whether the blood pressure of your classmates in your group is normal.

(2) Is there any difference in the systolic pressure measured by palpation or stethoscopy? Why?

	SBP/DBP(mmHg)	Pulse(beats/min)
Sport test		
before		
after (min)		
0		
1		
3		
5		
Body position change test		
decubitus		
Standing stance (min)		
0		
0. 5		
1		
3		
5		
7		

（3）What are the operational factors that influent the measurement accuracy of the blood pressure?

（4）Discuss the possible reason that cause the variety of the blood pressure and pulse after sport and body position change.

（5）Compared with a healthy man, what is the difference of the cardiovascular response in a man with heart failure or with sympathetic tonicity shortage after sport or body position change? Why?

（Ding Qilong）

实验二十九　希氏束电图

【实验目的】

通过希氏束电图的记录实验，了解希氏束电图各波的意义及其在临床诊断和实验研究中的作用。

【实验原理】

希氏束电图（his bundle electrogram，HBE）是一种应用特殊的导联方法和记录条件所获得的心电图，它能客观地反映心脏特殊传导系统中希氏束生物电活动的功能特征，在实验研究和临床检查中，具有一般心电图检查所无法取代的作用。

在心电图中，P－R间期代表从心房开始激动到心室开始激动所需要的时间，它包括兴奋在心房、房室结以及希氏束－浦肯野系统的传导时间，但在普通心电图上，PR段处于等电位线，记录不到电位变化，因而无法观察到上述各部分的传导功能。将心导管电极置于希氏束附近的心内膜处，即可记录到希氏束电图。常规的希氏束电图检查，是采用右心插管法，将导管经股静脉、腋静脉或颈外静脉插入右心室，也可自颈总动脉把导管插入主动脉根部以达到希氏束附近。前一种方法常用于临床，而后一种方法主要用于动物。

本实验选用颈总动脉插管，方法简便可靠。

【实验材料】

1. 器材　前置放大器1，双线示波器及照相机或记录仪，心导管电极1，动脉夹1，哺乳动物手术器械一套。

2. 药品　20%氨基甲酸乙酯，普萘洛尔，阿托品。

【实验方法】

1. 仪器连接与调试

（1）按图4－17示意连接仪器。

（2）仪器条件

①心导管电极：一般采用外径为0.9mm的无毒塑料管或硅橡胶管。

②前置放大器：需具有高低频滤波装置。

③记录仪走纸速度需达到 100～200mm/s。

④示波器：除可选用普通的 SBB-1 型双线示波器外，还可采用先进的记忆示波器，在屏幕上直接测量各参数。

（3）调整仪器参数

①前置放大器：记录心电图的前置放大器放大倍数为 1000 倍，时间常数为 1s，高频滤波为 100Hz，记录希氏束电图的前置放大器放大倍数为 1000 倍，时间常数为 0.001s，高频滤波为 300Hz。

②SBR-1 双线示波器上线显示标准导联 II 的心电图，总增益为 0.5mV/cm；下线显示希氏束电图，增益为 100μV/cm，扫描方式用上线前一心动周期 R 波进行自动触发，并适当调节扫描速度，使 P-R 间期能在荧光屏上显示出来。

2. 麻醉和固定 用 20% 氨基甲酸乙酯按 1g/kg 体重剂量经耳缘静脉注入，麻醉后将兔仰卧位固定在手术台上。

3. 记录 II 导联心电图 在右前肢和左下肢皮下插入注射针头作引导电极，经导线连至前置放大器，经放大后输入到双线示波器上线。

4. 心导管插入 在颈部正中做一长约 10cm 切口，分离出一侧颈总动脉 2～3cm 长，用线结扎其离心端，用动脉夹夹住近心端，在扎线与动脉夹之间剪一小口，将用肝素浸润过的心导管电极自切口插入，打开动脉夹，左手捏住动脉使血液不致漏出，右手推送心导管电极沿颈总动脉进入主动脉，将导管送入 15cm 左右即到达主动脉根部，此时再插会遇到阻力，并明显感到心脏的搏动。若电极导管进入 30cm 左右时还可以无阻力推进，则说明电极已进入腹主动脉，必须将电极导管退回到 10cm 处，转动方向，重新推送到主动脉根部，当感到有阻力和心脏搏动时，将导管电极后退约 0.5cm，即可将电极尾端连至前置放大器，再输入到 SBR-1 示波器的下线进行观察，此时下线上的波型对应 P 波为心房波（A 波），对应 R 波为心室波（V 波），在 V 波前约 30ms 处有一稳定的尖锐小波，波形呈单相、双相或三相，电压为 100～200μV，波宽 7～15ms，此波即为希氏束电位（图 4-18）。

5. 观察项目

（1）测量正常希氏束电图各项参数。①P-A 间期；②A-H 间期；③H-V 间期；④H 波持续时间（波宽）；⑤H 波的幅值（mV）。

（2）从耳缘静脉注射普萘洛尔（0.2mg/kg），待心率出现变化时重复测定上述五项指标并与给药前相比较。

（3）待普萘洛尔的效应消失后，心率基本恢复正常后，静脉注射阿托品（0.04mg/kg），当出现心率加快效应后测算上述五项指标。

【实验指导】

1. 预习要求

（1）希氏束电图各波和间期的含义（图 4-19）

A 波：位于心电图 P 波的中部，它是在房室结或希氏束部位所记录到的心房除极波。

H 波：位于 PR 段内，为一快速的单相、双相或三相电位，它代表希氏束的除极过程，随着记录部位的差异，尚可在 H 波之前记录到房室结电图（NE），而在其后记录到右束支电位（RBE）和左束支电位（LBE）。

V 波：是心室的除极波，其出现与 QRS 波基本一致。

P－A 间期：从体表心电图 P 波起点至希氏束电图 A 波开始的时间，称 P－A 间期。此间期代表窦性心律时从窦房结到房室结的传导时间，也就是激动在心房内传导的时间。

P－A 间期的正常值为 20ms。

A－H 间期：从希氏束电图 A 波的起点到 H 波开始的时间，称 A－H 间期，它代表激动在房室交界区（房－结区、结区、结－希区）传导的时间，正常值为 50～120ms，可因心动周期的长短和自律性的高低而有所变异。

H－V 间期：从 H 波的起点到 V 波起始部（相当于 QRS 波的开始）传导的时间，称为 H－V 间期，正常值为 25～55ms。H－V 间期代表激动自希氏束远端至浦氏纤维的传导时间。其中 H 波时矩为 15～20ms，代表激动在希氏束传导的时间。

（2）希氏束电图的实用意义

①确定传导阻滞发生的部位及其严重程度，指导应用心脏起搏器的类型及合理选择人工起搏方式和部位。

②早期发现隐匿性房室传导阻滞以利于采取预防性和治疗性措施。

③辅助鉴别室上性心动过速（伴室内差异性传导或束支传导阻滞）和室性心动过速，以指导抗心律失常药物的选择和应用。

④鉴别室性和室上性异位节律（伴室内差异性传导），以指导洋地黄或抗心律失常药物的应用，常见于服用洋地黄或急性心肌梗死患者。

⑤鉴别预激综合征的各种类型及发生机制，为其诊断和治疗提供依据。

⑥分析研究某些药物对心脏传导系统的电生理作用，为药物的选择和应用提供药理学基础。

2. 操作要点　插心导管时，一般插入 15cm 左右即达主动脉根部，此时感觉心导管有阻力和心脏搏动。通过示波器观察 H 波是否出现或是否典型，可采用示波照相的方式记录希氏束电图，或采用频响相配的记录仪描记下来。

3. 注意事项

（1）麻醉不宜太浅，冬季气温低注意保温，避免肌电干扰。

（2）要选择适当的心导管电极，不能太粗或太细。

（3）向主动脉根部推进心导管时动作要轻柔、缓慢，以免插破动脉或插入心室腔内。

（4）基线不稳或有干扰时，应排除后再进行记录。

4. 报告要点

（1）观测希氏束电图中各间期时矩，并与给药前后进行比较。

（2）讨论希氏束电图的临床和实验意义。

5. 思考题

（1）刺激迷走神经向心端，希氏束电图有何变化？为什么？

（2）正常情况下，交感神经对房室传导组织有何作用？对哪些组织的作用比较明显？对希氏束－浦肯野系统的作用是否明显？有何根据？

（3）引导记录希氏束电图的基本条件是什么？为什么？

（颜天华　刘冰冰）

29 His bundle electrogram

PURPOSE

To know the significance of every wave in His bundle electrogram and the uses in clinical diagnosis and scientific research by the experiment of recording His bundle electrogram.

PRINCIPLE

His bundle electrogram is an ECG that is recorded by a special lead method at special recording condition. It can express objectively the functional characteristics of His bundle in cardiac conduction system, so its role can't be replaced by common ECG examination in scientific research and clinical examination.

P – R interval is represent from the beginning of cardiac atrium's excitation to the beginning of cardiac ventricle's excitation, it consists of the interval for the conduction of activation in cardiac atrium, atrioventricular node and His bundle – Purkinje fiber. The potential difference can't be recorded because P – R interval is at the isoelectric level in common ECG, so the functional characteristics can't be observed at the above – mentioned sites. His bundle electrogram can be recorded when cardiac catheter electrode is placed the endocardium close to His bundle. Common His bundle electrogram examination is right heart intubation, one intubation is the catheter is inserted into right ventricle close to His bundle by femoral vein or axillary vein or external jugular vein, another is the catheter is inserted into the root of aorta close to His bundle by common carotid artery. The first intubation is used usually in clinical examination; the second is used in animal experiment.

The second intubation that is simple and reliable is used in the experiment.

MATERIALS

1. Equipments　preamplifier system, dual trace oscilloscope and camera (or recording system), cardiac catheter electrode, artery clamp, an operational tool for mammal.

2. Solutions　20% ethyl carbamate, propranolol, atropine.

3. Experimental object　rabbit.

METHOD

1. preparation of the recorder

(1) Refer to Fig. 4 – 17 and connect the devices.

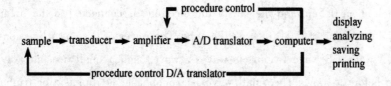

Fig. 4 – 17　abridged general view of guiding for His bundle electrogram

(2) conditions of the devices

①cardiac catheter electrode: harmless plastic tube or silica rubber vessel whose diameter is usually 0. 9mm.

②preamplifier system:It has the device.

③The chart drive speed of the recording system is close to 100,200mm/s.

④Oscilloscope:SBB – 1 model dual trace oscilloscope can be used or memory oscilloscope in whose screen the parameters can be measured directly can be used.

（3）Adjustment of device parameters

①preamplifier system:The amplifying power of preamplifier system that is used to record ECG is 1000 times, the time constant is 1s, the high – frequency of waves which are filtered is 100kHz. The amplifying power of preamplifier system that is used to record His bundle electrogram is 1000 times, the time constant is 0. 001s, the high – frequency of waves which are filtered is 300kHz.

②The top line of dual trace oscilloscope is used to show standard lead Ⅱ, the total gain is 0. 5mV/cm;The down line is used to show His bundle electrogram, the gain is 100μV/cm, the scanning is triggered by R wave of previous cardiac cycle on the top line, set the scanning speed properly to show P – R interval in the screen.

2. Anesthesia and fixation of the animal　　Inject 20% ethyl carbamate into the vein at the edge of rabbit ear with the dose of 1g/kg, secure the rabbit with its dorsal side down on the operation table after it is anesthetized.

3. Recording of standard lead Ⅱ　　Insert the tip of injection needles into the subcutaneous part of right forelimb and left lower limb as guiding electrode, connect it with the preamplifier by wires, amplify the signal and input it to the top line of dual trace oscilloscope.

4. Insertion of cardiac catheter　　Cut a 10cm hole in the middle of the neck, separate and expose unilateral common carotid artery to about 2 ~ 3cm length, bundle the distal side up with thread, clamp the proximal side with artery clamp, cut a small incision between the thread and the artery clamp, insert the cardiac catheter electrode that is soaked by heparin into the incision, grasp the proximal side to avoid the blood bleed with left hand and push the electrode into the aorta with right hand after aortic declamping. The electrode reaches to the boot of aorta when the electrode of 15cm length is in the blood vessel, the force of resistance can appear and heart beat can be touched if the electrode is pushed into the vessel continuously. If the electrode can be pushed smoothly when the electrode of 30cm length is in the blood vessel, the electrode is in the abdominal aorta. The electrode has to be back to the position where the electrode of 10cm length is in the blood vessel and is pushed to the boot of aorta again. When the force of resistance appears and heartbeat is touched, the electrode is back about 0. 5cm and the tail of the electrode is connected to the preamplifier. Input the signal to the down line of dual trace oscilloscope. The waves of the down line consist of P wave （atrium wave, A wave）, R wave （ventricle wave, V wave） and a small resistant wave at the point of about 30ms before V wave. The small wave is monophasic or diphasic or triphasic wave, the voltage is about 100 ~ 200μV, the width is about 7 ~ 15ms. The small wave is His bundle potential （Fig. 4 – 18）.

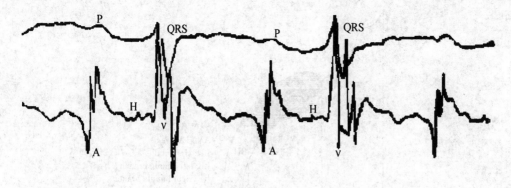

Fig. 4 – 18　His bundle electrogram

the top line is ECG,the down line is His bundle electrogram,A、H、V represents three potential respectively,

P、QRS represents the activation of the atrium、the ventricle

5. Observation items

（1）Measure the parameters of His bundle electrogram. ①P – A interval;②A – H interval; ③H – V interval;④width of H wave;⑤amplitude of H wave（mV）.

（2）Inject propranolol into the vein at the edge of rabbit ear with the dose of 0. 2mg/kg,measure the five parameters again when heart rate changes and compare them with the previous values.

（3）Inject atropine into the vein at the edge of rabbit ear with the dose of 0. 04mg/kg when the effect of propranolol on the heart rate is weak,measure the five parameters again when heart rate increases.

GUIDANCE

1. Preview

（1）Review the significance of all waves and intervals in His bundle electrogram（Fig. 4 – 19）.

A wave:The wave's position is at the middle of P wave,it represents the depolarization of atrial muscle recorded nearby the position of AV node or His bundle.

H wave:The wave's position is in the P – R segment,it is monophasic or diphasic or triphasic wave,it represents the depolarization of His bundle. When the position for recording changes,AV node electrogram can be recorded before H wave or right bundle branch electrogram and left bundle branch electrogram can be recorded after H wave.

V wave:The wave represents the depolarization of ventricular muscle,it is identical with QRS wave.

P – A interval:The interval is measured from the beginning of P wave in common ECG to the beginning of the A wave in His bundle electrogram,it represents the interval between the activation of the SA node and the AV node when cardiac rhythm is sinus rhythm,which is identical with the interval for the conduction of activation in the atrium. The normal value of P – A interval is 20ms.

A – H interval:The interval is measured from the beginning of the A wave in His bundle electrogram to the beginning of the H wave,it represents the interval for the conduction of activation in AV junction region. The normal value of A – H interval is 50 ~ 120ms,the value changes when cardiac cycle or auto – rhythmicity changes.

Fig. 4 – 19   denomination of the waves in His bundle electrogram the top figure
is cardiac conduction system the middle figure is
His bundle electrogram the down figure is ECG（lead – Ⅱ）

H – V interval：The interval is measured from the beginning of the H wave to the beginning of
the V wave，it represents the interval between the activation of distal His bundle and Purkinje fiber. The normal value of H – V interval is 25 ~ 55ms，it includes the time moment of H wave which
is 15 ~ 20ms. The time moment of H wave represents the interval for the conduction of activation in
His bundle.

（2）Practical significance of His bundle electrogram.

①Demonstrate the site where the conduction blocks and the block extent to guide to apply the
type of cardiac pacemaker and to select the way of artificial pacing and the site where artificial pacemaker is placed.

②Discover early latent atrioventricular block to apply prophylactic and remedial measures.

③Differentiate supraventricular tachycardia and ventricular tachycardia to guide to select and
apply antiarrhythmic drug. Supraventricular tachycardia accompanies with ventricular differential
conduction or bundle branches conduction block.

④Differentiate ventricular ectopic rhythm and supraventricular ectopic rhythm to guide to apply
digitalis and antiarrhythmic drug，which can help the patients who take digitalis or who has acute
myocardial infarction. Supraventricular ectopic rhythm accompanies with ventricular differential conduction.

⑤Differentiate the principle and various types of preexcitation syndrome to provide the information for diagnosis and therapy.

⑥Study and research electrophysiological effects of some drugs on cardiac conduction system to provide the pharmacological basis for the choice and application of drugs.

2. Manipulation　The cardiac catheter reaches to the boot of aorta when the cardiac catheter of 15cm length is in the blood vessel, the force of resistance can appear and heart beat can be touched if the electrode is pushed into the vessel continuously. Observe if H wave appears on the oscilloscope and if H wave is typical. Record His bundle electrogram by photography or recording system that matches the oscilloscope.

3. Notice

①The anesthesia shouldn't be shallow. Pay attention to keep warm in the winter. Avoid the interference of myopotential.

②Select suitable cardiac catheter electrode whose diameter shouldn't be too small or big.

③Push the cardiac catheter gently and slowly when the cardiac catheter is close to the boot of aorta to avoid breaking the aorta or entering in ventricular chamber.

④When the baseline is unstable or is interfered with, remove the interference before recording.

4. Report

(1) Measure the time moment of various intervals in His bundle electrogram. After injecting the drugs, measure the values again. Compare them with the previous values.

(2) Discuss the clinical and experimental significance of His bundle electrogram.

5. Questions

(1) When the proximal part of vagus nerve is stimulated, what is the changes of His bundle electrogram? Why?

(2) What effects the sympathetic nerve has on atrioventricular conduction tissue in normal condition? Which tissue the effects are obvious on? Are the effects obvious on His bundle and Purkinje fiber? Why?

(3) What is the elementary condition for recording His bundle electrogram? Why?

(Yan Tianhua　Liu Bingbing)

实验三十　家兔在体心脏单相动作电位的测定

【实验目的】

掌握家兔心外膜单相动作电位（monophasic action potential，MAP）的测定方法，并观察 MAP 的形态及其与心电图的对应关系。

【实验原理】

心肌动作电位在分析心脏活动中有较重要的意义，但玻璃微电极的细胞内记录方法，尚难用于较大动物在体心脏作较长时间的观察。MAP 是心肌细胞的局部电活动，通常使用吸引电极或接触电极记录。MAP 和跨膜动作电位（transmembrane action potential，TAP）的波形相似（图 4 – 20）。比较发现，MAP 虽然振幅较低，除极升支的时程较长，但其复极波形和时程与 TAP 十分相似，能比较准确地反映心肌细胞去极化过程的发生和整个复极化时相，是研究复极化时相变化的可信指标。

与 TAP 比较，MAP 主要具有以下特点。

1. MAP 的振幅较低 TAP 平均为 100 ~ 110mV，而家兔左室外膜 MAP 为 14 ~ 30mV，犬左室外膜为 35 ~ 55mV，心房的振幅则更低。

2. MAP 的间期与 TAP 间期很相近 兔左室外膜 $MAPD_{90}$ 一般为 150ms 左右（心率约为 200 次/分时），犬左室外膜 $MAPD_{90}$ 约为 190ms（心率约为 120 次/分时）。

3. MAP 去极化上升速率（dv/dt_{max}）较低（仅为 4V/s 左右） 这可能是由于电极的尖端较大，所接触的是多个心肌细胞，这些细胞的电活动在时间和空间上都是分散的和不同步的。

4. MAP 上升支出现内在偏转 这种去极化过程中出现的扭转是心室表面电图 QRS 波群所造成的，而偏转的程度在使用双极导管时较单极导管小。由于这种偏转，在 MAP 上无法得到静息电位、去极化最大上升速率的准确数值。

【实验材料】

1. 器材 哺乳动物手术器械一套，MAP 引导电极 1，微电极放大器，兔手术台 1，开胸器 1，双线示波器 1，示波照相机 1，二道生理记录仪 1。

2. 对象 家兔 1，雌雄不拘，体重 2 ~ 3kg。

3. 药品 生理盐水，20% 氨基甲酸乙酯。

【实验方法】

1. MAP 引导电极的制备 接触电极和吸引电极的制作方法见附录。实验前 1 小时将电极的引导部分浸入生理盐水中。

2. 仪器的连接与调节（图 4 – 21）

（1）将引导电极与微电极放大器的输入端连接，微放增益为 ×10。

（2）微放的输出端与示波器的上线连接，并与二道生理记录仪相连。示波器灵敏度为 100mV/cm，扫描速度视心率快慢及实验要求而定，一般选择 0.1s ~ 50ms/cm。

（3）心电图导联线与示波器下线相连，其灵敏度为 0.2V/cm，即可在示波器上得到心电图波形。同时连于二道生理记录仪。

（4）根据实验要求，分别调节二导生理记录仪的灵敏度及走纸速度，以同步描记 MAP 和心电图（ECG）波形。

3. 手术 将家兔以 20% 氨基甲酸乙酯（1g/kg，iv）麻醉后，背位固定于兔手术台上，于胸骨左缘第 3 ~ 4 肋间开胸，剪开心包膜，暴露心脏。注意保护胸膜，维持自然呼吸。

4. ECG 的引导 针形电极按常规导联方式刺入四肢皮下。

5. MAP 与 ECG 的观察与记录

（1）接触电极的引导 将接触电极弹性梁末端固定于微操纵器上，调节微操纵器，使电极引导部分与心外膜轻轻接触（单极电极引导时参考电极与胸壁皮肤相连），此时示波器上显示为心外膜电图波形，随着压力的增大，逐渐演变为 MAP 形态。

（2）吸引电极的引导 选择血管较少的心外膜安放电极，在电动泵的抽吸作用下（负压值16~47kPa），将电极吸附在心外膜上，即可记录出 MAP。单极引导时，Ag-AgCl 电极片作为无关电极置于颈部皮下。

（3）MAP 与 ECG 的同步记录　ECG 记录选用标准 Ⅱ 导联。在示波器上观察到满意的波形后，打开二道生理记录仪，可同步描记对应的 MAP 和 ECG 波形。也可用示波照相机同步拍照。

（4）波形的测量　MAP 的测量基本与 TAP 相同。典型的 MAP 包括去极化和复极化两个基本过程，并可将其区分为 0、1、2、3 和 4 五个相期。主要观察指标有三个：①MAPA 单相动作电位幅度；②$MAPD_{50}$ 为 MAP 复极达 50% 时的时程，能间接反应 AP 二期的变化情况；③$MAPD_{90}$ 为 MAP 复极达 90% 时的时程，可反应 AP 的总时程。

【实验指导】

1. 预习要求

（1）了解单相动作电位的特点。

（2）了解单相动作电位的记录方法，并复习跨膜动作电位的实验方法。

2. 操作要点

（1）接触电极记录时，电极对心肌的压力要适宜，压力过小不易记录到合格的波形或 MAP 振幅过低，压力过大则将影响心脏活动，造成心肌的局部损伤。

（2）吸引电极记录时，吸引的负压值在 16~47kPa 范围时，一般可记录持续 30~60 分钟的较稳定波形，负压过小不易吸牢；而负压过大时，起初振幅较大，但衰减较快。

（3）手术时切勿破损胸膜以维持自然呼吸。

（4）电极与心肌表面接触应尽量避开血管。

3. 注意事项

（1）必须控制好动物的麻醉深度。

（2）ECG 的针形电极应插入皮下，不可插入肌肉中，亦应防止脱落。

（3）心脏表面经常滴加保温生理盐水以保持湿润。

（4）注意动物及仪器的接地良好，以防干扰。

4. 报告要点

（1）单相动作电位的电生理特征及其波形的测量。

（2）心电图分析。

（3）注意 MAP 与 EGG 的对应关系，尤其是 MAFD 与心率的关系。

5. 思考题

（1）单相动作电位形成的特点及其与跨膜动作电位的异同点。

（2）心肌动作电位与心电图的对应关系如何？

附　单相动作电位引导电极的制备

（1）接触电极的制备　心外膜接触电极由弹性梁、Ag-AgCl 电极组成（图 4-22）。

1）弹性梁部分　弹性梁一般采用韧性材料制成，长、宽、厚分别为 150mm、5mm、0.5mm。一端（电极端）打一小孔，并通过此孔固定一长为 2cm，内径约为 1mm 的钢管，钢管外部绝缘。

2）Ag-AgCl 电极部分　两根直径约为 0.5mm 的银丝，其中一根的一端烧成球状，银丝外部绝缘。将二者镀以 AgCl，并行穿过钢管，银球裸露于管的顶端作为探测电极，另一根银丝裸端绕于银球上部的绝缘处作为参考电极。实验中，需在参考电极周围套一小块浸润生理盐水的海绵，参考电极由此与心脏良好接触。

制作单极电极时，仅在钢管内穿入一根乏极化银球电极即可。

（2）吸引电极的制备　吸引电极的引导部分为乏极化银丝，尖端直径约为0.1mm。其外套以长10~15cm，内径6mm塑料管。电极尖端突出塑料管口约0.5mm。实验时，在电动吸引泵的抽吸作用下，使塑料管内造成负压而将电极吸附于心外膜上。

（颜天华　刘冰冰）

30　Determination of monophasic action potential in rabbit heart *in vivo*

PURPOSE

To grasp the determination of monophasic action potential (MAP) in rabbit epicardium and to observe the shape of MAP to know the relation of MAP and ECG.

PRINCIPLE

Myocardial action potential is important to analyze heart activity. But it is difficult to observe myocardial action potential of major animal in vivo for a long time by intracellular recording. Glass microelectrode is used in intracellular recording. MAP is myocardial local electric action, so negative pressure electrode or contact electrode is used to record MAP. The shape of MAP is similar to TAP (transmembrane action potential) (Fig. 4 – 20). The shape and duration of MAP repolarization part is very similar to TAP though the amplitude of MAP is lower and the duration of MAP depolarization part is longer by comparing MAP with TAP. MAP can show correctly MAP depolarization and repolarization, so MAP is a reliable index to study and research the changes of repolarization phase.

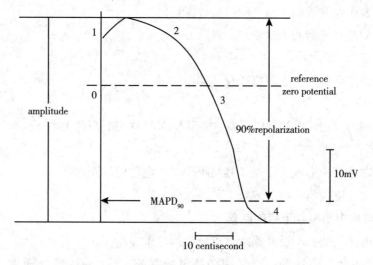

Fig. 4 – 20　the shape and the measure of MAP

MAP has the characteristics mainly by comparing with TAP.

1. The amplitude of MAP is lower than TAP　The amplitude of TAP is 100 ~ 110mV in average, the amplitude of MAP in Left ventricular epicardium of rabbit is 14 ~ 30mV, the amplitude of

MAP in Left ventricular epicardium of dog is 35 ~ 55mV, the amplitude of MAP in atrial epicardium of rabbit is lower than ventricular epicardium.

2. The interval of MAP is similar to TAP The D90 of MAP in Left ventricular epicardium of rabbit is 150ms in general when heart rate is 200bpm, the D90 of MAP in Left ventricular epicardium of dog is 190ms when heart beat is 120bpm.

3. The rise velocity of MAP is lower than TAP The rise velocity of MAP is about 4V/s. The reason may be the tip of electrode is large to result in the tip contact several cells, the electric action of every cell is not synchronous at time and dispersed in space.

4. The rise branch of MAP has intrinsic deflection The deflection in depolarization duration is caused by QRS waves of ventricular surface electrocardiogram. The extent of deflection is smaller when bipolar catheter is used than unipolar catheter. The values of resting potential and maximum rise velocity in MAP can't be obtained correctly because of the deflection.

MATERIALS

1. Equipments an operational tool for mammal, MAP guiding electrode, microelectrode amplifier, operation table for rabbit, open chest tool, dual trace oscilloscope, oscillographic camera, double – channel physiological recorder.

2. Solutions 20% ethyl carbamate, propranolol, saline.

3. Experimental object rabbit (male or female) whose weigh is 2 ~ 3kg.

METHOD

1. Preparation of MAP guiding electrode The preparation of contact electrode and negative pressure electrode refer to the appendix. The guiding part of negative pressure electrode is soaked in saline 1 hour before the experiment.

2. Preparation of the devices

(1) Connect the guiding electrode with the lead – in of microelectrode amplifier. The gain of microelectrode amplifier is " × 10".

(2) Connect the out put of microelectrode amplifier with the top line of dual trace oscilloscope and with double – channel physiological recorder. The sensitivity of oscilloscope is 100mV/cm, the scanning speed that is 0. 1s ~ 50ms/cm in general is determined by heart rate and experimental command.

(3) Connect the lead line of ECG with the down line of oscilloscope and with double – channel physiological recorder. When the sensitivity of oscilloscope is 0. 2V/cm, the waves of ECG appear in the oscilloscope.

(4) Set the sensitivity and chart drive speed of two channel respectively to record the waves of MAP and ECG synchronous according to experimental commands.

3. Preparation of the animal Anesthetize the rabbit by injecting 20% ethyl carbamate into the vein with the dose of 1g/kg, and secure the rabbit with its dorsal side down on the operation table, open the chest through 3rd, 4th rib gap at the left edge of breast bone, open the pericardium with scissors, expose the heart. Pay attention to protect the pleura and keep the rabbit breathing naturally.

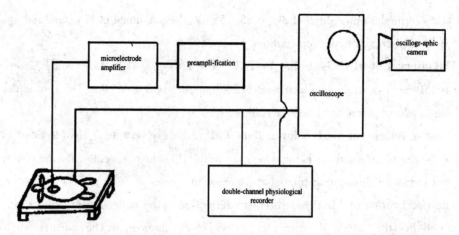

Fig. 4 – 21   abridged general view of the determination and recording device

4. Preparation of the ECG   Insert belonoid electrode into the subcutaneous part in four limbs according to common lead.

5. Observation and recording of MAP and ECG

(1) Connection of contact electrode

Fix the tip of elastic bridge in the contact electrode on the micromanipulator, set the micromanipulator to keep the guiding of the electrode in contact with the epicardium slightly (keep reference electrode in contact with the skin of chest wall when monopolar electrode is connected). The waves of epicardium electrocardiogram are showed on the top line of oscilloscope. As the pressure increases, the shape of the waves changes to the shape of MAP gradually.

(2) Connection of negative pressure electrode

Place the electrode at the epicardium with less blood vessels, keep the electrode in contact with the epicardium through suction of electric pump (the value of negative pressure is $16 \sim 47 kPa$), then record MAP. When monopolar electrode is connected, Ag – AgCl electrode is placed at the subcutaneous part in the neck as indifferent electrode.

(3) recording synchronous of MAP and ECG

ECG is recorded from standard lead II. Turn on double – channel physiological recorder to record synchronous the waves of MAP and ECG after good waves appear on the oscilloscope, or take some pictures synchronous with oscillographic camera.

(4) Measure of some indexes

Measure of some indexes in MAP is same to TAP generally. A typical MAP includes two parts: depolarization part andrepolarization part, and MAP can be separated to five phases: 0 phase, 1 phase, 2 phase, 3 phase, 4 phase. The main indexes are three: ①MAPA, amplitude of MAP. ②$MAPD_{50}$, duration when repolarization of MAP reaches to the extent of 50%. The index can reflect indirectly the changes of 2 phase in MAP. ③$MAPD_{90}$, duration when repolarization of MAP reaches to the extent of 90%. The index can reflect the changes of the duration of MAP.

GUIDANCE

1. Preview

(1) Know the characteristics of MAP.

（2）Know the recording of MAP and review the methods of transmembrane action potential.

2. Manipulation

（1）The pressure of the electrode on cardiac muscle must be suitable when turn on the contact electrode. If the pressure is weaker, good waves can't be recorded or amplitude of MAP is lower. If the pressure is stronger, heart action may be affected and local injury of cardiac muscle may be caused.

（2）The recording that stable waves appear can last 30 ~ 60min when the value of negative pressure is 16 ~ 47kPa. If the pressure is weaker, the contact is not stable. If the pressure is stronger, amplitude of MAP is large at the beginning, but it decreases more quickly.

（3）Do not injury the pleura to keep the rabbit breathing naturally when operating on the rabbit.

（4）Avoid contacting the electrode with blood vessel when the electrode contacts with the surface of cardiac muscle.

3. Notice

（1）Control the degree of anesthesia when the animal is anesthetized.

（2）Insert belonoid electrode of ECG into the subcutaneous part, avoid inserting into the muscle, prevent them from dropping.

（3）Wet the surface of the heart occasionally by dripping warm saline on it.

（4）Keep the animal and the devices connecting well with the ground to prevent from interference.

4. Report

（1）Discuss electrophysiological characteristics of MAP and measure of some indexes in MAP.

（2）Analyze the electrocardiogram.

（3）Discuss the relation of MAP and ECG, discuss the relation of MAPD with heart rate.

5. Questions

（1）What are the main points in the formation of MAP? What is the same and different points comparing with the formation of transmembrane action potential?

（2）Discuss every part of MAP and the corresponding part of ECG.

APPENDIX

Preparation of guiding electrode for MAP

（1）Preparation of contact electrode　Epicardium contact electrode consists of elastic bridge and Ag – AgCl electrode.

1）elastic bridge　Elastic bridge is made from ductile material, its length、width、thickness is 150、5、0. 5mm respectively. Punch a hole at the electrode tip, secure a steel pipe in the hole. The length of the steel pipe is 2cm, the bore is 1mm. The outside of the steel pipe is dielectric.

2）Ag – AgCl electrode　There are two silver wires whose diameter is 0. 5mm. A tip of a wire is burned and its shape changes to globular shape, insulate the outside of the wire, electroplate two wires with AgCl, go straight through the steel pipe with two wires concurrently. The silver ball is exposed at the top of the pipe as detecting electrode. The tip of another wire circle the insulator above the silver ball as reference electrode. Surround the reference electrode with the sponge that is soaked in saline to keep the reference electrode in contact with the heart.

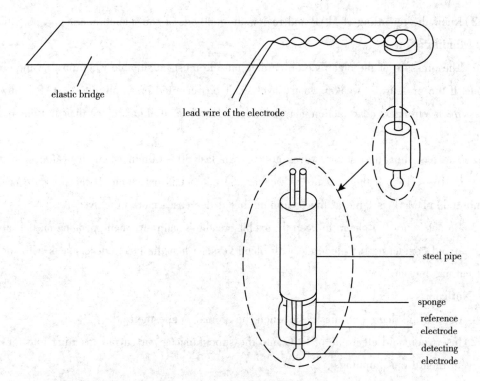

elastic bridge

lead wire of the electrode

steel pipe

sponge

reference electrode

detecting electrode

Fig. 4 – 22   abridged general view of epicardium contact electrode

Go straight through the steel pipe with only a non – polarizable electrode whose tip is silver ball when making monopolar electrode.

（2）Preparation of negative pressure electrode   The guiding part of negative pressure electrode is non – polarizable silver wire. The diameter of the tip in the wire is 0. 1mm. The wire is encased in the plastic tube, the length of plastic tube is 10 ~ 15cm, the bore of plastic tube is 6mm. The tip of the electrode is about 0. 5mm over the opening of the plastic tube. Keep the electrode in contact with the epicardium through suction of electric pump in the experiment because the pressure in the plastic tube is negative pressure.

（Yan Tianhua   Liu Bingbing）

实验三十一   蛙肠系膜微循环的观察

【实验目的】

本实验目的是观察肠系膜血管内血流状况，以了解微循环各组成部分的结构和血流特点。

【实验原理】

微循环是指微动脉和微静脉之间的血液循环，是组织与血液进行物质交换的直接场所，由微动脉、后微动脉、毛细血管前括约肌、真毛细血管网、微静脉、通血毛细血管和动 – 静脉吻合支等部分组成。其中小动脉、微动脉管壁厚，管腔内径小，血流速度快，血流方向是从主干向分支，有轴流（血细胞在血管中央流动）现象；小静脉、微静脉管壁薄，管

扫码"学一学"

腔内径大，血流速度慢，无轴流现象，血流方向是从分支向主干汇合；而毛细血管管径最细，仅允许单个血细胞依次通过。

【实验材料】

1. 器材 显微镜、有孔的软木蛙板、蛙类手术器械、大头针、吸管、注射器。

2. 溶液 20%氨基甲酸乙酯（乌拉坦）溶液、任氏液。

3. 对象 蛙（或蟾蜍）。

【实验方法】

1. 取蛙一只，以20%的氨基甲酸乙酯进行尾骨两侧的皮下淋巴囊注射，剂量为200mg/kg，10～15min进入麻醉状态。

2. 用大头针将蛙腹位（或背位）固定在蛙板上，于腹部侧方做3～4cm的纵行切口，轻轻拉出一段小肠，将肠系膜展开，用大头针数枚固定在有孔的软木蛙板上（图4-23）。

3. 在低倍显微镜下，分辨小动脉、小静脉和毛细血管，观察其中血行的速度、特征以及血细胞在血管内流动的形式。

［附］ 蛙舌微循环的观察 用小镊子将蛙舌自口腔内拉出，以大头针将舌头边缘固定于板孔周围，于显微镜下观察微循环的情况。

【实验指导】

1. 预习要求 预习微循环的组成及其功能的有关理论。

2. 操作要点

（1）手术切口在下腹部一侧，待麻醉完全后进行。

（2）固定肠系膜时，动作要轻，以防出血，影响观察。

3. 注意事项

（1）手术操作要仔细，避免出血造成视野模糊。

（2）固定肠系膜不要牵引过紧，以免影响血管内血液流动。

（3）为防止干燥要经常以任氏液湿润肠系膜。但任氏液也不必加得太多。

4. 报告要点 比较镜下小动脉、小静脉、毛细血管的血流特征及血管口径、管壁的特征。

5. 思考题

（1）实验中，如何区分小动脉、小静脉和毛细血管？

（2）血管中血流各有什么特点？动脉中的血流为什么有轴流、壁流之分？

（丁启龙）

31　Observation of the mesenteric microcirculation in toad

PURPOSE

The purpose of the experiment is to understand the structure of each part and characteristic of blood current in microcirculation by observing the condition of blood flow in mesenteric blood vessel.

PRINCIPLE

Microcirculation is blood circulation between arteriole and venule, and is the direct location of material exchange between tissue and blood. It includes arteriole, metarteriole, precapillary sphincter, true capillary network, venule, capillary with flowing blood, and arterial – venous anastomose branch etc. In small artery and arteriole, with thick wall and small calibre, the velocity of the blood current is quick, and the blood current with the axial flow phenomenon (blood cell flow at the central of blood vessels) is from the stem to the branch. In the small vein and venule, with thin wall and large calibre, the velocity of blood current is slow, and the bloodcurrent with no axial flow phenomenon is from the branch to the stem. The capillary has the smallest calibre, and only allows single blood cells to pass one by one.

MATERIALS

1. Equipments   Microscope, soft wooden frog plank with a small hole, frog surgical apparatus, pin, pipette, syringe.

2. Solutions   20% ethyl carbamate (urethane), Ringer's solution.

3. Object   Frog (or toad).

METHODS

1. Take a toad, inject 20% ethyl carbamate (urethane) with 0.1 ml /10g body weight into the subcutaneous lymphaticcapsule near the coccyx. After about 10 ~ 15 mins, the toad enters into the anaesthetic state.

2. Fix the toad in the decubitus (or the supine position) on the plank, cut a 3 ~ 4 cm incision at one side of its belly, and pull out a section of the small intestine. And then unfold the mesentery; fix it on the soft wooden frog plank with some pins (Fig. 4 – 23).

3. Under the low time microscope, distinguish the small artery, the small vein and the capillary, and observe the speed of blood current, the characteristic and the flow manner of blood cells in blood vessels.

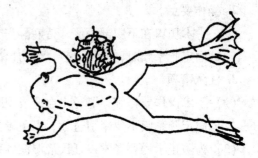

Fig. 4 – 23   The fixing method of
the mesentery in toad

[Attachment]   Observation of the microcirculation of frog tongue

Pull out the frog tongue from the mouth with small forceps, fix the border of tongue around the plank hole with pins, and observe the circumstance of microcirculation under the microscope.

GUIDANCE

1. Preview   Learn the composition and the function of microcirculation and the relevant theories before class.

2. Manipulation

(1)The surgical cut is at one side of hypogastrium; the cut should be operated after the toad has been anesthetized completely.

(2) Fix the mesentery carefully in order to prevent from bleeding so as not to affect observation.

3. Notices

(1) Be careful in the operation, in order to avoid bleeding.

(2) Don't pull tightly when fixing the mesentery, in order to avoid affecting the blood flow in small blood vessel.

(3) Often wet the mesentery with Ringer's solution in order to prevent it from drying, but not too much.

4. Report Compare characteristics of arteriole, venule and capillary in the blood current, the calibre of blood vessels and the wall under a microscope.

5. Questions

(1) How to distinguish the small artery, small vein and capillary in the experiment?

(2) What are the characteristics of the blood current in the blood vessel? Why are there the two different blood flow manners (axial flow and wall flow) in small artery?

(Ding Qilong)

实验三十二 兔减压神经放电

【实验目的】

观察减压神经传入冲动的发放特征以及动脉血压变动与减压神经传入冲动发放的相互关系，从而加深对减压反射的认识，并了解减压神经放电的引导记录方法。

【实验原理】

绝大多数哺乳类动物主动脉弓压力感受器的传入神经纤维参与迷走神经进入延髓，兔的主动脉弓压力感受器传入纤维自成一束，与迷走神经和颈交感神经干伴行，称为减压神经，其传入中枢的冲动对动脉血压的升降有监控作用。动脉血压升高时其传入冲动增加，冲动到达心血管中枢后，使迷走中枢的紧张性加强，由迷走神经传至心脏的冲动增多；同时，使心交感中枢和交感缩血管中枢紧张性减弱，由心交感神经传至心脏，缩血管神经传至血管平滑肌的冲动减少，于是心搏减慢，血管舒张，外周阻力减小，使动脉血压保持在较低的水平。反之，动脉血压降低，其传入冲动减少或停止，对中枢的作用减轻，动脉血压又可升高。因此，减压反射是一种负反馈调节，它的生理意义在于维持动脉血压相对稳定。本实验学习记录神经放电的基本方法，并观察放电和动脉血压间的相互关系。

【实验材料】

1. 器材 BL-420F 生物信号采集与分析系统，引导电极（直径 0.2mm 银丝，两极间距 2mm 左右），电极固定架，哺乳动物手术器械，兔手术台，动脉套管，注射器（2ml、10ml、20ml 各 1）。

2. 溶液 20%氨基甲酸乙酯，1：10000去甲肾上腺素，1：10000乙酰胆碱，生理盐水，液状石蜡。

3. 对象 家兔。

【实验方法】

1. 动物麻醉与固定 按1g/kg体重剂量经兔耳缘静脉缓慢注射20%氨基甲酸乙酯麻醉，将麻醉动物仰卧位固定在兔手术台上，颈部放正拉直，开亮手术台底部灯以保温。

2. 手术 剪去颈前部兔毛，在颈部正中切开皮肤约10cm，分离皮下组织及肌肉，暴露气管，在甲状软骨下约第三或第四环状软骨水平做倒"T"切口，向肺方向插入气管套管后用棉线将其扎紧。

沿气管两侧小心分离降压神经，在其下穿一根经过任氏液浸润的细线，轻轻提起，滴上液状石蜡（38~40℃），以防干燥而损伤神经。同时进行颈总动脉插管。

3. 记录系统的连接与仪器调试

（1）记录电极通过屏蔽导线输入到BL-420F第1通道上，记录降压神经放电，BL-420F输出接监听器（可选）。地线接在动物手术切口处，仪器外壳也应接地。

（2）颈总动脉插管通过压力换能器输入到BL-420F第3通道上，记录血压变化。

（3）进入BL-420F，生理，减压神经放电，参数设置为：SR=2~10ms（内部采样周期为0.05ms），横向压缩1：4，通道1增益500~1000倍，滤波10kHz，时间常数0.01s。也可用"通用四道记录仪"，此时，2道应设为对1通道进行直方图处理。

（4）安置引导电极 用银丝弓引导电极将降压神经轻轻勾起。注意神经不可牵拉过紧，并使引导电极悬空，不要触及周围组织。

4. 观察项目

（1）记录血压正常时降压神经放电情况，观察放电与心搏、血压间的关系。

（2）向耳缘静脉注射1：10000去甲肾上腺素0.5ml，观察减压神经放电频率和幅度的变化及动脉血压的变化。

（3）待血压恢复后，向耳缘静脉注射1：10000乙酰胆碱0.3ml，观察减压神经放电频率和幅度的变化及动脉血压的变化。

【实验指导】

1. 预习要求

（1）复习血压的神经-体液调节，重点复习减压反射的调节过程及其生理意义。

（2）复习BL-420F生物信号采集与分析系统的操作应用。

2. 操作要点

（1）减压神经的分离要准确，在确定减压神经之前，应保持血管神经束的自然位置关系，在结缔组织内寻找减压神经。

（2）引导电极要用铂或银丝（直径0.2mm）制成，两极间距为2mm左右，不可用铜丝，引导电极短路或断路，可突然出现交流干扰。

3. 注意事项

（1）仪器和动物都要接地，并注意适当屏蔽。

（2）麻醉不宜太浅，以免动物挣扎，产生肌电干扰和拉伤神经。

（3）分离神经时动作要轻，分离后及时滴加温热液状石蜡。

（4）保持神经与引导电极接触良好；引导电极不可触及周围组织，以免带来干扰。

4. 报告要点

（1）总结减压神经放电的特征。

（2）总结减压神经放电与动脉血压的关系，并绘制血压 – 放电频率关系曲线。

5. 思考题

（1）减压神经放电的基本波形有何特点？

（2）以实验结果证明反射具有负反馈特征，说明其调节过程和意义。

（颜天华　刘冰冰）

32　Discharge of depressor nerve in rabbit

PURPOSE

To observe the characteristics of depressor nerve discharge and the relationships between depressor nerve discharges and changes in arterial pressure, in order to have more knowledge of depressor reflex and learn the methods of recording the discharge of depressor nerve.

PRINCIPLE

The afferent nerve fiber located at pressure receptor of aortic arch in most mammal joins the vagus nerve reaching to medulla oblongata. But the afferent nerve fiber in rabbit is different, which is an independent tract, accompanying the vagus nerve and the stem of sympathetic nerve. It is called depressor nerve. The impulse of depressor nerve reaching to the center can regulate arterial pressure. When arterial pressure rises, the afferent impulses of depressor nerve reaching cardiovascular center are increased, which can strengthen the tension of vagus center and cause the increase of the impulses to heart from vagus nerve ; At the same time, the afferent impulses of depressor nerve can weaken the tension of sympathetic center and vasoconstrictor center. This results in the decrease of the impulses of sympathetic nerve reaching to heart and the impulses of vasoconstrictor nerve reaching to vascular smooth muscle. So heart rate becomes slow, blood vessel is relaxed, peripheral resistance is decreased and thus arterial pressure maintains low lever. On the contrary, when arterial pressure decreases, the afferent impulses of depressor nerve are decreased or ceased, of which action on the center is weakened and arterial pressure rises again. Therefore, the reflection of depressor nerve is a negative feedback, and it physiologically maintains the stability of arterial pressure relatively. In the experiment, we try to learn the methods of recording the discharges of depressor nerve and observe the relationship between depressor nerve discharge and changes in arterial pressure.

MATERIALS

1. Equipments　BL – 420F biological signal acquisition and analysis system, Guiding electrode (silver wire: 0. 2mm diameter, 2mm spacing of two tips), electrode fixing frame, operational plate for mammal, rabbit board, arterial cannula, injector (2ml, 10ml, 20ml)

2. Solutions　20% ethyl carbamate, 1 : 10000 noradrenaline, saline, liquid paraffin, 1 : 10000 acetylcholine.

3. Experimental object　rabbit.

METHOD

1. Anesthesia and fixation of the animal　Inject 20% ethyl carbamate into vein in ear slowly with the dose of 1g/kg, and secure the rabbit with its dorsal side down on the board, then turn on the lamp under the board to keep the rabbit warm.

2. Operation　First cut off the hair in front of the rabbit's neck, and cut a 10cm hole in the middle of the skin, then separates muscle and subcutaneous tissue to expose the windpipe. Now make a upside – down "T" incision at the third or fourth cricoid cartilage under thyroid cartilage, and insert tracheal cannula toward the lung, then bundle it up tightly with cotton thread.

Separate carefully depressor nerve, and put a piece of thread under the nerves and raise it carefully, while dripping some warm liquid paraffin on the thread, so as to prevent the nerve from injury. In the meantime, insert arterial cannula into common carotid artery to record blood pressure.

3. Connection and adjustment of recording system

(1) Connect recording electrode to the first channel of the recording system by shield cable, so as to record discharge of depressor nerve, and connect the system to audiomonitor (optional). The incision is connected with groundwire and the shell of the equipments must be connected with the ground.

(2) Connect arterial cannula with the third channel of the system so as to record the blood pressure.

(3) Open the BL – 420F the parameter is as the follows: SR = 2 ~ 10ms (interior sampling period is 0.05ms), the ratio of compression is 1 : 4, gain of the first channel is 500 ~ 1000, filtering: 10kHz, time constant is 0.01s. "general 4 channels recorder" can also be used. When it is used, two channels should be setted to one channel for managing with histogram.

(4) Set guiding electrode: tick off depressor nerve slightly with guiding electrode made of silver. Avoid stretching strongly, and suspending guiding electrode in midair (do not have it touched the surrounding tissue).

4. Observation Items

(1) Record discharge of depressor nerve when blood pressure is normal in order to observe the relationship between the discharge and the heart beat or blood pressure.

(2) Inject 0.5ml noradrenaline (1 : 10000), to observe changes in discharge frequency and discharge range of depressor nerve, and observe changes in blood pressure.

(3) After blood pressure comes to normal, inject 0.3ml acetylcholine (1 : 10000), to observe changes in discharge frequency and discharge range of depressor nerve, and changes in blood pressure.

GUIDANCE

1. Requirements for Preparation

(1) Review nervous – humoral regulation of blood pressure, focusing on the regulation of depressor nerve and its physiological significance.

(2)Review the use of BL – 420F biological signal acquisition and analysis system.

2. Requirements for Manipulation

(1)Separate depressor nerve accurately. Before the nerve is found, keep naturalthe position of blood vessel and nerve tract, and look for depressor nerve in connective tissue.

(2)Guiding electrode is made of silver wire or platinum wire (its diameter is 0. 2mm), and the distance of its two tips is about 2mm. If guiding electrode is a copper one, interference of alternating current will come unexpectedly when the circuit of guiding electrode is shorted or is turn – out.

3. Notice

(1)Connect equipments and animals with the ground, and shield them to avoid electric interference.

(2)Corneal and withdrawal reflexes should not be obvious (because the animal is not properly anesthetized), which avoids moving of the animal that can cause myoelectric interference and injury of some nerves.

(3)Separate the nerves softly, and drip warm liquid paraffin in time once the nerves are separated.

(4)The connection of nerve and guiding electrode should be well; guiding electrode should not be connected with surrounding tissue to avoid electric interference.

4. Requirements for Report

(1)Write down characteristics of discharge of depressor nerve.

(2)Write down relationship between the blood pressure and the discharge of depressor nerve, and then plot the relationship of the both.

5. Consideration Problems

(1)What is the characteristic of the discharge of the depressor nerve?

(2)Prove that the reflection is a negative feedback, and try to account for the procedure of the regulation and significance of the reflection.

(Yan Tianhua Liu Bingbing)

第五章　呼吸系统

Respiratory system

实验三十三　家兔呼吸运动的调节

【实验目的】

本实验是观察多种刺激因素对家兔呼吸运动（呼吸频率、节律、幅度）的影响，并分析其作用机制。

【实验原理】

呼吸运动是呼吸中枢节律性活动的反应。在不同生理状态下，呼吸运动所发生的适应性变化有赖于神经系统的反射性调节，其中较为重要的有呼吸中枢、肺牵张反射以及外周化学感受器的反射性调节。因此，体内外各种刺激，可以直接作用于中枢部位或通过不同的感受器反射性地影响呼吸运动。

【实验材料】

1. 实验仪器　BL-420F 生物信号采集与分析系统，哺乳动物手术器械，兔手术台，玛利氏气鼓张力换能器，气管插管，注射器（20ml、10ml），50cm 长的橡皮管，纱布，粗、细棉线，装有 N_2、CO_2 及 O_2 的气囊。

2. 溶液　20% 氨基甲酸乙酯，3% 乳酸，生理盐水。

3. 对象　兔（体重 $1.8 \sim 2.2kg$）。

【实验方法】

1. 麻醉与固定　由兔耳缘静脉注射 20% 氨基甲酸乙酯（$1 \sim 1.2g/kg$），待兔麻醉后仰卧位固定于手术台上。

2. 手术　剪去兔颈前部的毛，沿颈部正中线切开皮肤 $5 \sim 7cm$，用止血钳钝性分离颈部肌肉，暴露气管。把甲状软骨以下的气管与周围组织分离，在气管下放置一粗棉线备用。在甲状腺下面的气管上做一"⊥"型切口。插入气管插管，用粗棉线将气管结扎固定。分离两侧迷走神经，在神经下穿线备用。手术完毕后用温热生理盐水纱布覆盖手术伤口部位。

3. 呼吸运动描记

（1）膈肌运动描计法　在剑突下方沿腹白线做 3cm 左右的切口，辨认剑突内侧面附着的两块膈小肌，仔细分离剑突与各小肌之间的组织并剪断剑突（注意压迫止血）；此时用弯针钩住剑突软骨，使游离的膈小肌和张力换能器（量程为 25g）相连接，由 BL-420F 生物信号采集与分析系统描记呼吸运动曲线（图 5 – 1）。此种描记法可反映呼吸频率、呼吸深度以及呼吸停止状态。缺点是在动物移动或稍有挣扎之后，基线变化较大，不得不再次调整描记系统。

（2）气鼓描记法 将气管插管的一个侧管用适当粗细的橡皮管连于玛利氏气鼓之铁管上，将玛利氏气鼓与张力换能器相连（图 5 – 2）。用电脑观察呼吸运动，并将呼吸运动曲线打印出来。此种描记方法基线稳，一般不受动物挣扎移动的影响，能很好地反映动物的呼吸频率，但在某种情况下却不能很真实地反映呼吸深度，这主要是由于气鼓底盘可能限制了橡皮鼓膜的下移。此外，刺激呼吸中枢或观察某种反射活动，常可使呼吸停止在呼气或吸气状态，此种状态无法用引导气管插管侧管气流的气鼓描记法真实地反映出来，因为不管呼吸停止在何种状态，呼吸曲线都是在中间划出一条直线，因此气鼓描记法不宜于进行这一类实验观察。

（3）胸内压描计法 将腰椎穿刺针用橡皮管与水压检计相连，由肋间斜刺入胸膜腔，观察水柱随呼吸频率变化及幅值的改变（图 5 – 3）（具体操作步骤可参见胸内负压测定实验）。此描计法不仅基线平稳，而且比较忠实的反映呼吸运动的频率、呼吸深度以及呼吸停止状态。

4. 观察项目

（1）吸入气中 CO_2 浓度增加时对呼吸运动的影响 将气管插管侧管开口端与装 CO_2 气囊上的橡皮管口相对，稍稍松开气囊上的螺丝夹，使一部分 CO_2 随吸气进入气管。观察吸入高浓度 CO_2 后呼吸运动有何变化。

（2）缺 O_2 对呼吸运动的影响 将气管插管侧管开口端与装 N_2 气囊的橡皮管口相对，打开 N_2 气囊上的螺丝夹，使一部分 N_2 随吸气进入气管，观察吸入 N_2 后呼吸运动有何变化。

（3）增大气道阻力对呼吸运动的影响 待呼吸平稳后，部分阻塞一侧气管插管，观察呼吸有何变化。

（4）无效腔增大对呼吸运动的影响 在气管插管侧管连接一长 50cm 的橡皮管，使无效腔增大，观察对呼吸运动的影响。

（5）血液中酸性物质增多对呼吸运动的影响 由兔耳缘静脉较快地注入 3% 乳酸 2ml，观察呼吸运动的变化过程。

（6）肺牵张反射的观察与分析 在气管插管的一个侧管上，用橡皮管连一 20ml 以上的注射器，里面先装好约 20ml 空气，描记一段对照呼吸曲线，然后在吸气相迅速夹闭气管插管的另一侧管，并向肺内注入约 20ml 的空气，使肺处于持续扩张状态，观察呼吸运动的变化。之后开放夹闭之侧管，使动物呼吸恢复。然后在呼气相再次夹闭此侧管，并立即从肺内用注射器抽出一定量气体，使肺处于萎陷状态，观察呼吸运动的变化。之后开放夹闭之气管插管的侧管，使动物呼吸恢复。以上实验可重复进行观察，待现象明确后，切断两侧迷走神经，描记迷走神经切断前后呼吸运动的变化。然后再依上法重复上述实验，比较切断迷走神经前后的实验效果。

用不同频率的电刺激，刺激迷走神经的向中端，可以模拟上述充气与排气刺激。低频（$8 \sim 50$ 次/秒）刺激常使呼吸抑制，类似肺持续充气，使呼吸停止在呼气状态；而高频刺激常使呼吸加强，相当于排气刺激，有时可使呼吸停止在吸气状态。引起以上呼吸效果的具体刺激频率还与刺激强度和麻醉深浅有关。

【实验指导】

1. 预习要求

（1）复习呼吸节律形成机制。

（2）复习呼吸的反射性调节及化学因素对呼吸的调节。

2. 操作要点

（1）膈肌运动描记法记录呼吸时，游离剑突的剪口应在剑突与胸骨体连接处（剑突骨柄）。使剑突软骨与胸骨完全分离。提起剑突，可见剑突随膈肌的收缩自由运动。

（2）气鼓描记法记录呼吸运动时，气管插管大小要与气管直径相近。可在与外界相通的气管插管上加接一小段（要尽量短些）橡皮管，调节此管的口径而增加气道阻力，这可使描记曲线幅度增大。

3. 注意事项

（1）膈肌运动描记法记录呼吸运动时，游离剑突片应与滑轮及连接线在一条线上，使力量比较集中，且连接线不宜过长，使其有一定紧张度，否则影响描记。游离剑突时剪口不可过深，以防气胸形成。同时切忌剪断附着于剑突后方的膈小肌。

（2）气鼓描记法记录呼吸运动时，气鼓上的乳胶膜捆扎不宜太紧或太松。一般要求吸气时气鼓膜内陷不要触及鼓底，而且不论在呼气或吸气，杠杆都有活动余地。装有各种气体的气囊，开口不能直接套在气管插管的侧管上，以免加大死腔和附加窒息因素而影响实验结果。

4. 报告要点

（1）描记呼吸运动曲线图。

（2）根据实验结果结合理论分析以下几点：①吸入气中 CO_2 浓度增加及吸入纯 N_2 缺氧时对呼吸运动的影响，并阐明机制。②增大气道阻力及解剖无效腔对呼吸运动的影响，并阐明机制。③静脉注射乳酸对呼吸运动的影响，并阐明机制。④迷走神经在维持节律性呼吸中起的作用。

5. 思考题

（1）什么麻醉颈动脉体后，再吸入 CO_2 和纯 N_2 时，对呼吸运动的影响不同？

（2）中等强度刺激一侧迷走神经向中端，呼吸运动会不会发生变化？

（李运曼）

33 Regulation of respiratory movement in rabbit

PURPOSE

To observe the effects of stimulating factors on respiratory movement in rabbit（frequency, rhythm and range of respiratory）to and analyze mechanisms.

PRINCIPLE

Respiratory movement is the reflect of rhythmical movement of respiratory center. In different physiological conditions, adaptive changes happened in respiratory movement are depended on the reflex adjustment of nervous system, in which the reflex adjustments of respiratory center and peripheral chemoreceptor and the pulmonary stretch reflex are more important than others. So all the stimulating factors, no matter be given by vivo or by vitro, can change respiratory movement directly through affecting on the center or reflex through different peripheral chemoreceptors.

MATERIALS

1. Equipments　BL – 420F biological signal acquisition and analysis system, Surgical tools, operating table for rabbit, Mary's tambour tensile transducer, tracheal cannula, syringe, rubber tube (50cm), gauze, thread, N_2, CO_2 and O_2 ballonet.

2. Solutions　Urethan 20%. Lactic Acid 3%. 0.9% NaCl.

3. Object　Rabbit, body weight: 1.8 ~ 2.2kg.

METHODS

1. Anesthesia and fixation　20% Urethan (1 ~ 1.2g/kg) was injected into the vein in the rabbit's ear. And then fix the rabbit on the operation table in supine body position when the rabbit was anesthetized.

2. Operation　Shear the hairs on neck; cut down the skin along the middle line, separate trachea with hemostats until trachea under the thyroid cartilage is detached from nearby constitutions. Cut down trachea and insert the Y tracheal cannula, then fix the trachea with lines. Detach pneumogastric nerve, and put thread under it. When the operation was done, cover the wound with warm gauze soaked by normal saline.

3. Record of respiratory movement

(1) record of movement of diaphragm: make a 3cm incisions along the linea alba abdominis under the xiphoid, identify the two small diaphragms attached with inter surface of the xiphoid, dissociate the tissue between two small diaphragms and xiphoid carefully and cut the xiphoid off; then hook the cartilage of xiphoid to make the dissociated small diaphragm connected with tensile transducer (25g), record the curves of respiratory movement (Fig. 5 – 1). This record can reflect the respiratory frequency, the respiratory range. When rabbit moves or struggles slightly, the change of baseline may be changed, So it has to be adjusted again.

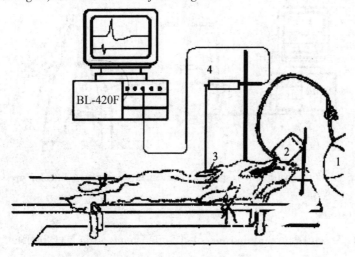

Fig. 5 – 1　Instruments for recording respiratory movement

1. CO_2 ballonet 2. beaker 3. diaphragmatic muscle 4. tensile transducer

（2）Record of tambour：connect a lateral pip of tracheal cannula with the iron tube of Mary's tambour through a proper rubber tube. Connect Mary's tambour and tensile transducer as Fig. 5 – 2. Record respiratory movement with BL – 420F，and then print the results. In this method，the baseline is steady and not be effected by animal's action in general. It can reflect respiratory frequency well，but it cannot reflect respiratory range correctly in some condition，which is mainly because the bottom of the tambour may restrict rubber drum membrane's movement. In addition，when respiratory centrum is stimulated or respiratory movement is observed，respiration is stopped in state of expiration or inspiration. This state cannot be reflected really by the record of tambour，because no matter which state respiration is stopped，the respiratory curve is a straight line. So this record is not fit for observations of this kind of experiments.

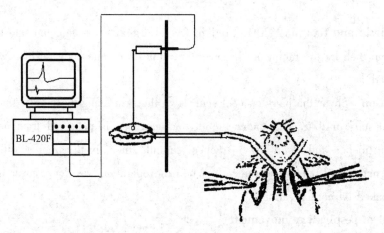

Fig. 5 – 2　Recording respiratory movement of rabbit with tambour

（3）Record of thoracic interior pressure：Connect a puncture needle and a pressure transducer with a rubber tube. Stick the needle into thoracic cavity between ribs，and then observe the change of the pressure in the cavity when respiratory frequency and the change of range（Fig. 5 – 3）. This method with a steady baseline can reflect respiratory frequency，respiratory range and respiratory state.

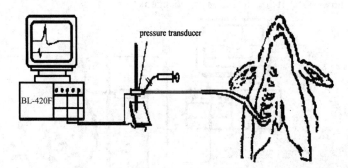

Fig. 5 – 3　Observation of respiratory movement by thoracic interior pressure

4. Observing items

（1）Effect of CO_2 on respiratory movement：The peristome of the CO_2 ballonet was aimed to another opening of the tracheal cannula，then open screw clip on the CO_2 ballonet to make some CO_2 into trachea.

(2)Effect ofO_2 lack on respiratory movement: The peristome of the N_2 ballonet was aimed to another opening of the tracheal cannula, then open screw clip on the N_2 ballonet to make some N_2 into trachea.

(3)Effect of tracheal resistance on respiratory movement: When respiratory is steady, block one side of tracheal cannula and observe the changes of respiration.

(4)The changes of respiratory movement when dead space enlarges: Block one side of tracheal cannula and record a curve of respiratory movement, then connect a 50cm rubber tube with the other one to make dead space enlarge. Observe the changes of respiratory movement.

(5)Effect of acid substances in blood on respiratory movement: After 3% Lactic Acid 2ml was injected fast into vein in the rabbit, observe the changes of respiratory movement.

(6)Observe and analyze the pulmonary stretch reflex.

a. Connect a 20ml syringe, which is full of air beforehand with one branch of tracheal cannula with a rubber tube. Record the contrast respiratory curve, then close the other branch quickly in the phase of expiration. Inject about 20ml air, make the lung expand constantly, observe the changes. Then open the closed branch to make the rabbit recover respiration. Close the branch in the expiration phase again, deflate some air from lung immediately, and then observe the changes. Open the branch to make the rabbit's respiration recover. This experiment can be donerepeatedly. When phenomena are clear, cut off vagus nerve both sides and record the changes of respiratory movement. Repeat the experiment and compare the results.

b. Stimulation on the tip of vagus nerve toward nerve center can simulate stimulation of the inflation and exhaustas described previously. The low frequency stimulation (8～50times/s) often restrains respiration and makes the respiration stop in expiration state, like the constant lung inflation; The high frequency stimulation often enhances respiration and makes the respiration stop in inspiration state, like the constant lung exhaust. The specific frequencies, which cause the respiratory effects, are relevant to stimulating intensity and narcotic depth.

GUIDANCE

1. Preview

(1)Review the mechanism of respiratory rhythm to form.

(2)Review the respiratory reflex adjustment and adjustment caused by chemical factors.

2. Manipulation

(1)Tracing of movement of muscle of diaphragm: The cut of xiphoid should be the place where xiphoid and mesosternum connected. Xiphoid cartilage and sternum should be separated completely.

(2)Tracing of tambour: The size of tracheal cannula should be suitable. And a short rubber tub can be added to strengthen resisting force of airway.

3. Notices

(1)Tracing of movement of muscle of diaphragm: The free xiphoid should be in line with pulley and lines; the line should not be too long; the cut should not be too deep. Avoid not cutting off small muscles of diaphragm under xiphoid.

(2)Tracing of tambour: Latex coat should not be too tight or too loose.

4. Reports

（1）Record curve of respiratory movement

（2）Analyze the points as follows according to experiment results.

a. Effect on respiratory movement when CO_2 and N_2 concentrate rise in inhalation air and its mechanism.

b. Effect on respiratory movement when tracheal resistance rises and its mechanism.

c. Effect on respiratory movement when acid substances in blood rise and its mechanism.

5. Questions

（1）Why the effects on respiratory movement are different when CO_2 and N_2 are given?

（2）Will respiratory movement change when middling stimulation to the centrum – toward tip of vagus nerve?

（Li Yunman）

实验三十四　膈神经放电

【实验目的】

学习神经放电的记录方法，同时加深对呼吸运动调节的认识。

【实验原理】

呼吸肌属于骨骼肌，其活动依赖膈神经和肋间神经的支配。呼吸运动的节律来源于呼吸中枢。膈神经放电是指经引导电极记录的膈神经上的电信号，与膈肌放电相似。

【实验材料】

1. 器材　哺乳动物手术器械一套，兔台，气管插管，BL – 420F 生物信号采集与分析系统（或前置放大器、示波器、监听器），引导电极，呼吸换能器（可选），固定支架，注射器（30ml、20ml），玻璃分针。

2. 溶液　20% 氨基甲酸乙酯，生理盐水，液状石蜡，CO_2 气体，尼可刹米注射液。

3. 对象　兔。

【实验方法】

1. 手术操作

（1）麻醉和固定　20% 氨基甲酸乙酯（5ml/kg）自耳缘静脉注射麻醉后，取仰卧位固定在兔台上。

（2）剪去颈部兔毛，自胸骨上端向头部做一正中切口，约10cm。分离皮下组织、肌肉及气管，做气管插管。分离颈部两侧的迷走神经，穿线备用。

（3）一侧颈外静脉和胸锁乳突肌之间用止血钳向深部分离，可见到较粗的臂丛神经向后外方行走。在臂丛的内侧有一条较细的膈神经横过臂丛神经并和它交叉，向后内侧行走，从斜方肌的腹缘进入胸腔。用玻璃分针将膈神经分离 1~2cm，在神经的外周端穿线备用。

做好皮兜，注入38℃的液状石蜡，起保温、绝缘和防止神经干燥的作用。将膈神经钩在悬空的引导电极上，避免触及周围组织，以减少干扰。

2. 仪器的连接与调试 膈神经放电信号接 BL－420F 通道1，BL－420F 输出接监听器（可选）。地线接在动物手术切口处。仪器外壳均应接地。

若同时记录呼吸曲线，则换能器接 BL－420F 通道4。

进入 BL－420F，生理→膈神经放电，参数设置为：SR＝2～10ms（内部采样周期为0.05ms），横向压缩1∶4，通道1增益500～1000倍，滤波10kHz，时间常数0.01s。也可用"通用四道记录仪"，此时，2道应设为对1道进行直方图处理。

3. 观察项目

（1）观察膈神经放电与呼吸运动的关系，注意膈神经的放电形式及其通过监听器所发出的声音与吸气相的关系（图5－4）。

（2）吸入气中 CO_2 浓度增加对膈神经放电的影响。将充有 CO_2 的球胆对准气管插管的开口，使动物吸入 CO_2，观察膈神经放电和呼吸运动的变化。

（3）兔耳缘静脉注入稀释的尼可刹米1ml（内含50mg），观察膈神经放电和呼吸运动的变化。

（4）切断一侧迷走神经干后，观察膈神经放电和呼吸运动有何变化。再切断另一侧迷走神经，观察膈神经放电的变化。

【实验指导】

1. 预习要求

（1）学习呼吸节律的形成机制。

（2）学习呼吸的反射性调节机制。

（3）学习化学因素对呼吸的调节作用。

2. 操作要求

（1）准确寻找膈神经并在实验过程中保护好膈神经。

（2）适当调节时间窗，使直方图更加明显。

3. 注意事项

（1）分离膈神经动作要小心仔细。

（2）也可不做皮兜，但要用温液状石蜡棉条覆盖在神经上。

（3）注意动物和仪器的接地要可靠。

（4）注意区别放电频率与呼吸频率。

4. 实验报告 剪下打印的膈神经放电图并粘贴在实验报告本上，根据实验结果分析讨论其机制。

5. 思考题

（1）吸入 CO_2，膈神经的放电有何变化？是通过什么途径实现的？

（2）静脉注射尼可刹米以后，膈神经放电有何变化？为什么？

（3）切断两侧迷走神经干后，呼吸运动的频率、深度和膈神经放电各有何改变？为什么？

（王秋娟）

34　Discharge of phrenic nerve

PURPOSE

The purpose of this experiment is to learn the recording method of nerve discharge and to cognize the modulation in respiratory movements.

PRINCIPLE

Breath muscles, as parts of skeletal muscles, are dominated by phrenic nerve and intercostal nerve. Rhythm of respiratory movement comes from respiratory center. Discharge of phrenic nerve is defined as the electrical signal recorded by the introductory electrode. The discharge forms of midriff muscle and the electric signal of midriff muscle are similar.

MATERIALS

1. Equipments　BL – 420F biological signal acquisition and analysis system (or preamplification, oscilloscope, audiomonitor), Operative instruments for mammal, operative table for rabbit, tracheal cannula, guiding electrode, respiratory converter, fixing cradle, syringe (30ml, 20ml, 1ml), glass separating needle.

2. Solutions　20% ethyl carbamate, physiological saline solution, liquid olefin, CO_2 gas, nikethamide injection.

3. Object　Rabbit.

METHODS

1. Surgical operation

(1) Anesthesia and fixation　Injecting 20% carbamic acid into the scapha vein of the rabbit to anesthetize the rabbit. After disappearance of cornea reflex and muscle tension, the rabbit can be fixed on the operating table in supine position.

(2) Trachea intubation and nerves separation　Shear coated hair of rabbit neck, make a incision of 10cm on the middle line of neck skin, separate subcutaneous tissue and muscle, trachea, insert the Cannula into trachea and fix it with a crude cotton thread. Separate the pneumogastric nerves (vagus) on both laterals of trachea, put a cotton thread under vaguses for availability.

(3) Exposure phrenic muscle and insert the needle electrode　Separate between external jugular vein and sternocephalicus muscle to profundus tissue. Find the thick brachial plexus trunk with a rear and lateral direction and the medial midriff nerve that is relatively thinner, transverse by brachial plexus trunk, with a rear and medial direction, and advance into thoracic cavity from the inferior edge of trapezius muscle. Use the grass needle to separate 1 ~ 2cm phrenic nerve and put a thread under its peripheral end. Make a skin bag and fill it with liquid olefin (38℃) to keep the nerve warm, moist and insulated. Fix phrenic nerve with an inducting electrode and avoid it to contact with surrounding tissue. Connect a ground lead to the incision skin to decrease interference current.

2. Instruments connection and debugging　Connect the needle – inducing electrode with channel 1 on BL – 420F panel. BL – 420F output and stethophone are linked (optional). Ground lead is connected to the operated incision.

To record the breath curve at the same time, the tension transducer is connected to channel 4 on BL – 420F panel.

The user interfaces of BL – 420F, physiology and discharge of phrenic nerve are opened one by one. Parameters intercalation: SR = 2 ~ 10ms (sampling cycle inside computer is 0.05ms), compress rate in landscape orientation: 1 ： 4, channel 1 plus: 500 ~ 1000, filter: 10kHz, time constant: 0.01s. When Common Four Channels Recorder is chosen, channel 2 in BL – 420F may be intercalate as histogram.

3. Observe items

(1) Observe the discharge form of phrenic nerve and the relationships between the discharge and breath. Pay attention to the association of inhale phase and sounds in monitor (Fig. 5 – 4).

(2) After the rabbit inbreathes CO_2 gas (deposited in a rubber globe), observe the changes of phrenic nerve discharge and respiration.

(3) Inject nikethamide 1ml (including nikethamide 5mg) into the marginal vein of the rabbit ear and observe the changes in phrenic nerve discharge and respiration.

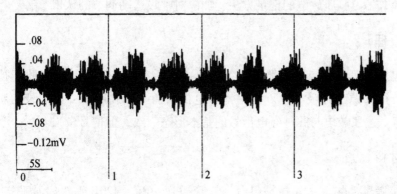

Fig. 5 – 4　Discharge of phrenic nerve

(4) Cut off a vagus, observe waves of the discharge and respiration. Recut the other vagus, observe waves of the discharge and respiration.

GUIDANCE

1. Preview

(1) Learn the mechanism of respiratory rhythm.

(2) Learn the reflex mechanism in respiratory modulation.

(3) Learn the mechanism of chemical factors in respiratory modulation.

2. Manipulation

(1) Find the phrenic nerve accurately and protect it properly.

(2) Regulate the time window appropriately and then make the histogram more obvious.

3. Notices

(1) Be careful in nerve separation.

(2) Cotton thread saturated with warm liquid olefin will also do if not choosing skin bag.

(3) Do fix the line to ground.

(4) Pay attention to the distinction of discharge rhythm and respiratory rate.

4. Report　Cut the printed curves of midriff muscle discharge in this experiment and stick it to

the report. Analyze and discuss the experiment result.

5. Questions

（1）Are there any changes in discharge of phrenic nerve while breathing in CO_2 and what is the mechanism of it?

（2）Are there any changes in discharge of phrenic nerve while injecting nikethamide？Why?

（3）Are there any changes in rhythm and depth of respiratory movement，or phrenic nerve discharge while cutting the bilateral vagus nerves？Why?

（Wang Qiujuan）

实验三十五　膈肌放电

【实验目的】

通过实验，学习膈肌放电的记录方法，加深对呼吸运动调节的认识。

【实验原理】

呼吸肌包括肋间肌和膈肌，都属于骨骼肌，其活动依赖于膈神经和肋间神经的支配，呼吸运动的节律来源于呼吸中枢。利用针形电极，插入到膈肌中，所记录的肌肉电活动，称为膈肌放电。膈肌放电与膈神经电信号的基本形态一致，但信号较强。

【实验材料】

1. 器材　哺乳动物手术器械，兔台，气管插管，BL－420F 生物信号采集与分析系统（或前置放大器、示波器、监听器），引导电极，呼吸换能器，固定支架，注射器（30ml、20ml、1ml），玻璃分针。

2. 溶液　20%氨基甲酸乙酯，生理盐水，液状石蜡，CO_2气体，尼可刹米注射液。

3. 对象　兔。

【实验方法】

1. 手术操作

（1）用20%氨基甲酸乙酯（乌拉坦）自兔耳缘静脉注射麻醉后，取仰卧位将其固定在兔台上。

（2）颈部正中切口，分离气管，进行气管插管并用粗棉线固定。分离颈部两侧与颈总动脉伴行的迷走神经，穿线备用。

（3）在胸骨下端正中做一切口，找到剑突并用止血钳向外拉，暴露与之相连的"小膈肌"。将两根带有绝缘套的针形电极（用针灸针制作）插入小膈肌，并用动脉夹固定在剑突上。

2. 仪器的连接与调试　膈肌放电信号接 BL－420F 通道 1，BL－420F 输出接监听器（可选）。地线接在动物手术切口处。若同时记录呼吸曲线，则换能器接 BL－420F 通道 4。

进入 BL-420F，生理，膈肌放电窗口。参数设置为：SR=2~10ms（内部采样周期为 0.05ms），横向压缩 1:4，通道 1 增益 400~1000 倍，滤波 10kHz，时间常数 0.01s。也可用"通用四道记录仪"，此时 2 通道设为直方图处理。

3. 观察项目

（1）观察膈肌放电的基本形态（图 5-5），电活动与机械活动之间的关系。

（2）将充有 CO_2 的球胆对准气管插管地开口，使动物摄入 CO_2，观察膈肌放电和呼吸运动的变化。

（3）兔耳缘静脉注入稀释的尼可刹米 1ml（内含 5mg），观察膈肌放电和呼吸运动的变化。

（4）切断一侧迷走神经后，呼吸及膈肌放电有何变化？再切断另一侧迷走神经，观察膈肌放电的变化。

（5）刺激一次迷走神经中枢端，观察膈肌放电和呼吸运动的变化。

【实验指导】

1. 预习要求 预习参与呼吸运动的肌肉及呼吸运动的调节机制。

2. 操作要点

（1）两根引导电极要插入到膈肌的肌肉中。

（2）适当调节时间窗，以使直方图比较明显。

3. 注意事项

（1）针形引导电极除尖端外要做绝缘处理。

（2）针形引导电极要适当固定，以防脱落。

4. 报告要点 对实验结果记录图做适当修剪后贴在报告本上，并对实验结果进行分析讨论。

5. 思考题

（1）膈肌放电的幅度和频率与呼吸之间的关系如何？

（2）刺激迷走神经中枢端，引起膈肌放电和呼吸变化的机制是什么？

（丁启龙）

35 Discharge of midriff muscle

PURPOSE

After learning the recording method of midriff muscle discharge, we can know the mechanism of respiratory regulation deeply.

PRINCIPLE

As parts of skeletal muscles, breath muscles including midriff muscle and intercostal muscles belong to the skeletal muscles. Their movements are controlled by midriff nerve and intercostal nerve. Rhythm of breath comes from breath centrum in medulla.

Discharge of midriff muscle is defined as the electrical signal recorded by the needle electrode inserted to midriff muscle. The discharge forms of midriff muscle and the electric signal of midriff nerve are similar, but the former electric signal is stronger.

MATERIALS

1. Equipments Operating instruments for mammal, operating table for rabbit, trachea cannula, BL – 420F biological signal acquisition and analysis system (or former amplifier, oscillograph, stethophone), needle inducting electrode, tension transducer, fixing bracket, syringe (30ml, 20ml, 1ml), glass needle for separation.

2. Solutions 20% ethyl carbamate, physiological saline solution, liquid olefin, CO_2 gas, nikethamide injection.

3. Object Rabbit.

METHODS

1. Surgical operation

(1) Injecting 20% ethyl carbamate into the scapha vein of the rabbit for anesthetizing the rabbit. After disappearance of cornea reflex and muscle tension, the rabbit is laid on its back and fixed on the operational table.

(2) Incise a cut on the middle line of neck skin, separate trachea, insert the cannula into the trachea and fix it with a crude cotton thread.

Separate the pneumogastric nerves (vagus) accompanied with common carotid arteries on both laterals of the trachea, put a cotton thread under each vagus.

(3) Cut an incision on the skin and muscle in the middle of upper abdomen. Expose midriff muscle with a hemostat. Insert two needle electrodes with insulated cover into the midriff muscle in different position and fix them with artery nips respectively.

2. Instruments connection and debugging

Connect the needle induction electrodes with channel 1 on BL – 420F panel. BL – 420F output may be linked with a stethophone. The ground lead is connected to the incision. To record the breath curve at the same time, a tension transducer may be connected with channel 4 on BL – 420F panel.

The manipulation interfaces of BL – 420F, the window of physiology and discharge of midriff are opened one by one. Parameters: SR = 2 ~ 10ms (sampling cycle inside computer is 0.05ms), Compress rate in landscape orientation: 1 : 4, Channel 1 gain: 400 ~ 1000, Filter: 10kHz, Time constant: 0.01s. When Common Four Channels Recorder is chosen, channel 2 in BL – 420F may be intercalated as histogram.

3. Observing items

(1) Observe the discharge waves of midriff muscle (Fig. 5 – 5) and the relationships between the discharge and respiration.

(2) After the rabbit inbreathes CO_2 gas (deposited in a rubber globe), observe waves of the discharge of midriff muscle and respiration.

(3) Inject nikethamide injection 1ml (containing nikethamide 5mg) into the scapha vein of the rabbit, then observe waves of the discharge and respiration.

(4) Cut off a vagus, observe waves of the discharge and respiration. Cut off the other vagus and observe waves of the discharge and respiration.

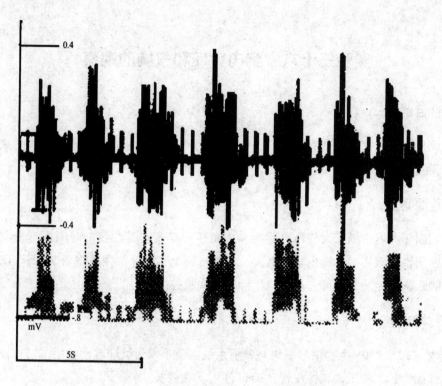

Fig. 5 – 5　The discharge waves of midriff muscle

（5）Stimulate the end of vagus near centrum, observe waves of the discharge and respiration.

GUIDANCE

1. Preview　Learn the knowledge of muscles taking part in breath and the mechanism regulating respiration.

2. Manipulation

（1）Two leading electrodes must be inserted into the abdomen of midriff muscle.

（2）It is appropriate to regulate the time window and then make the histogram more obvious.

3. Notices

（1）All the needle recording electrodes must be insulated but the tip.

（2）The needle record electrodes must be fixed.

4. Report　Cut the printed curves of midriff muscle discharge in this experiment and stick it to the report. Analyze and discuss the experiment result.

5. Questions

（1）What is the relationship between the range and frequency of midriff muscle discharge and the respiration?

（2）What is the mechanism of the variation of midriff muscle discharge and respiration after stimulating the end of vagus near centrum?

（Ding Qilong）

实验三十六　胸内负压和气胸的观察

【实验目的】

本实验是直接观察家兔平静呼吸及在呼吸运动变化时胸内负压的变化。同时观察人工气胸、胸膜腔与外界相通及胸膜腔内压力与大气压相等时，胸内负压即消失。

【实验原理】

胸膜腔内压力通常低于大气压，称为胸内负压。正常时其数值随呼吸深度而变化。在胸膜腔的密闭性被破坏时，胸内负压消失。如果将腰椎穿刺针头用橡皮管与水检压计相连，穿刺针头刺入胸膜腔后，即可通过水检压计观察胸膜腔内压力的变化。

【实验材料】

1. 器材　BL-420F生物信号采集与分析系统，兔手术台，哺乳动物手术器械。腰椎穿刺针，气管插管，水检压计和橡皮管，20ml注射器和针头。

2. 溶液　20%氨基甲酸乙酯，生理盐水。

3. 对象　兔。

【实验方法】

1. 麻醉与固定　以20%氨基甲酸乙酯（1～1.2g/kg）注入兔耳缘静脉，待其麻醉后仰卧位固定于兔手术台上。

2. 手术　剪去颈部和右侧胸部的毛。在颈部做正中线切开，分离出气管，插入气管插管，以棉线固定。

将腰椎穿刺针用橡皮管连接水检压计，检压计内的水中可略加染料，以便读出水柱的高度（图5-3）。在兔胸腋前线的第五肋骨上缘，将针头顺肋骨方向斜插入胸腔，如见水检压计的水柱面下降并随呼吸而升降，即表示已插入胸膜腔内。用胶布将针尾固定于胸部皮肤上，以防针头移位或滑出。

如需同时记录呼吸运动，可在兔胸骨剑突下方的皮肤上穿一根细线，打结后将线尾悬挂于张力换能器（量程为25g）的悬梁上，将呼吸时的机械变化转换成电信号，经接线输入至BL-420F输入端，进行放大和记录。

3. 观察项目

（1）平静呼吸时的胸内压　记录平静呼吸运动2～3分钟。待呼吸运动曲线平稳后，从水检压计上读出胸内负压的数值，并对照呼吸运动曲线，比较吸气时和呼气时胸内负压有何不同？

（2）加强呼吸运动的效应　将气管插管的一侧管接一短橡皮管后，予以夹闭；在另一支侧管上接一根50cm长的橡皮管，以增大深呼吸的无效腔，使呼吸加深加快。观察并记录深呼吸时的胸内压数值，此时的胸内压与平静呼吸时有何不同？

（3）憋气的效应　在吸气末和呼气末，分别堵塞或夹闭气管插管。此时动物虽有力呼吸，但不能呼出或吸入外界气体，处于用力憋气的状态。观察并记录此时胸内压变动的最大幅度，胸内压是否可高于大气压？

（4）气胸及其影响　先从上腹部切开腹壁，将内脏下推，可观察到膈肌运动，然后沿第七肋骨上缘切开皮肤，用止血钳分离肋间肌，造成一长约1cm的贯穿胸壁创口，使胸膜腔与大气相通而形成气胸。观察肺组织是否萎陷；胸内压是否仍低于大气压并随呼吸而升降？用手术刀扩大创口并剪去5~6cm长的一段肋骨，此时胸内压又有何变化？

【实验指导】

1. 预习要求
（1）复习胸内压概念及胸内负压形成机制。
（2）复习气胸概念及气胸时胸内负压的改变。

2. 操作要点
胸腔内插管检测胸内压时，穿刺针斜面应朝向头侧，针体沿肋骨上缘与水平面保持一定角度（45°），首先用较大力量穿透皮肤，然后控制力量缓慢插入。用手指抵住胸壁以防刺入过深，直至手感通过胸膜，同时水检压计液面呈负值后，固定针尾于胸部皮肤上。

3. 注意事项
（1）用穿刺针时不要插得过猛和过深，以免刺破肺组织和血管，形成气胸和血胸。
（2）形成气胸后可迅速封闭漏气创口，并用注射器抽出胸膜腔内气体，此时胸内压可重新呈现负值。若发生血胸，应及时查找出血点并结扎止血。
（3）如果针头刺入胸壁已相当深，仍未见水面波动，应停止刺入。这时将针头转动一下，或稍微摆动一下角度。如仍无效，应拔出针头，检查是否针口被组织碎片或血块堵塞，疏通后重做。

4. 报告要点
（1）记录各项实验的胸内压值，以毫米水柱表示（mmH_2O）。
（2）描述观察到的现象，并解释发生这些现象的原因。

5. 思考题
（1）平静呼吸时，胸内压为什么始终低于大气压？
（2）在什么情况下，胸内压会是正压？

（李运曼）

36　Observation of intrathoracic negative pressure

PURPOSE

To observe the changes of intrathoracic negative pressure when rabbit's respiratory movement changes and the disappearance of intrathoracic negative pressure in artificial pneumothorax.

PRINCIPLES

The pressure inside pleural cavity is called intrathoracic negative pressure, which is usually lower than atmospheric pressure. Its numeric value would change when respiratory range changes. Intrathoracic negative pressure will disappear whenpleural cavity is broken. Connect lumbar ver-

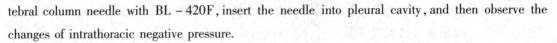

tebral column needle with BL – 420F, insert the needle into pleural cavity, and then observe the changes of intrathoracic negative pressure.

MATERIALS

1. Equipments BL – 420F biological signal acquisition and analysis system, Surgical instruments, operating table for rabbit, tracheal cannula, syringe, rubber tube, puncture needle, water manometer.

2. Solutions Urethan 20%. Saline.

3. Object Rabbit.

METHODS

1. Anesthesia procedure and fixation Inject 20% urethan (1g/kg) into vein of the rabbit's ears and fix it on operation table in supine body position when the rabbit was anesthetized.

2. Operation Shear the hair on neck and right chest. Cut down skin along the middle cervical line and separate trachea with hemostats. Cut down trachea and insert the tracheal cannula, and then fix the trachea with threads.

Connect a puncture needle with a pressure transducer that is inputted to BL – 420F. Insert the needle into pleural cavity at the fifth costa in pectoral axillary front line. Fix the end of needle on skin with a sticking plaster.

Cut through the skin below xiphoid with a strip of thread and hung the thread to a tensile transducer (25g)'s stick to record respiratory movement. Then input the signal to BL – 420F.

3. Observing items

(1) Intrathoracic pressure at eupnea Record respiratory movement at eupnea for 2 ~ 3 minutes. Measure intrathoracic negative pressures by BL – 420F after the curve of respiratory movement goes stable and then compares the difference of intrathoracic negative pressure between inspiration and expiration.

(2) The effect of augmented respiratory movement: Connect a short rubber tube with a branch of the tracheal cannula and shut it. Connect a 50cm rubber tube with another branch of tracheal cannula in order to deepen and speed up respiration by enlarging the dead space of deep breath. Observe and record value of intrathoracic negative pressures at deep breathing. Compare the difference of intrathoracic negative pressures between at deep breathing and eupnea.

(3) The effect of breathholding: Block or shut the tracheal cannula at the end of inspiration and expiration. Though the rabbit makes an effort to breathe, it cannot exhale or inhale air from environment in the state of breathholding. Observe and record the maximum range of variation of intrathoracic negative pressure. Whether intrathoracic negative pressure is higher than atmospheric pressure or not?

(4) Pneumothorax and its influence: When cut open abdominal wall from upper abdomen and push splanchna down, the movement of phrenic muscle can be observed. Cut open skin along superior border of the seventh rib and separate intercostal muscle with hemostat to make a 1cm wound running through chest wall through which air can go into pleural cavity. Pneumothorax is formed. Observe whether lung collapse happens; whether intrathoracic pressure is lower than atmos-

pheric pressure and varies with respiration. Enlarge the wound and cut a segment of rib for 5 ~ 6 cm with operating scalpel. What is the change of intrathoracic pressure?

GUIDANCE

1. Preview

(1) Review the conception of intrathoracic pressure and the mechanism of intrathoracic negative pressure.

(2) Review the conception of pneumothorax and the change of intrathoracic negative pressure at pneumothorax.

2. Manipulation

When measuring intrathoracic pressure by cannula in thoracic cavity, puncture needle ram should face to head and needle body along superior border of rib should keep a certain angle (45°) to transverse section. Make an effort to penetrate skin and then control strength to let the needle go slowly. Press chest wall with figure to prevent sticking too deeply until the needle feels passing through pleura. Fix the tail of needle on skin of chest.

3. Notices

(1) Do not insert puncture needle too fast and too deeply in case of cutting lung and vessel with the result of pneumothorax or hemathorax.

(2) If pneumothorax happens, block the wound quickly and draw out air from pleural cavity with syringe. Intrathoracic pressure can recover negative. If hemathorax happens, hemorrhagic spots should be found in time and ligatured.

(3) If the needle is fairly deep in chest wall, stick should be stopped. Then turn around needle little or change the angle slightly. If it does not work, the needle should be pulled out and examed. If fragments of tissue or blood clot block the needle, clear it out and redo.

4. Reports

(1) Record value of intrathoracic pressure in every experiment.

(2) Describe Phenomena observed and give out the cause.

5. Questions

(1) Why is intrathoracic pressure lower than atmospheric pressure all the time at eupnea?

(2) Under what case intrathoracic pressure is positive pressure?

(Li Yunman)

第六章　消化系统

Digestive system

实验三十七　离体肠肌运动

【实验目的】

观察胃肠平滑肌的一般特性及肾上腺素、小鼠肾上腺水溶性提取物和乙酰胆碱对离体兔肠的作用，并掌握温血动物离体器官的实验方法。

【实验原理】

消化道平滑肌与骨骼肌、心肌一样，具有肌肉组织共有的特性，如兴奋性、传导性和收缩性等。但消化道平滑肌又有其特点，即兴奋性较低，收缩缓慢，富有伸展性，具有紧张性、自动节律性，对化学、温度和机械牵张刺激较敏感等。这些特点对维持消化道内一定压力，保持胃肠等一定的形态和位置，适合于消化道内容物的理化变化具有生理意义。这些特点在整体内受中枢神经系统和体液因素的调节。为观察哺乳动物消化道平滑肌的特性，必须给予离体肠肌以接近于在体情况的适宜环境。本实验以台氏液作灌流液，其离子成分和 pH 与哺乳动物的体液相似。在整个实验过程中，灌流液的温度基本恒定在 37℃ 左右，并不断向灌流液输入氧气。

【实验材料】

1. 器材　BL-420F 生物信号采集与分析系统，张力换能器，超级恒温水浴，哺乳动物手术器械，小乳钵，氧气发生器或氧气球胎，铁站架，烧杯（100ml、250ml），滴管，表面皿，浴槽，玻棒，注射器（1ml），橡皮管，蛇形冷凝管及冷凝管夹，试管及试管夹，棉线。

2. 溶液　台氏液，生理盐水，1∶10000 乙酰胆碱，1∶10000 肾上腺素，0.1mol/L NaOH 溶液。

3. 对象　兔，小白鼠。

【实验方法】

1. 准备　装好实验装置，用超级恒温水浴调温至（37±0.5）℃。

2. 离体兔肠制备

（1）用木槌猛击兔头部使其昏迷后，立即剖开腹腔，找到胃幽门与十二指肠交界处，在十二指肠起始端扎一线，剪取十二指肠、空肠，放入室温已经 O_2 饱和的台氏液内备用。

扫码"学一学"

扫码"看一看"

（2）剪取约2cm长的一段小肠，轻轻冲洗，以除去肠内容物。边洗边通入O_2。冲洗后在其两端肠壁对角部位各穿一条线结扎，上线与张力换能器的应变梁相连，下线固定于浴槽底部。放入台氏液，并立即通入O_2，适应20min。

3. 小鼠肾上腺水溶性提取物的制备　取小鼠1只，处死后剖腹取两侧肾上腺，放入小乳钵内，碾碎后加生理盐水2ml，静置20min备用。

4. 观测项目

（1）观察平滑肌的节律性活动并记录一段正常曲线后，往浴槽内加入1：10000的肾上腺素1～2滴，观察肠管的紧张性及收缩情况。

（2）放出浴槽内液体，用台氏液换洗三次，待恢复正常后，在浴皿中加小鼠肾上腺提取液1ml，观察肠管活动有何变化。待作用出现后，放掉浴槽内液体，用台氏液换洗三次。

（3）取两支试管，一管加入肾上腺提取物1ml，另一管加入生理盐水1ml和1～2滴1：10000肾上腺素，再在两管中各加入0.1mol/L NaOH 1～2滴，在沸水浴中加热3min，待冷至37℃左右时，分别加入浴槽中，观察对肠管的作用有无变化。

（4）放掉浴槽内的液体，用台氏液换洗3次，待恢复正常后，加入1：10000乙酰胆碱1～2滴，观察肠管活动有何变化。

【实验指导】

1. 预习要求　复习消化道平滑肌的生理特性及胃肠道平滑肌的受体分布等内容。

2. 操作要点　注意掌握制备离体兔肠及制备小鼠肾上腺提取物的方法。

3. 注意事项

（1）加药前必须准备好更换用的37℃台氏液。

（2）每次加药出现效果后，必须立即更换浴槽内的台氏液并冲洗3次，待肠肌恢复正常活动后再观察下一项目。

（3）浴槽内台氏液一定要高出标本，并在实验中保持同一高度。

（4）实验中始终要通入O_2，气泡量不要太多，以每秒2～3个为宜。气泡过多会影响记录。

（5）加碱不可过多，因碱本身对肠管平滑肌也是一种化学刺激。

（6）取兔肠及兔肠穿线时，尽可能不用金属及手指触及。

4. 报告要点　用配有文字说明的记录曲线表达实验结果。根据结果讨论平滑肌的生理特性及平滑肌的神经体液性调节。

5. 思考题

（1）本实验是否可用麻醉剂麻醉动物后取肠？

（2）哺乳类动物离体组织器官实验时，需控制哪些条件？

（3）在本实验中，消化道平滑肌的生理特点主要表现在哪些方面？试对实验项目中观察到的现象给予解释。

（4）加入乙酰胆碱后再加入阿托品，肠段活动受到抑制，为什么？

（郭青龙）

37　Movement of intestine muscle *in vitro*

PURPOSE

Observe general characteristics of gastrointestinal smooth muscle in rabbit. And observe the effect of adrenalin, water – dissolve extract that was obtained from adrenal grand of mice and ACh on rabbit's intestine in vitro. Master the experiment method of organ of warm – blood animal in vitro.

PRINCIPLE

The properties of smooth muscle in digestive tract are the same as skeletal muscle and myocardium, such as excitability, conductivity and contractility. Smooth muscle in digestive tract also has its specific characteristics, such as lower excitability, slow contraction, extension, tension, auto – rhythmicity, sensitivity to stimulators of chemistry, temperature and mechanical stretch. This is important to maintain pressure in digestive tract, keep certain form and position of gastrointestinal tract, and suit to physical and chemical change of substance in digestive tract. These characteristics are also adjusted by central nervous system and humoral factors in vivo. Intestine muscle in vitro must be put in suitable environment that is near to in vivo in order to obverse characteristics of smooth muscle in digestive tract of mammal. Tyrodo's solution is selected as infusingsolution in the experiment because ion component and pH in it are similar to humor. Control infusing solution temperature at about 37℃ and input oxygen to Tyrodo's solution constantly during the experiment.

MATERIALS

1. Equipments　BL – 420F biological signal acquisition and analysis system, tension transducer, super homoeothermic water bath, operating instruments of toad, dropper, mortar and pounder, oxygen generator or oxygen balloon, coiled condenser and condenser clamps, iron support, beaker (100ml, 250ml), glass stick, bath dish, bath tube, syringe (1ml), test tube and holder, rubber tube, cotton thread.

2. Solutions　Tyrodo's solution, 0.9% NaCl, 1 ∶ 10000 adrenalin, 1 ∶ 10000 ACh, 0.1mol/L NaOH.

3. Objects　Rabbit, mouse.

METHODS

1. Emplace experimental device and set the temperature of super homoiothermic water bath at 37 ± 0.5℃.

2. Preparation of a rabbit's intestine sample in vitro

（1）Beat the head with a mallet to make rabbit coma, then open its abdominal cavity. Ligate the initiation of dodecadactylon with a thread after finding boundary between stomach pylorus and dodecadactylon, then take dodecadactylon and jejunum and put them into Tyrodo's solution saturated with O_2 in room temperature.

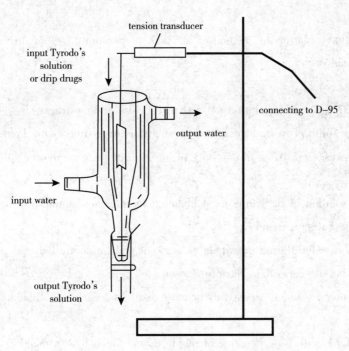

Fig. 6 – 1   The instrument for intestine in vitro

(2) Cut a small intestine about 2cm and wash it with Tyrodo's solution to get rid of intestinal materials. Do not forget to add O_2 during washing. Ligate resptectively at both opposite angles of the length of intestine wall with thread and needle after cleaning. Superior thread is connected with the strain patch of a tension transducer, and inferior thread is fixed in bottom of the bath tube. Infuse Tyrodo's solution and input O_2 into the bath tube for 20 minutes.

3. Preparation of water dissolving extract of adrenal gland of a mouse   Take two adrenals of a sacrificed mouse, put it into a mortar. Add 2ml normal saline to the mortar after adrenals have been milled and then lay it up for 20minutes.

4. Observational items

(1) After observing and recording rhythmic movement of smooth muscle, add adrenalin (1 : 10000) 1~2 drops to bath tube. Observe tension and contraction of the intestine.

(2) Discharge fluid in bath tube and clean it for three times with Tyrodo's solution. Add the dissolving extract of adrenals (1ml) to bath tube and observe the changes of intestine activity. Discharge the fluid in bath tube and then wash it for three times with Tyrodo's solution.

(3) Add extract of adrenal gland (1ml) to one test tube and physiological saline (1ml) with adrenal (1 : 10000) 1~2 drops to another. Then add 0.1mol/L NaOH 1~2 drop to each test tube. Persevere the two test tubes in boiling water for 3 minutes. After temperature decreased to about 37℃, put fluid in test tube to the bath tube. Observe the effect on the intestine.

(4) Discharge the solution fluid in bath tube and clean it for three times with Tyrodo's solution. Add ACh (1 : 10000) 1~2 drops to the bath tube and observe the changes of intestine activity.

GUIDANCE

1. Preview   Review physiological characteristics of smooth muscle and receptor distribution in digestive tract.

2. Manipulation　Master the method of intestine preparation of rabbit in vitro and extract of adrenal gland of mouse.

3. Notices

（1）Prepare 37℃ Tyrodo's solution for exchange before adding drugs.

（2）Exchange solution in bath tube and clean it for three times with Tyrodo's solution after the effect of drug was seen. After the activity of intestine muscle recovered, please observe next item.

（3）Tyrodo's solution in bath tube must higher than intestine sample and be controlled at the same height during the experiment.

（4）O_2 must be added during the whole experiment and be controlled at $2 \sim 3$ O_2 bubbles per second. Excessive bubble may affect recording result.

（5）Alkali cannot be added excessively because alkali is a chemical stimulation to smooth muscle of intestine.

（6）When taking or ligating intestine of rabbit, do not touch it with metal or finger.

4. Report　Descript the result of experiment with recording curve that has letter interpretation. Discuss physiological characteristics of smooth muscle and adjustment of nerve and humoral factors to smooth muscle.

5. Questions

（1）Whether can the intestine of rabbit be taken after animal was anesthetized in the experiment?

（2）What conditions are required in vitro experiment for tissues and organs of mammalian?

（3）What are the main physiological characters of smooth muscles in digestive tract in this experiment? Explain the phenomena observed in the experiment.

（4）Atropine inhibits the activity of intestine after ACh is added. Why?

（Guo Qinglong）

实验三十八　兔胆汁分泌的调节

【实验目的】

本实验以细塑料管直接插入胆总管引流胆汁，观察胆汁分泌以及迷走神经、胰泌素和胆盐对胆汁分泌的影响。

【实验原理】

胆汁由肝细胞不断分泌，经肝管流出。在非消化期，由于胆总管括约肌收缩，阻止胆汁排入十二指肠，故胆汁流入胆囊贮存。当进食开始后，通过神经和体液调节，一方面促进肝细胞分泌胆汁，另一方面促进胆囊收缩和胆总管括约肌舒张，从而将胆汁排入十二指肠。胆汁分泌不仅受神经控制，还受激素控制。刺激迷走神经可使胆汁分泌，胰泌素能引起胆汁分泌增加。

【实验材料】

1. 器材 兔手术台，哺乳动物手术器械，电刺激器，注射器（10ml 和 5ml），细塑料管，小烧杯，保护电极。

2. 溶液 生理盐水，20% 氨基甲酸乙酯，粗制胰泌素。

3. 对象 兔。

【实验方法】

1. 麻醉 经兔耳缘静脉注射 20% 氨基甲酸乙酯（1g/kg），麻醉后仰卧位固定于兔手术台上。

2. 颈部手术 颈部剪毛，沿颈正中线切开皮肤，分离左侧迷走神经（因左侧迷走神经支配肝脏），穿线备用。

3. 腹部手术 腹部剪毛，沿剑突下正中线切开皮肤，切口长约 10cm，打开腹腔。沿胃幽门端找到十二指肠，在十二指肠上端的背侧可见一黄绿色较粗的肌性管即胆总管（图 6-2）。

4. 胆总管插管 在近十二指肠处仔细分离胆总管（注意避免出血），在其下穿一丝线。在靠近十二指肠处的胆总管上，向胆囊方向剪一小口，插入细塑料管，用丝线结扎固定。塑料管插入胆总管后，立即可见绿色胆汁从插管流出。如果不见有胆汁流出，则可能塑料管插入胆总管周围组织，需取出重插。注意插入的塑料管应与胆总管相平行。

5. 收集胆汁 用小烧杯收集胆汁备用。待胆汁流出的速度稳定后开始观察。

6. 观察项目

（1）观察正常胆汁分泌，计每分钟胆汁分泌的滴数。

（2）用中等强度和频率的电刺激，间断刺激左侧颈迷走神经，观察胆汁分泌速度有何变化。

（3）静脉缓慢注射稀胆汁（用生理盐水将流出的胆汁稀释 1 倍）4ml，观察胆汁分泌速度有何变化。

（4）静脉缓慢注射粗制胰泌素 4~6ml，观察胆汁分泌的变化。

【实验指导】

1. 预习要求

（1）复习胆汁分泌、贮存及胆汁的生理功能。

（2）复习胆汁分泌的神经和体液调节。

（3）复习胰泌素的产生部位及生理功能。

2. 操作要点

（1）在分离胆总管时，要避免损伤与其伴行的血管、神经，如有出血，应及时止血。

（2）粗制胰泌素的制备法 取兔十二指肠，将肠腔冲洗干净，纵向剪开肠壁，平铺板上，刮下黏膜。将黏膜置研钵中研磨，并添加 0.5% HCl 10~15ml。将研成的稀浆倒入烧杯中，再加 0.5% HCl 100ml，煮沸 10~15min。随即加入 10% NaOH 中和至中性，并用滤纸过滤，滤液中即含有胰泌素，置冰箱 4℃ 保存备用。

3. 注意事项

（1）打开腹腔后，用温生理盐水纱布覆盖切口保温。

（2）胆总管切口应尽量靠近十二指肠一侧。

（3）胆总管插管方向与胆总管的走向保持平行，不能扭转。

4. 报告要点　列表小结实验结果并加以分析。

5. 思考题

（1）胆总管插管后，即刻有胆汁流出，速度很快，随后减慢并趋稳定，怎样解释这一现象？

（2）刺激左侧迷走神经，通过哪些机制影响肝胆汁分泌？

（3）胆汁中什么成分影响肝胆汁分泌？正常生理条件下它通过什么途径影响胆汁分泌？

（4）正常生理条件下，胰泌素通过什么途径影响胆汁分泌？

（吴玉林）

38　Regulation of bile secretion in rabbits

PURPOSE

To observe bile secretion and the effects of vagus nerve, secretin and bile salt on bile secretion by draining bile through a fine plastic tube inserted into common bile duct directly.

PRINCIPLE

Bile is excreted by hepatocytes continuously and is drained out by hepatic ducts. Owing to the contraction of sphincter of common bile duct in the interdigestive stage, bile is prevented from excreting into duodenum and stored up in gallbladder. Since the beginning of eating, hepatocytes are promoted to excrete bile. On the other hand, the contraction of gallbladder and the relaxation of sphincter of common bile duct are facilitated, thus bile is excluded into duodenum by neural and humoral regulation. The secretion of bile is controlled not only by nerves, but also by hormones. Bile can be secreted by the stimulation of vagus nerves. Bile secretion is also obviously increased by secretin.

MATERIALS

1. Equipments　Operating table for rabbit, operating instruments, Electrostimulation apparatus, Syringe (10ml, 5ml and 1ml), Fine plastic tube, Beaker, Protective Electrode.

2. Solutions　Saline, 20% Ethyl Carbamate, Manufactured Secretin.

3. Object　Rabbit.

METHODS

1. Anesthesia　The rabbit is anesthetized with 20% Ethyl Carbamate before surgery. The injection volume is 1g/kg for intravenous route by posterior auricular vein. After anesthesia, the rabbit is fixed on the rabbit operation table on its back.

2. Operation on Neck　The rabbit is sheared on the neck, and the skin of neck is slitted along the midline. The liver is governed by the nervous ramification of the vagus nerve on the left, so the latter is dissociated and is available by introducing a piece of silk under it.

3. Operation on abdominal region   The rabbit is sheared on the abdomen. The skin is slitted along the midline below the xiphoid, and the incision is about 10cm long. The abdominal cavity is opened. The duodenum can be found at the end of pylorus, and the common bile duct, a major muscular duct which is yellow and green can be seen on the back of the superior extremity of duodenum.

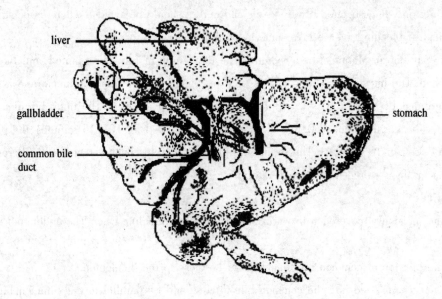

Fig. 6 – 2   Anatomical position of common bile duct in rabbit

4. Intubation of common bile duct   The common bile duct close to the duodenum is dissociated and is available by introducing a piece of silk under it. The bleeding should be avoided. A minor incisionis opened on the common bile duct close to the duodenum. A fine plastic tube is inserted into it and is fixed by ligaturing. Green bile flows out soon after insertion of the tube into common bile duct. If there is no bile flowing out, it is possible that the tube is inserted into the peripheral tissues of common bile duct. So the tube should be taken out and inserted again. To pay attention, the inserted tube should be parallel to the common bile duct.

5. Collection of bile   The bile is collected and is stored with beaker. Please observe until the bile flow out in stable speed.

6. Observation items

(1) Please observe the normal bile secretion, and count the dribbling bile per minute.

(2) Please observe what changes happen in the speed of bile secretion when discontinuous stimulating the vagus nerve on the left with medium intensity and frequency.

(3) Please observe what changes happen in the speed of bile secretion when injecting 4ml dilute bile (the outflow bile is diluted with saline by single volume) intravenously.

(4) Please observe what changes happen in the speed of bile secretion when injecting 4 ~ 6ml secretin intravenously.

GUIDANCE

1. Preview

(1) Please review the knowledge on bile secretion, bile storage and the physiological functions

of bile.

(2)Please review the knowledge on the neural and humoral regulation of bilesecretion.

(3)Please review the knowledge on the producing sites of secretin and the physiological functions of secretin.

2. Manipulations

(1)The injury of associated blood vessels and nerves should be avoided when dissociating common bile duct. If bleeding, please take some hemostatic measures in time.

(2)Preparation of Manufactured Secretin: The duodenum of rabbits is gained, and the enterocoel is washed. The intestine is slitted and is tiled on the board. The mucous membrane is scraped off and is grinded. 0.5% HCl 10 ~ 15ml is added into it when grinding. The thick liquid is poured down into the beaker. It is added 0.5% HCl 100ml and is boiled for 10 ~ 15 minutes, the pH being adjusted to 7.0 with 10% NaOH. The liquid is filtered with filter paper at last. The filtered liquid containing secretin is stored in the refrigerator.

3. Notices

(1)The incision is covered with warm bandage dipped in saline when The abdominal cavity is opened.

(2)The incision of common bile duct should be close to the duodenum.

(3)The tube inserted into the common bile duct should be parallel to the common bile duct, and cannot be twisted.

4. Report　Please make a list in order to summarize and analyze the results of the experiment.

5. Questions

(1) How to explain this phenomenon that bile flows out fast soon after the intubation of common bile duct, the speed is lessened and inclines to be stable?

(2)What is the mechanism which bile secretion is affected by when stimulating the vagus nerve on the left?

(3)Which ingredients in the bile influence bile secretion? And how they affect bile secretion under the normal physiological condition?

(4)How secretin affects bile secretion under the normal physiological condition?

(Wu Yulin)

第七章　泌尿系统

Urinary system

实验三十九　尿生成的影响因素

扫码"学一学"

【目的要求】

通过本实验观察一些因素对尿量及尿的成分的影响，并分析其影响机制。

了解尿的收集方法，学习输尿管插管或膀胱插管技术。

【实验原理】

尿生成过程包括肾小球的滤过及肾小管与集合管的重吸收和分泌作用。肾小球滤过作用的动力是有效滤过压，而有效滤过压的高低主要取决于肾小球毛细血管血压、血浆胶体渗透压和囊内压。正常情况下，囊内压不会有什么变化。肾小球毛细血管血压主要受全身动脉血压的影响，当动脉血压在 $80 \sim 180 \mathrm{mmHg}$ 范围内变动时，由于肾血流的自身调节作用，肾小球毛细血管血压均能维持在相对稳定水平。但当动脉血压高于 $180 \mathrm{mmHg}$ 或低于 $80 \mathrm{mmHg}$ 时，肾小球毛细血管血压就会随血压变化而变化，肾小球滤过率也发生相应变化。另外，血浆胶体渗透压降低，会使有效滤过压增高，肾小球滤过率增加。影响肾小管、集合管泌尿功能的因素，包括肾小管溶液中溶质浓度和抗利尿激素等。肾小管溶质浓度增高，可妨碍肾小管对水的重吸收，因而使尿量增加；抗利尿激素可促进肾小管与集合管对水的重吸收，导致尿量减少。

【实验材料】

1. 器材　BL-420F 生物信号采集与分析系统，血压换能器，保护电极，兔手术台，哺乳动物手术器械，气管插管，动脉插管，动脉夹，10ml 量筒，记滴器，膀胱插管或输尿管插管，棉线，丝线。

2. 溶液　5% 枸橼酸钠，20% 氨基甲酸乙酯，1∶10000 去甲肾上腺素，呋塞米，生理盐水，25% 葡萄糖，垂体后叶素，0.6% 酚红（酚磺酞），10% NaOH，斑氏试剂。

3. 对象　家兔。

【实验方法】

1. 麻醉与固定　用20% 氨基甲酸乙酯 $1 \sim 1.2 \mathrm{g/kg}$ 剂量给兔耳缘静脉缓慢注射，麻醉后将兔仰卧位固定于兔手术台上。

2. 颈部手术　剪去颈前部兔毛，在颈前正中做一长 4cm 的切口，分离气管并做气管插管，而后分离左侧颈总动脉和右侧迷走神经，在其下各穿两根线备用，手术完毕后用生理盐水纱布覆盖创面。

3. 腹部手术 剪去下腹兔毛，从耻骨联合向上沿中线做一长约 4cm 的切口，沿腹白线切开腹壁，用手轻轻将膀胱移出腹腔外便可以进行插管。插管方法有以下两种。

（1）输尿管插管导尿 认清输尿管进入膀胱背侧部的位置，细心分离出一侧输尿管，先在靠近膀胱处穿线结扎，再在离此结扎线约 2cm 处穿一条线备用，用眼科剪在管壁上剪一斜向肾侧的小口，向肾方向插入充满生理盐水的细塑料管，用缚线结扎固定，见图 7 - 1。将此导尿塑料管放入 10ml 量筒记录尿流量或记录尿滴（滴/分）。

（2）膀胱插管导尿 进行插管时先认清输尿管在膀胱的开口位置，在两输尿管口水平连线中点的（膀胱背壁）正下方，选择血管最少处做一约 0.7cm 的纵行切口，立即将充满生理盐水的膀胱插管插入膀胱，并继续向膀胱顶部移动插管。直至两输尿管口水平连线中点的稍下方，但不能高于两输尿管口水平线的位置，以免扎线时将输尿管口扎住，没有尿液流出（也可将膀胱插管正对一侧输尿管口）。然后用粗棉线将膀胱插管头端及其周围的膀胱组织一起扎住，这样不仅将尿道在膀胱开口扎住，防止尿液自尿道外漏，而且仅保留膀胱顶部的一小部分，使尿液容易将容积较小的膀胱充满而经膀胱插管流出。膀胱插管插好后将其上的弹簧夹松开，插管另一端放在低于膀胱的位置，并连接量筒，记录尿流量。手术完毕后用温生理盐水纱布覆盖腹部伤口。

4. 记录血压 于左颈总动脉插入充满抗凝剂（枸橼酸钠溶液）的动脉插管，动脉插管连接至血压换能器，后者连接微型计算机输入端，进行血压记录，仪器使用详见实验二十七。

5. 观察项目

（1）静脉注射 38℃ 生理盐水 30ml，观察血压和尿量的改变。

（2）静脉注射 1：10000 去甲肾上腺素（NE）0.5ml，观察血压和尿量的变化。

（3）取 2 滴尿液做尿糖定性试验，然后静脉注射 25% 葡萄糖 5ml，观察尿量有何变化。当尿量显著变化时，取流出的尿液再做一次尿糖定性试验，观察有无尿糖。

（4）结扎并剪断右侧迷走神经，用中等刺激强度（10V 左右）的电脉冲间断刺激其外周端，频率为 8~16Hz，时间一般为 1min，每次持续 5s，间隔 3s，观察尿量变化。

（5）静脉注射呋塞米 5mg/kg（10mg/ml），观察尿量有何变化。

（6）静脉注射 0.6% 的酚红 0.5ml，用盛有 10% NaOH 溶液的培养皿收集尿液，计算从注射酚红到尿中出现酚红所需的时间（酚红在碱性溶液中呈红色）。通常注射酚红 5 分钟后，尿中即有酚红出现。

（7）静脉注射垂体后叶素 2U，观察尿量有何变化。

将上述结果填入表 7 - 1。

【实验指导】

1. 预习要求

（1）复习肾血流量的自身调节。

（2）复习肾小球的滤过功能、肾小管与集合管的泌尿功能及其影响因素。

（3）复习尿的浓缩与稀释机制。

（4）复习 BL - 420F 生物信号采集与分析系统。

（5）复习家兔动脉插管及神经血管分离的操作方法。

2. 操作要点

（1）耳缘静脉注射麻醉药时前半量可稍快一些，后半量一定要缓慢推注，以免推注过快导致家兔死亡。

（2）动脉插管 将左侧颈总动脉分离2～4cm长，穿双线备用，颈总动脉近心端夹动脉夹，离心端结扎，用眼科剪在距动脉夹1.5～2cm处剪一小斜口，插入动脉插管，并用缚线将其结扎固定，此详细过程见家兔动脉血压调节实验。

（3）膀胱或输尿管插管 膀胱插管或输尿管插管内要充满生理盐水，并将管内气泡驱逐干净。

（4）BL－420F生物信号采集与分析系统使用方法见家兔血压实验。

3. 注意事项

（1）实验前给家兔用导尿管向兔胃灌入20ml清水，以增加其基础尿流量。

（2）做膀胱插管时，操作要轻柔，以免膀胱受刺激而缩得很小，增加插管难度（若作输尿管插管，则要防止血凝块堵塞插管或因扭曲而阻断尿液的流通）。

（3）手术创口不宜过大，防止动物体温下降，影响实验。

（4）各项实验的顺序是，在尿流量增多的基础上进行减少尿生成的实验。

（5）本实验经兔耳缘静脉给药，故应注意保护好该静脉，开始时应从其末梢端注射，这样，一条耳缘静脉可以多次注射；亦可于耳缘静脉插一头皮针，用于多次静脉给药。

（6）必须等到上一个实验项目作用基本消失后，再进行下一个实验项目。

（7）如同时记录血压，其注意事项同血压调节实验。

4. 报告要点

（1）将各项结果填入表7－1，并分析各项结果的产生机制。

表7－1 若干因素对尿量的影响

影响因素	尿量（滴/分钟）		变化率（%）	血压（mmHg）		变化率（%）
	对照	实验		对照	实验	
生理盐水30ml						
1∶10000NE 0.5ml						
25%葡萄糖20ml						
刺激右侧迷走神经						
呋塞米0.5ml/kg体重						
垂体后叶素2U						

（2）在本实验中，哪些因素可影响肾小球的滤过，哪些因素影响肾小管和集合管的重吸收和分泌。

5. 思考题

（1）本实验刺激迷走神经为何选用右侧而很少用左侧？

（2）电刺激迷走神经观察尿量变化实验中，应注意什么？

（3）静脉注射1∶10000去甲肾上腺素（NE）后，有时尿量变化不大，是何原因？

（4）为什么注射垂体后叶素后，尿量可出现先多后少的现象？

（5）全身动脉血压升高，尿量一定增加；血压降低，尿量一定减少，这话对吗？为什么？

（6）测定酚红排泄时间的生理意义是什么？

［附］

尿糖定性试验：预先在试管中加入斑氏试剂1ml，再加尿液2滴，在酒精灯上加热煮沸片刻，冷却后观察尿液和沉淀的颜色。如由原来的绿色溶液变为黄色或砖红色，即为尿糖试验阳性，表示尿中有糖。

（李运曼）

39　Factors influencing urine formation

PURPOSE

To observe influencing factors on urine volume and some components in urine and then analyze the mechanisms.

To understand the way to collect urine, and to learn the usage of ureter cannula or bladder cannula.

PRINCIPLES

The procedure of urine formation includes the filtration in renal glomerulus, the reabsorption and excretion in renal tubule and collecting duct. The dynamic of filtration in renal glomerulus is effective filtration pressure. There are 3 main factors that can affect it: glomerular capillary pressure, plasma colloid osmotic pressure and pressure inside bladder. Pressure inside bladder little changes in general. Glomerular capillary pressure is influenced by arterial pressure all over the body. When arterial pressure is 80 ~ 100mmHg, it will maintain in a relative steady level, but when arterial pressure is high above 180mmHg or below 80mmHg, glomerular capillary pressure will change and the rate of filtration in renal glomerulus will change too. In addition, the decreasing of plasma colloid osmotic pressure will raise effective filtration pressure and the rate of filtration in renal glomerulus.

Factors that can influence the procedure of excreting urine in renal tubule and collecting duct mainly include the concentration of solution and antidiuretic in renal tubule. The augmentation of the concentration of solution in renal tubule can restrain the reabsorption of water in renal tubule and enlarge urine volume. The antidiuretic can promote the reabsorption of water in renal tubule and collect duct and decrease urine volume.

MATERIALS

1. Equipments　BL – 420F biological signal acquisition and analysis system, surgical instruments, operating table for rabbit, pressure transducer, shielded electrode, artery cannula, artery clamp, 10ml measuring cylinder, drop recorder, bladder cannula or ureter cannula

2. Solutions　sodium citrate 5%, urethan 20%, 1 : 10000 noradvenaline (NE), furosemide, saline, 25% glucose, pituitrin, 0.6% phenolsulfonphthalein, 10% NaOH, Benedict reagent.

3. Object　rabbit.

METHODS

1. Anesthesia procedure and fixation i. v. 20% Urethan (1 ~ 1.2g/kg) into the rabbit's ears and fix it on operation table in supine body position when the rabbit was anesthetized.

2. Operation Shear the hair on neck, cut open skin along the middle cervical line and separate trachea with hemostats. Cut down trachea and insert the tracheal cannula, then fix the trachea with thread, separate the aorta of lateral portion of neck and right side of vagus nerve, penetrate two threads. When operation is done, cover the wound with warm gauze soaked by Saline.

Shear the hair on inferior belly, make a 4cm wound upward along middle linefrom pubic symphysis. Cut open abdominal wall along linea alba abdominis, move the bladder outside by hand. Then insert the cannula. There are 2 methods to do this.

(1) Ureter cannula Identify clearly the dorsalis place of bladder where ureter enter, and then separate a side of ureter. At first, the ureter is ligated near the bladder, and then a thread is passed through the ureter at the 2cm near the ligation. Make a cut on the ureter wall with eye scissors. A plastic tube with full of saline is inserted toward the kidney and is fixed. Connect the plastic tube with drop recorder; record the flow of urine (d/min) on drum kymograph with signal magnet. (Fig. 7 – 1) If there is no drop recorder for use, you can connect directly the tube with cylinder and compute the urine flow.

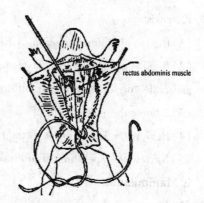

rectus abdominis muscle

Fig. 7 – 1   instrument of ureter cannula

(2) Cannulation of Bladder cannula identify clearly the opening of ureter in bladder. Make a 0.7cm longitudinal cut in a place where there is few blood vessels right under the middle point of the horizontal line between the two orifices. Make sure that the orifices are not ligated. Then ligate the end of bladder cannula and constitution together with cotton threads. This can not only prevent urine from leaking out, but also make it easy for urine to fill fully with bladder and outflow. After plugging the cannula and decamping alligator clamp, place the other end below the bladder and connect it with drop recorder or cylinder, record the urine flow. Cover the wound with warm gauze soaked by saline after operation.

Record the blood pressure; insert an arterial cannula full of anticoagulant (sodium citrate) in left common carotid artery. Record blood pressure with drum kymograph. Record the urine flow, stimulating signal and intervals with three signal magnet. If the two – tract recording equipment takes the place of drum kymograph, connect the arterial cannula with blood pressure transducer that is connected with the lead – in of blood pressure amplifier.

3. Observing items

(1) i. v. 38℃ saline 30 ml. Observe the change of blood pressure and urine volume.

(2) i. v. 1 : 10000 NE 0.5 ml. Observe the change of blood pressure and urine volume.

(3) Take 2 drops of urine and do the qualitative experiment of glucose in urine. i. v. 25% glucose 5ml, observe the change of urine volume. When urine volume changes markedly, take the urine

and do the qualitative experiment of glucose in urine again. Is there any glucose in urine?

(4)Ligate and cut off vagus nerve in right side, give it peripheral stimulation with 10V electric pulse discontinuously for a minute. Each stimulation should keep 5 seconds and there should be 3 seconds intermission between each time. Observe the changes of urine volume.

(5)i. v. franyl 0. 5ml/kg. Observe the change of urine volume.

(6)i. v. 0. 6% phenolsulfonphthalein 0. 5ml, collect urine into a petri dish with some 10% NaOH inside. Compute the time from injection to the appearance of phenolsulfonphthalein in urine.

(7)i. v. pituitrin 2U. Observe the change of urine volume.

GUIDANCE

1. Preview

(1)Review the autoregulation of RBF.

(2)Review the mechanism of glomerular filtration, the reabsorption and excretion in renal tubule and collecting duct and their influencing factors.

(3)Review the mechanism of concentration and dilution of urine.

(4)Review the usage of two – tract recording equipment and stimulator.

(5)Review the operation of arterial cannula in rabbit and free nerve and blood vessel.

2. Manipulation

(1)Intravenous injection   the injection should be fast in initiation and after that be slowly to prevent the rabbit from dying.

(2)Arterial cannula   free a 4cm left branch of common carotid artery, cut through two threads, close artery clamp at the end of near – heart end. Ligate the other end, make a little inclined wound with eye scissors 1. 5~2cm distance between. Plug the cannula in, and fix it with threads.

(3)Bladder cannula or ureter cannula   fill the cannula with saline, and don't leave any bubble in it.

3. Notices

(1)Feed the rabbit with vegetables before experiment, or perfuse 20ml water in its stomach to increase its elementary urine volume.

(2)During the procedure of bladder cannula, please operate gently to prevent from bladder contracting.

(3)The wound should not be too large. Otherwise, the animal's temperature will decrease.

(4)The sequence of experiment is: decrease the urine formation in the base of the urine flow increasing.

(5)During the intravenous injection, the injection should start in the end of vein.

(6)Don't do the next entry until one entry is over.

4. Reports

(1)Fill results in table 7 – 1 and analyze the mechanisms.

(2)What can influence glomerular filtration and what will influence the reabsorption and excretion in renal tubule and collecting duct in this experiment?

5. Questions

(1) We stimulate the right vagus nerve but not the left. Why?

(2) What should be noticed in electric stimulation?

(3) The volume of urine sometimes does not change remarkably after i. v. 1 : 10000 NE. Why?

(4) The volume of urine is earlier than it afterward after i. v. pituitrin. Why?

(5) Someone says: if the blood pressure rises, the urine volume certainly rises, ifthe blood pressure declines, the urine volume certainly reduces. Is it right or wrong? Why?

(6) What is the physiological meaning of measuring excretive time of phenolsulfonphthalein?

Supplement

add Benedict reagent 1ml in a test tube beforehand, then add 2 drops urine in, boil the solutions inside the test tube on alcohol burner for a while. Observe the color of urine and deposit when it is cold. If the solution's color changes from green to yellow or brick red, the experiment is positive and indicates that there are some glucose in urine.

(Li Yunman)

实验四十 家兔膀胱的神经调节

【实验目的】

观察刺激支配膀胱的神经所引起的反应，从而了解膀胱排尿活动的神经调节。

【实验原理】

膀胱的功能是暂时储存尿液和快速地将积聚的尿液经尿道排出体外。膀胱和尿道括约肌的功能受神经系统调节，有三对神经与排尿活动有关：①盆神经（副交感神经），它的兴奋可使逼尿肌收缩、内括约肌弛缓，促进排尿，是支配膀胱的主要神经；②腹下神经（交感神经），它的兴奋可使逼尿肌松弛（此作用很弱），内括约肌收缩，阻抑尿的排放；③阴部神经（躯体神经），其传出冲动能引起外括约肌收缩，从而阻止尿的排出。在这些神经中，还混有起自膀胱和（或）尿道的感觉纤维。膀胱的胀满感主要由盆神经中的感觉纤维传入，从而引起排尿反射。由于在排尿活动中，副交感神经起主要作用，交感神经作用比较次要，故刺激支配膀胱的神经时（盆神经和腹下神经），通常出现盆神经受刺激的效应。

【实验材料】

1. 器材 兔手术台，哺乳动物手术器械，刺激器，保护电极，铁架台。

2. 溶液 20%氨基甲酸乙酯，生理盐水。

3. 对象 兔。

【实验方法】

1. 麻醉与固定 用20%氨基甲酸乙酯按1~1.2g/kg体重剂量注入兔耳缘静脉，待动物麻醉，将兔背位交叉仰卧位固定于兔手术台上。

2. 手术

（1）剪去下腹部兔毛，在靠近耻骨联合上缘，沿正中线做一长约4cm的切口，沿腹白线剪开腹壁及腹膜，暴露膀胱，用手将膀胱轻轻移出腹外，在膀胱下面垫一块温生理盐水纱布。

（2）在膀胱底部两侧找到输尿管，分布于膀胱壁上的神经（包括盆神经和腹下神经）沿膀胱两侧的输尿管与血管伴行，见图7-2。用玻璃分针小心将一侧血管及神经从膀胱壁上分离1.5cm，穿线后提起，用钩形保护电极将血管与神经一起钩住，然后给予电刺激（刺激强度10~20V，频率8~16Hz，波宽2~5ms），观察膀胱反应，通常出现盆神经兴奋的效应。

【实验指导】

1. 预习要求

（1）复习膀胱及尿道的神经支配，即膀胱逼尿肌、尿道内括约肌、尿道外括约肌分别受什么神经支配。

（2）复习膀胱排尿的神经反射调节过程。

2. 操作要点

（1）认清两侧输尿管在膀胱的开口位置，细心分离神经血管。

（2）刺激神经时，时间不要过长，以免神经疲劳。一般一次刺激时间为10s。

（3）做手术切口时，皮肤、肌肉及腹膜应分层切开，不能用力过大一刀将三层组织切开，以免切破膀胱。

3. 注意事项

（1）分离神经应用玻璃分针，禁用金属器械碰触神经，以免损伤。

（2）静脉注射麻药时，量要准确，并要缓慢推注，以角膜反射消失、四肢肌肉松弛为最适麻醉标准。

4. 报告要点　写出电刺激盆神经和腹下神经所引起的膀胱反应，并对其进行分析讨论。说明膀胱排尿的神经反射调节过程。

5. 思考题

（1）膀胱的神经调节与排尿的关系。

（2）在膀胱排尿过程中，起主要作用的是哪种神经？为什么？

（3）膀胱内的压力是随膀胱内的尿量增多而增加的，这句话对吗？

（李运曼）

40　The nervous regulation of bladder in rabbit

PURPOSE

Stimulate the nerves that govern the bladder. Observe the response; get to know the nervous regulation of bladder.

PRINCIPLES

The function of bladder is storing urine temporarily and ejecting accumulating urine quickly. The function of bladder and sphincter of urethra is regulated by nervous system. There are 3 pairs of nerves related with micturition: (a) pelvicganglia. If it is excited, it can contract detrusor, relax internal sphincter, and promote the micturition. And it is the main nerve that governs the bladder. (b) Hypogastric nerves. If it is excited, it can relax detrusor, contract internal sphincter, and stop the micturition. (c) Pudendal nerve. Its impulse can contract external sphincter, then restrain micturition. There are some sensory fibers originating from bladder and urethra in these nerves. The feeling of expansion mainly conducts in sensory fibers and causes urine reflection. Because parasympathetic nerve play a more important role than sympathetic nerve in micturition, the effect of stimulating pelvic ganglia often appears when the nerves that govern the bladder are stimulating.

MATERIALS

1. Equipments　Operating instruments, operating table for rabbit, stimulator, shield electrode, iron stand

2. Solutions　Urethan 20%. Saline.

3. Object　Rabbit.

METHODS

1. Anesthesia procedure and fixation　i. v. 20% Urethan (1 ~ 1. 2g/kg) to the rabbit's ears and fix it on operation table in supine body position when the rabbit is anesthetized.

2. operations　Shear the hair on inferior belly, make a 4cm wound upward along middle line from pubic symphysis. (Fig. 7 – 2) Cut open abdominal wall along linea alba abdominis, move the bladder outside by hand. Find the ureter in both sides in the bottom of the bladder. The nerves walk with blood vessel along the ureter. Separate a 1. 5cm nerve and blood vessel from the bladder wallcarefully with glass hook. Pass a thread through and raise it. Hook nerves and blood vessels with shield electrode, stimulate them with electricity. The method: continuous A, 10 ~ 20V, 8 ~ 16 Hz, 2 ~ 5 ms. Observe the effect.

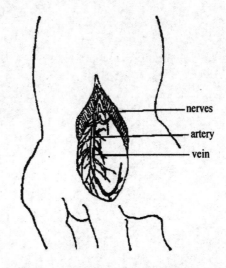

Fig. 7 – 2　**the distribution of blood vessel and nerves of bladder in rabbit**

GUIDANCE

1. Preview

(1) Reviews the governance of nerves in the bladder and urethra.

(2) Review the nervous reflex regulation of bladder in micturition.

(3) Review the operation of stimulator.

2. Manipulation

（1）Recognize the opening of ureter in the bladder. Free the nerves and blood vessel carefully.

（2）Operate the stimulator rightly. Be sure that the stimulator is connected with the earth to prevent the electric induction from taking place. Check the output of stimulator beforehand after connecting the wires. Push the START button, if the light is not bright, check the line to make sure that it is not a short circuit or the electrode does not meet. If it is, clear it. Don't stimulate the nerves for a too long time. The proper time is 10 seconds.

（3）Cut off the skins, muscles and peritoneum level by level.

3. Notices

（1）Don't free nerves with metal tools.

（2）When i. v. Urethan, the quantity should be exact, and the injection should be slow.

4. Report

Write down the reflect caused by stimulating the pelvic ganglia and hypogastric nerves. Analyze it. Illustrate the procedure of the nervous reflex regulation of bladder in micturition.

5. Questions

（1）The relation between micturition and nervous regulation of bladder.

（2）During the procedure of micturition, which nerve takes the important part? Why?

（3）The pressure inside the bladder increases when the urine volume increases. Is this right?

(Li Yunman)

第八章 内分泌与生殖系统

Endocrine and reproductive system

实验四十一 胰岛素的生理作用

扫码"学一学"

【实验目的】

观察注入大量胰岛素所引起的小白鼠惊厥反应及葡萄糖的解救作用，以了解胰岛素的生理作用。

【实验原理】

胰岛素由胰腺的胰岛细胞分泌，它能促进肝细胞、肌细胞对葡萄糖的摄取、贮存和利用。细胞摄取葡萄糖后，一方面将其转化为糖原贮存起来，或在肝细胞内转变成脂肪酸并转运到脂肪组织中贮存；另一方面促进葡萄糖的氧化，生成高能磷酸化合物如 ATP，作为细胞的能源。由于胰岛素能促进葡萄糖的贮存和利用，因此腹腔注射大量胰岛素后，可使血糖浓度降低。血糖浓度过低可使组织细胞内可利用的糖缺乏，特别是脑组织内的糖贮备很少，仅靠血糖来供应能量，故对血糖变化非常敏感。当血糖低于 2.8mmol/L 时，中枢神经系统可出现先兴奋后抑制以致昏迷的现象，称为"胰岛素休克"，表现为流汗、流涎、共济失调、惊厥、死亡。如果在出现惊厥时，立即腹腔注入葡萄糖溶液，脑功能可恢复正常，症状缓解。

【实验材料】

1. **器材** 注射器（1ml），温度计，烧杯（800ml、1000ml），5 号针头。
2. **溶液** 胰岛素（4U/ml），20% 葡萄糖。
3. **对象** 小白鼠。

【实验方法】

1. 实验前将小鼠饥饿 24 小时。做好标记后，分别腹腔注射胰岛素 0.5ml（2U）。注射完毕将小鼠放于 800ml 烧杯中，以盛有温水（39℃）的 1000ml 烧杯作为水浴保温。观察小鼠活动。

2. 待小鼠发生惊厥时，取一只小鼠腹腔注入 20% 葡萄糖 1ml，另一只作对照，观察结果。可见注入葡萄糖的小鼠被救活，另一只则死亡。

【实验指导】

1. **预习要求** 复习有关胰岛素的分泌调节及其生理功能。
2. **操作要点** 小鼠腹腔注射，一般应左手持鼠，右手持注射器，注入部位于小鼠左下腹部，刺入后要回抽，无血或其他液体回流才可注入。

3. 注意事项

（1）动物在实验前必须饥饿 24h。

（2）动物要注意保温。

（3）20％的葡萄糖要预先吸入注射器，待惊厥出现立即注入。

4. 报告要点 详细描述注射胰岛素后小鼠出现的各种症状及急救和未急救小鼠表现的异同，分析其机制。

5. 思考题 胰岛素有哪些生理功能？体内影响其分泌的主要因素是什么？

（李运曼）

41　Physiological effect of insulin

PURPOSE

Observe the convulsion of mice when a great mount of insulin was administered. And to observe the saving function and physiological function of insulin.

PRINCIPLES

Insulin is secreted by Islet cell in pancreas. It can promote hepatocyte and muscle cell to absorb, store and utilize the glucose. There are two transformative ways after the glucose is absorbed. One is that glucose transforms to glycogen and is stored or transformed to fatty acid in liver cells. Then it is transported to fatty tissue and stored. The other way is that to promote the oxidizing of glucose to form energy – rich phosphate, such as ATP, to be the energy source for cells. I. p. a great mount of insulin may decrease the concentration of blood sugar because insulin can promote the storage and utilization of glucose. If the concentration of blood sugar is too low, the blood sugar available in histocyte will be lack, especially in the brain. Because there is few glucose stored in the brain, the brain depends on the blood sugar to supply the energy. It is very sensitive to the change of blood sugar. When the blood sugar is lower than 2. 3mmol/L, the coma called insulin shock, which causes previous stimuli and later suppression in central nervous system, will take place. It will cause sweating, drooling, incoordination, convulsion and death. If i. p. glucose as soon as the convulsion takes place, the brain function will recover and the symptom will relieve.

MATERIALS

1. Equipments Syringe, thermometer, beaker, needle (5 type).

2. Solutions Insulin (4U/ml), 20％ glucose.

3. Object Mice.

METHODS

1. Stop feeding the mice 24 hours before experiment. Mark them. I. p. insulin 0. 5ml (2U) respectively. Put the mice into an 800ml beaker after injection; keep temperature with a 1000ml beaker with 39℃ water inside. Observe the mice's move ment.

2. When the convulsion takes place, take one mouse and i. p. 20％ glucose 1ml, take another to

contrast. Observe the results. The mouse that was injected glucose will be saved and the other will die.

GUIDANCE

1. Preview　Review the adjustment and physiological effect of insulin.

2. Manipulation　During the procedure of i. p. the mice, hold the mouse with left hand, and hold the syringe in your right hand. The needle is inserted in the left lower part where it is not likely to penetrate the liver and chest.

3. Notice

（1）The animal must have been hungry for 24 hours before experiment.

（2）Keep the animal warm in the experiment.

（3）20% glucose should be prepared beforehand. If the convulsion takes place, inject it immediately.

4. Report　Describe the symptoms happen in mice after injecting insulin detailed and explain their mechanisms.

5. Question

What are the physiological functions of insulin? What are the main factors influencing its secretion in vivo?

（Li Yunman）

实验四十二　小鼠雄性腺切除对附性器官的影响

【实验目的】

观察雄性小鼠睾丸切除后对附性器官的影响，以了解内分泌腺对机体的重要性。

【实验原理】

睾丸具有产生精子和分泌雄性激素（睾丸酮）两项重要生理功能。睾丸酮主要由间质细胞分泌，其生理作用除了促进精子的生成与发育以外，还促进雄性附性器官的发育和成熟，并维持附性器官的正常生理功能。如睾丸切除以后，其附性器官精囊腺会逐渐萎缩，功能减弱。

【实验材料】

1. 器材　剪刀，镊子，蛙板，棉球，丝线。

2. 药品　碘酒棉球，75%酒精棉球，乙醚。

3. 对象　雄性小白鼠（体重29～30g）。

【实验方法】

1. 将小白鼠用乙醚麻醉，仰卧在蛙板上。用碘酒棉球及75%酒精棉球消毒会阴。在肛门及生殖器之间做1cm的横切口，用镊子分离皮下组织，在腹壁稍加压，睾丸即从创口露出。将其根部连同周围皮肤结扎，切除睾丸。

2. 术后饲养两周，然后解剖小白鼠，观察精囊腺的变化，并与正常雄性小鼠比较，看有何差异。

【实验指导】

1. 预习要求 复习有关睾丸的生理功能及其调节作用。

2. 操作要点 切除睾丸是本实验的关键步骤。两侧睾丸均要切除，以免结果不明显。

3. 注意事项 切除睾丸前后要彻底消毒会阴部，防止术后感染；切除睾丸之前，要将其根部与其周围的皮肤用线扎紧，以防出血。

4. 报告要点 根据观察对比的结果，结合理论讨论性腺的生理功能。

5. 思考题 雄激素有哪些生理功能？

（吴玉林）

42　Effects of removal of testes on accessory genital organs in mice

PURPOSE

To understand the importance of endocrine glands on organisms, the testes are removed in male mice to observe the effects of testes on accessory genital organs.

PRINCIPLE

The testes have two important physiological functions: producing sperms and secreting androgenic hormone (testosterone). Testosterone is excreted mainly by interstitial cells, which can promote the production and development of sperms. Besides it can promote the development and maturity of male accessory genital organs, and also maintain their normal physiological functions. After the removal of androgenic glands (testis) in mice, the accessory genital organs, such as seminalvesicle, will atrophy gradually, and their function will fail.

MATERIALS

1. Equipments Scissors, Forceps, Frog Operation Table, Medical Cotton, Silk.

2. Solutions Tincture of Iodine, Alcohol, diethyl ether.

3. Objects Mice (male, BW25 ~ 30g).

METHODS

1. The mouse is anesthetized with ethyl ether during surgery and is fixed on the frog operation bench with lying on its back. The perineum is disinfected with medical cotton dipped in tincture of iodine and alcohol. The transection is made between the anus and the reproductive organ, which is 1cm long. The subcutaneous tissues are separated with forceps. The abdominal wall is compressed slightly and the testis is exposed from the incision. The radicular part of testis is ligatured with its peripheral cutis. The testis is excised.

2. The postoperative mouse is raised for two weeks and is dissected. The changes of its seminal

vesical are observed and are compared with that of the normal male mouse to determine. Weather or not there are any differences between them?

GUIDANCE

1. Preview　Please review the knowledge on the physiological functions and the regulating function of testis.

2. Manipulations　Removal of testis is the key step in this experiment. Both testes should be-excised in order to avoid undefined results.

3. Notice　In order to prevent the postoperative infection, the perineum should be disinfected thoroughly not only before but also after the operation. Before the removal of testis, the radicular part of testis and its peripheral cutis should be ligated tightly to prevent bleeding.

4. Report　According to the results observed and compared, discuss the physiological functions of gonads considering the theories.

5. Questions　What are the physiological functions of androgenic hormone?

(WuYulin)

第九章　实验设计

Experiment design

【目的要求】

使学生通过对实验课题的设计，熟悉进行实验所必需的基本要求与一般程序，以达到训练其解决实际问题的能力，并使学生经历一次科学研究素质的训练。

【实验步骤】

1. 选题　根据教师提出的实验课题任选一题，学生自己提出课题经教师同意也可。

2. 拟定实验方案　根据已学过的生理学理论知识和实验技能，在现有实验室条件下，通过查阅有关文献资料，拟定一个详细的实验方案，并交教师审阅。

【实验设计内容】

1. 课题名称。
2. 目的要求：本实验最后所要达到的目的。
3. 基本原理：实验设计理论的依据与思路。
4. 动物、器材与药品。
5. 方法与步骤：实验方法、实验项目或观察内容、指标，每一步实验可能出现的结果。

【实验设计的基本原则】

1. 科学性　在设计实验时，必须有足够的科学依据，要以前人的实验或自己的实验为基础，而不是随意设想。例如某化学物质对离体心脏的影响，首先通过查阅资料，了解这种化学物质对心脏是否有影响（如心率快慢、收缩力强弱等），为什么会有这些影响，以此为依据，便可设计出观察指标明确，选材准确，有的放矢，科学性强的实验。

2. 严谨性　实验设计要严谨，要使需要说明的问题无懈可击，这就需设置对照实验（包括某一处理前的正常对照或对照组），这样便于实验前后或组间比较，以观察某因素对某器官的生理活动是否有影响。例如观察某因素对呼吸频率的影响时，必须记录施加某因素前的呼吸频率，而后在给予某因素后记录呼吸频率，并对实验前后呼吸频率给予比较，是否有显著差异。

3. 实验条件的一致性　在实验过程中，除预处理因素以外，其他实验条件必须保持前后一致，不能在实验过程中随意变动，只有在实验条件完全一致的情况下，才能反映出处理因素对实验结果的影响。

4. 可重复性　任何实验不能仅进行一次便作为正式结果，必须要足够实验次数，才能判断实验结果的可靠性，如果各次实验结果比较接近，可以减少重复次数。但由于本实验设计不是系统的科学研究，所以应力求在减少人力、物力和时间的条件下，取得理想结果。

5. 动物敏感性　首先根据实验内容确定所选动物的种类，因为某种动物可能对某种生理反应最为敏感，而另一种动物就不够敏感。如猫的呕吐反应较为敏感，而大鼠则缺乏这种反应，所以应选择猫来研究呕吐反应。另外，还要注意动物品种的选择，如同是大鼠，有的品种容易形成某种病理模型，有的则不容易。因此在选择动物时需要参考前人的经验，查阅有关文献。

6. 指标合理性　实验指标的选择应注意合理性，即所选指标是否代表所研究的现象。如利用小鼠做避孕研究，如果选用性周期变化作为指标是不合适的。因为性周期可能不受影响而仍具有避孕效果，若选择怀孕率作为指标就合乎情理了。

【实验的准备与实施】

根据实验设计的内容进行实验准备工作，包括仪器的安装与检测，药品的配制，实验动物的准备等。按照实验设计的方法与步骤，严格进行手术或标本制备，并完成实验的全过程。实验过程中做好观察、记录、实验资料的收集，并对实验结果进行处理分析，最后写出完整的实验报告。实验报告以论文格式书写，内容包括前言、方法、结果、讨论、参考文献及摘要。

【课题举例】

课题选择的内容应根据本实验室的条件、科学研究的方向而定，主要包括以下几方面。

1. 验证基本理论。

2. 实验技术的革新，即用新方法、新技术研究某器官的生理功能。

3. 学生实验中遇到的某些疑难问题，可列为课题，通过实验研究，以求解决。

下面列举几题，仅供参考。

（1）动脉血压与尿量的关系。

（2）温度对离体肠管活动的影响。

（3）某一化学物质对心肌不应期的影响。

（李运曼）

Requirement

Students are required to familiarize the basal requirement and general procedure which the experiment requires, through the design of experimental task, to get to be trained to have the ability of solving practical problems, and to undergo a training of scientific research quality.

Experimental procedure

1. Selecting the subject　Students can select any one of the experimental subjects, which the teachers pose, or pose the subjects themselves, which must be agreed to by the teacher.

2. Formulating the experimental scheme　On the base of physiological theory and experimental skill which have been studied, under the condition of the current laboratory, through finding up the relative literature, a detailed experimental scheme is formulated, which ought to be checked and approved by the teacher.

Experiment designing contents

1. The name of subject

2. Requirement: The purpose that the experiment finally gets to

3. Basal principle: The basis and reason of the experiment designing theory

4. Animals、equipment and medicine

5. Method and steps: Experimental method、subject or observing contents、index, as well as the result that every step may arise.

Basal principle of the experiment designing

1. Scientific nature   Ample scientific basis must be provided when designing the experiment. It should be on the base of previous or own experiment, not conceive randomly. Such as the influence of some chemical material to the heart in vitro, first through finding up literature, knows about whether this material has influence to the heart (such as the heart rate. contracting power etc) or not, and why.

According to this, the experiment can be formulated, which has the explicit observing index, accurate materials and powerful scientific nature.

2. Rigorism   Experiment designing must be rigorous and have no mistakes to the problems which are required to explain, so control experiment must be set (including some pretreated normal control or control group), which is convenient to compare the index before and after experiment or inter − group, to observe if some factor has influence on some factor to respiratory frequency, the respiratory frequency must be recorded before exerting the factor, and then the frequency after exerting the factor. At last the respiratory frequency can be compared before and after experiment to see if there is significant difference.

3. Accordance of the experimental condition   During the experiment, the other experimental condition must remain according before and after experiment except the wanted treating factor, and can't be changed randomly. The influence of the treating factor to the experimental result only can be reflected under the completely according experimental condition.

4. Repetition   Any experiment can't be the formal result by only once. The reliability of the experimental results must be judged through enough times. If every experimental results is very close, the repeating times can be reduced. But as this experiment designing is not systematic scientific research, the ideal results can be achieved under the condition of reducing manpower, material and time as much as we can.

5. Sensitivity of animals   At first, to decide which kind of animal should be selected according to our experiment. Because some animal may be sensitive to certain physical reactions while some others may not. For example cat has sensitive vomit reaction while rat lacks. So we should choose cats in vomit experiment. Otherwise we should pay attention to the breed of animals. As rats, a special breed is easy to form special pathology model, and other breeds are difficult. When choosing animals, we should consult experience before and refer to relevant literature.

6. Rationality of index   The index we choose should be reasonable. That is to say these index should represent phenomena we research. For example, it isn't appropriate to select the variety of sexual cycle as our index, when we choose mice as our experiment animal in contraception experiment. Because some chemicals without any influence on mice sexual cycle which have had contraceptive effect. So it's reasonable if we have taken the rate of conceived as index.

Preparation and implement

We make our preparation in terms of experiment plan, including installation and measurement of instruments, confection of drug and preparation of animals. We must perform operations or prepare samples strictly, according to the method and process in plan, and complete the whole experiment. In this course we should observe, record, collect and analyze result, get an integrated report. The report should write in form of thesis, including forward, method, result, discussion, reference and summary.

Topic for example

The content of our experiment must be chosen according to the condition of our lab and the direction of our scientific research, mainly including following aspects:

1. To verify basic theory.

2. Innovation of experiment technique, namely adopting new method and new technique to study physiological function of apparatus.

3. The problem emerging from student experiments could be our research topic, and be solved through experiment research.

Giving several examples for consult only.

(1) The relationship between blood pressure of artery and urine amount.

(2) The effect of temperature on gut movement of Guinea pig in vitro.

(3) The effect of a kind of chemical on refractory period of myocardium.

(Li Yunman)

附　录

附录一　常用生理溶液的配制

在进行离体组织或器官实验时，为了维持标本的"正常"功能活动，必须尽可能地使标本所处的环境因素与体内相近似。这些因素主要包括电解质成分、渗透压、酸碱度，甚至个别营养物质、温度。这样的溶液称为生理代用液或生理溶液。

在生理实验中，常用生理溶液有生理盐水、任氏液、乐氏液（Locke）及台氏液（Tyrode）。各种生理溶液的成分见表1。

表1　常用生理溶液成分（g）

	NaCl	KCl	CaCl$_2$	NaHCO$_3$	NaH$_2$PO$_4$	MgCl$_2$	葡萄糖
任氏液（两栖类用）	6.5	0.14	0.12	0.2	0.01	—	2.0
乐氏液（哺乳类用）	9.0	0.42	0.24	0.1~0.3	—	—	1.0~2.5
台氏液（哺乳类用）	8.0	0.2	0.2	1.0	0.05	0.1	1.0
生理盐水							
两栖类	6.5~7.0	—	—	—	—	—	—
哺乳类	9.0	—	—	—	—	—	—

注：上述溶液均各加蒸馏水至1000ml。

以上代用液不仅电解质的晶体渗透压与体液相同，而且几种离子的比例，O$_2$与葡萄糖的含量以及缓冲力也与体液相同，用这样的代用液能长久地保持离体组织或器官的功能。

代用液不宜久置，应临用时配制，为了方便配制，最好事先配好代用液所需各种成分较浓的基础液，到用时按所需量取基础液置于量瓶中，加蒸馏水到定量刻度即可（表2）。在配制溶液前应烘干药品，然后精确称量。注意在加入电解质成分时，应先将其他成分基础液混合，并加入蒸馏水后再加氯化钙基础液，同时要边加边搅匀，以免产生不溶解的磷酸钙，使溶液混浊。另外葡萄糖应在临用前加入，以免滋长细菌。配制成的代用液要测定其酸碱度，pH应在7.2~7.8之间。

表2　配制生理溶液所需的基础溶液及其容量（ml）

	NaCl (20%)	KCl (10%)	CaCl$_2$ (10%)	NaH$_2$PO$_4$ (1%)	MgCl$_2$ (5%)	NaHCO$_3$ (5%)	葡萄糖 (g)	蒸馏水
任氏液	32.5	1.1	1.2	1.0	—	4.0	2.0	加至
乐氏液	45.0	4.2	2.4	—	—	4.0	1.0~25	1000ml
台氏液	40.0	2.0	2.0	5.0	2.0	20.0	1.0	

1　Frequently used solution dispensation

It must make specimen in order to remain specimen's normal function. It must be in fit environment like in vitro, which environment includes electrolyte, osmotic pressure, nutrition and temperature. These solutions are called frequently used solution of dispensation.

Frequently used solution of dispensation includes saline、Locke and Tyrode. These normal solutions of dispensation have same crystal pressure.

Tab 1　Component of frequently used physio – solutions（g）

	NaCl	KCl	CaCl$_2$	NaHCO$_3$	NaH$_2$PO$_4$	MgCl$_2$	Glucose
Ringer（amphibians animals）	6.5	0.14	0.12	0.2	0.01	—	2.0
Locke（mammal）	9.0	0.42	0.24	0.1~0.3	—	—	1.0~2.5
Tyrode（mammal）	8.0	0.2	0.2	1.0	0.05	0.1	1.0
Saline							
amphibians animals	6.5~7.0	—	—	—	—	—	—
mammal	9.0	—	—	—	—	—	—

Remarks：The solutions above must be added to 1000ml with distilled water.

The ratio of several ion, O$_2$ and glucose is the same as body fluid. So normal solution of dispensation can make tissue organ living.

Tab 2　Basal solution and volume of phsio – solutions（ml）

	NaCl (20%)	KCl (10%)	CaCl$_2$ (10%)	NaH$_2$PO$_4$ (1%)	MgCl$_2$ (5%)	NaHCO$_3$ (5%)	Glucose (g)	Distilled water
Ringer	32.5	1.1	1.2	1.0	—	4.0	2.0	Add to 1000ml
Locke	45.0	4.2	2.4	—	—	4.0	1.0~25	
Tyrode	40.0	2.0	2.0	5.0	2.0	20.0	1.0	

Normal solution of dispensation can't be deposited for long, it must confect when we need. In order to dispense convenience, we can dispense every dense basic solution, which are needed when using Normal solution of dispensation, mete basic solution, add distilled water until we require. Before dispensing solution, drug should be drying, weight be exactitude. When we add electrolyte, the other basic solution be mixed, then add distilled water and calcium chloride, at the same time mill in order to solute calcium phosphate and make the solution clear. In addition glucose is added just before use, because it can grow bacterium. Normal solution of dispensation's acidity is from 7.2 to 7.8.

附录二　常用实验动物的一些生理常数

表3　常用实验动物的一些生理常数

指标	小白鼠	大白鼠	豚鼠	家兔	猫	狗
适用体重（kg）	0.018~0.025	0.1~0.2	0.3~0.6	1.5~2.5	2~3	5~15
寿命（年）	1.5~2.0	2.0~2.5	6~8	5~7	6~10	10~15
性成熟年龄（月）	1.2~1.7	2~8	4~6	5~6	10~12	10~12
孕期（日）	20~22	21~24	65~72	30~35	60~70	58~65
平均体温（℃）	37.4	38.0	39.5	39.0	38.5	38.5
呼吸（次/分）	136~216	100~150	100~150	55~90	25~50	20~30

237

续表

指标		小白鼠	大白鼠	豚鼠	家兔	猫	狗
心率（次/分）		400~600	250~400	180~250	150~220	120~180	100~200
血压（mmHg）		115	110	80	105/75	130/75	125/70
血量（ml/100g 体重）		7.8	6.0	5.8	7.2	7.2	7.8
红细胞（百万/mm³）		7.7~12.5	7.2~9.6	4.5~7.0	4.5~7.0	6.5~9.5	4.5~7.0
血红蛋白（g%）		10.0~19.0	12.0~17.5	11.0~16.5	8.0~15.0	7.0~15.5	11.0~18.0
血小板（千/mm³）		60~110	50~100	68~87	38~52	10~50	10~60
白细胞总数（千/mm³）		6.0~10.0	6.0~15.0	0~12.0	7.0~11.3	14.0~18.0	9.0~13.0
白细胞分类（%）	嗜中性	12~44	9~34	22~50	26~52	44~82	62~80
	嗜酸性	0~5	1~6	5~12	1~4	2~11	2~24
	嗜碱性	0~1	0~1.5	0~2	1~3	0~0.5	0~2
	淋巴	54~85	65~84	36~64	30~82	15~44	10~28
	大单核	0~15	0~5	3~13	1~4	0.5~0.7	3~9

2　Some physio – constants of frequently used animals

Tab 3　Some physio – constants of frequently used animals

Index		Mouse	Rat	Guinea pig	Rabbit	Cat	Dog
Suitable weight(kg)		0.018~0.025	0.1~0.2	0.3~0.6	1.5~2.5	2~3	5~15
life span(years)		1.5~2.0	2.0~2.5	6~8	5~7	6~10	10~15
Age of sexual maturity(months)		1.2~1.7	2~8	4~6	5~6	10~12	10~12
gestation period (days)		20~22	21~24	65~72	30~35	60~70	58~65
average temperature (℃)		37.4	38.0	39.5	39.0	38.5	38.5
respiration(times/min)		136~216	100~150	100~150	55~90	25~50	20~30
Heart rate (times/min)		400~600	250~400	180~250	150~220	120~180	100~200
Blood pressure(mmHg)		115	110	80	105/75	130/75	125/70
blood volume(ml/100gBW)		7.8	6.0	5.8	7.2	7.2	7.8
erythrocyte(million/mm³)		7.7~12.5	7.2~9.6	4.5~7.0	4.5~7.0	6.5~9.5	4.5~7.0
ferrohemoglobin(g%)		10.0~19.0	12.0~17.5	11.0~16.5	8.0~15.0	7.0~15.5	11.0~18.0
thrombocyte (thousand s/mm³)		60~110	50~100	68~87	38~52	10~50	10~60
Total leucocyte(thousand s/mm³)		6.0~10.0	6.0~15.0	0~12.0	7.0~11.3	14.0~18.0	9.0~13.0
Leucocyte type (%)	neutrophilia	12~44	9~34	22~50	26~52	44~82	62~80
	acidophila	0~5	1~6	5~12	1~4	2~11	2~24
	asophilia	0~1	0~1.5	0~2	1~3	0~0.5	0~2
	lymph	54~85	65~84	36~64	30~82	15~44	10~28
	monocyt	0~15	0~5	3~13	1~4	0.5~0.7	3~9

附录三　常用血液抗凝剂

1. 草酸钾　常用于供检验用血液样品之抗凝。在试管内加饱和草酸钾溶液 2 滴，轻轻敲击试管，使溶液分散到管壁四周，置 80℃ 以下的烘箱中烤干（如烘烤温度过高，草酸钾将分解为碳酸钾而失去抗凝作用）。这样制备的抗凝管可使 3～5ml 血液不致凝固。供钾、钙含量测定的血样不能用草酸钾抗凝。

2. 肝素　取 1% 肝素溶液 0.1ml 于试管内，均匀浸湿试管内壁，放入 80～100℃烘箱烤干。每管能使 5～10ml 血液不凝。

市售的肝素注射液每毫升含肝素 12500U（相当于肝素钠 125mg），应置冰箱中保存。

3. 枸橼酸钠　3.8% 的枸橼酸钠溶液 1 份，可使 9 份血液不致凝固，用于做红细胞渗透脆性实验等。做急性血压实验时，则用 5%～7% 的枸橼酸钠溶液。

3 Frequently used anticoagulant

1. Potassium oxalate　It is usually used as anticoagulant in blood samples for testing. Add 2 drops of saturated potassium oxalate solution to tube, shock the tube softly to disperse the solution around the wall, and then heat to dryness in the oven under 80℃ (Potassium oxalate will decompose to potassium carbonate and lead disfunction in high temperature). 3～5ml of blood in this tube will not coagulate. Potassium oxalate cannot be used in the blood samples for determination of potassium and calcium.

2. Heparin　Add 0.1ml of 1% heparin solution to a tube, soak the inter wall equally, and then heat to dryness in the oven under 80～100℃. 5～10ml of blood in this tube will not coagulate.

Soled heparin parenteral solution contains 12500U heparin per milliliter (correspondent to 125mg sodium heparin). Stored in refrigerator.

3. Sodium citrate　9 folds of blood will not coagulate with 1 fold of 3.8% Sodium citrate. The solution is used for osmosis fragility of erythrocyte. 5%～7% Sodium citrate is used in the acute pressure experiment.

附录四　几种易变质药物溶液的配制与保存

1. 氯乙酰胆碱　本品在一般水溶液中易水解失效，但在 pH4 的溶液中则比较稳定。如以 5% 的 NaH_2PO_4 溶液配成 0.1% 左右的氯乙酰胆碱存液，用小瓶分装，密封后在冰箱中存放，约可保持药效 1 年。临用前用生理盐水稀释至所需浓度。

2. 盐酸肾上腺素　本品在溶液中容易氧化失效。如溶液为碱性，则破坏更快。因此只能以生理盐水稀释，不能以任氏液或台氏液稀释，盐酸肾上腺素的稀释液一般只能存数小时。如在溶液中添加微量（10^{-4}mol/L）抗坏血酸，则其稳定性可显著提高。

3. 水杨酸毒扁豆碱　本品在水溶液中氧化变质，在制剂中宜适当添加抗氧化剂。取水杨酸毒扁豆碱 0.1g 及亚硫酸氢钠 0.05g，加水至 100ml，制成 0.1% 的水杨酸毒扁豆碱溶液，用棕色瓶贮存，约可保持药效 1 周，如发现溶液呈粉红色，即不可用。

4. 催产素及垂体后叶素　它们在水溶液中也易变质失效。但如以 0.25% 的醋酸溶液配制，用小瓶分装，密封后置冰箱中保存（4℃左右，不宜冰冻），约可保持药效 3 个月。临用前用生理盐水稀释至适当浓度。如发现催产素或垂体后叶素溶液出现沉淀，即不可用。

4 Dispensation and conservation of some kinds of drug solution apt to deteriorate

1. Chlovidize acetylcholine　Chlovidize acetylcheline is inclined to be hydrolyzed and become invalid in aqueous solution, but remain fairly stable in solution whose pH is 4. For example, if dispense 1% acecolex reservoir with 5% solution of NaH_2PO_4, pack into small bottles, seal up and preserve in refrigerator, the effect of reservoir can be kept for about 1 year. Dilute to the density required with NS before using.

2. Hydrochloric adrenaline　Hydrochloric adrenaline is apt to be oxidized and lose efficacy in solution. The oxidization will accelerate when in alkaline solution. So it must be diluted by NS and can't by Ringer's and Tyrode's solution. The diluent of hydrochloric adrenaline can be preserved for hours. Adding trace ascorbic (10^{-4} mol/L) can improve the stability of the solution remarkably.

3. Eserine salicylate　Eserine salicylate can be oxidized and go bad easily. So antioxidant should be added in the agent. The 1% solution of eserine salicylate can be made up by taking 0.1g eserine salicylate and 0.05g NaHSO3, then adding to 100ml with water. The effect of this solution that is conserved in brown bottles can be kept for 1 week. Don't use if solution becomes pink.

4. OXT and pituitrin　OXT and pituitrin are easy to go bad and become efficiency, but if it is dispensed with 0.25% acetic acid, packed into small bottles, sealed up and conserved in refrigerator (4℃ or so, don't be freeze), the effect can be kept for 3 months. Dilute to proper density before using. Don't use if sediment was founded in the solution.

附录五　常用计量单位

根据《中华人民共和国法定计量单位》的规定，本书采用法定计量。表4是本书常用的计量单位及其代表符号。

表4　常用计量单位表

量的名称	单位名称	单位符号	备注
长度	米，厘米 毫米，微米	m, cm mm, μm	
质量	千克，克，毫克	kg, g, mg	千克即公斤
时间	天（日），时，分； 秒，毫秒，微秒	d, h, min； s, ms, μs	
速度	米/秒，厘米/秒 毫米/秒	m/s, cm/s mm/s	
体积	升，毫升	L（l），ml；	$1ml = 1cm^3 = 1000mm^3$
电阻	兆欧，千欧 欧［姆］	MΩ, kΩ Ω	
电压，电位	伏［特］，毫伏 微伏	V, mV μV	
频率	千赫，赫［兹］	kHz, Hz	
物质的量	摩［尔］	mol	
压力	毫米汞柱 毫米水柱 帕	mmHg mmH$_2$O Pa	$1mmHg = 133.322Pa$ $1mmH_2O = 9.806Pa$

（李运曼）

5　Frequently used metric units

The book uses legal metric units according to the Legal Measures of the People's Republic of China. Frequently used metric units and their symbols are in Table 6.

Tab 4　Metric units

Unit Type	Unit Name	Symbol	Remarks
Length	meter, centimeter	m, cm	
	millimeter, micrometer	mm, μm	
Mass	kilogram, gram, milligram	kg, g, mg	
Time	day, hour, minute;	d, h, min;	
	second, milli − second, microsecond	s, ms, μs	
Velocity	meter/second, centimeter/second	m/s, cm/s	
	Millimeter/second	mm/s	
Volum	liter, millilitre	L (l), ml	$1\,ml = 1\,cm^3 = 1000\,mm^3$
Electrical resistance	megohm, kilo − ohm	MΩ, kΩ	
	Ohm	n	
Voltage: potential	volt, millivolt	V, mV	
	Micro − volt	μV	
Frequency	Kilohertz, hertz	kHz, Hz	
Amount of Substance	Mole	mol	
pressure	millimetres of mercury	mmHg	$1\,mmHg = 133.322\,Pa$
	Millimeters of water	mmH$_2$O	$1\,mmH_2O = 9.806\,Pa$
	Pascal	Pa